Clinical Notes
for the
FRCA

For Maddie

Commissioning Editor: Timothy Horne/Jeremy Bowes
Development Editor: Nicola Lally
Project Manager: Annie Victor
Designer: Stewart Larking
Illustration Manager: Bruce Hogarth
Illustrator: Gillian Richards

THIRD EDITION

Clinical Notes
for the
FRCA

Charles D. Deakin
MA MD MB BChir FRCP FRCA FERC

Consultant Anaesthetist

Shackleton Department of Anaesthetics

Southampton University Hospital NHS Trust

Southampton

UK

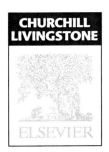

CHURCHILL LIVINGSTONE

ELSEVIER

Edinburgh   London   New York   Oxford   Philadelphia   St Louis   Sydney   Toronto 2011

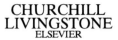

CHURCHILL LIVINGSTONE
ELSEVIER

First edition 1996
Second edition 2000
Third edition 2011

ISBN : 978-0-7020-3525-8

British Library Cataloguing in Publication Data
A catalogue record for this book is available from the British Library

Library of Congress Cataloging in Publication Data
A catalog record for this book is available from the Library of Congress

your source for books, journals and multimedia in the health sciences

www.elsevierhealth.com

Working together to grow libraries in developing countries

www.elsevier.com | www.bookaid.org | www.sabre.org

ELSEVIER   BOOK AID International   Sabre Foundation

The Publisher's policy is to use **paper manufactured from sustainable forests**

Transferred to Digital Printing in 2011

Contents

12. Equipment 398

13. Reports 421

Appendix 445

Index 543

Preface

Since the first edition of this book in 1996, both clinical anaesthesia and the associated Royal College of Anaesthetists' (RCoA) examinations have progressed significantly. Clinical anaesthesia has advanced considerably in many areas with emphasis on improving the patient experience. New drugs and techniques have refined and improved the delivery of anaesthesia, and the avalanche of guidelines and reports have focused on improving clinical standards and reducing morbidity and mortality. The RCoA Primary and Final FRCA examinations have both undergone revision and restructuring.

This third edition is completely rewritten and improves on the successful first two editions by incorporating these changes and improving many areas of the original book. All anaesthetic literature has been extensively reviewed to distil the important details, particularly those relevant to the exam, while aiming to keep the text detailed but concise. Summaries of guidelines and reports of relevance to clinical anaesthesia and the FRCA examinations have also been updated, together with references for key areas.

While this text has areas of interest for most anaesthetists, all of it is of relevance to those sitting the FRCA exams – to whom I wish every success.

C.D.D.   January 2011

Abbreviations

AAG	α_1 acid glycoprotein
AAGBI	Association of Anaesthetists of Great Britain and Ireland
ACE	Angiotensin converting enzyme
ACh	Acetylcholine
ACS	Abdominal compartment syndrome
ACTH	Adrenocorticotrophic hormone
ADH	Antidiuretic hormone
AIO	Ambulance incident officer
AKI	Acute kidney injury
ALS	Advanced life support
ANS	Autonomic nervous system
Ao	Aorta
APTR	Activated partial thromboplastin time ratio
ARDS	Acute respiratory distress syndrome
ATLS	Advanced trauma life support
A-V	Atrioventricular
BBB	Blood–brain barrier
BMI	Body mass index
CABG	Coronary artery bypass graft
cAMP	Cyclic adenosine monophosphate
CBF	Cerebral blood flow
CCF	Congestive cardiac failure
cGMP	Cyclic guanosine monophosphate
CMR	Cerebral metabolic rate
CMV	Cytomegalovirus
CNS	Central nervous system
CO	Cardiac output
COPD	Chronic obstructive pulmonary disease
CPAP	Continuous positive airway pressure
CPP	Coronary perfusion pressure
CPR	Cardiopulmonary resuscitation
CVA	Cerebrovascular accident (stroke)
CVP	Central venous pressure
CVS	Cardiovascular system
CPR	Cardiopulmonary resuscitation
CXR	Chest X-ray
DAG	Di-acylglycerol
DIC	Disseminated intravascular coagulation
DO_2	Oxygen delivery
dTC	Tubocurarine
ECG	Electrocardiograph
ECMO	Extracorporeal membrane oxygenation

EEG	Electroencephalogram
ETT	Endotracheal tube
FEV_1	Forced expiratory volume in 1 s
FFP	Fresh frozen plasma
FRC	Functional residual capacity
FSH	Follicle-stimulating hormone
FVC	Forced vital capacity
GA	General anaesthetic
GDP	Guanosine diphosphate
GFR	Glomerular filtration rate
GH	Growth hormone
GI	Gastrointestinal
GTN	Glyceryl trinitrate
GTP	Guanosine triphosphate
Hb	Haemoglobin
HbF	Fetal haemoglobin
HT	Hydroxytryptamine
ICP	Intracranial pressure
ICS	Intraoperative cell salvage
IE	Infective endocarditis
IHD	Ischaemic heart disease
i.m.	Intramuscular
INR	International normalized ratio
IP_3	Inositol triphosphate
IPPV	Intermittent positive pressure ventilation
IUGR	Intrauterine growth retardation
i.v.	Intravenous
IVC	Inferior vena cava
JVP	Jugular venous pressure
LA	Local anaesthetic
LA	Left atrium
LH	Luteinizing hormone
LMWH	Low-molecular-weight heparin
LPA	Left pulmonary artery
LPV	Left pulmonary vein
LV	Left ventricle
LVEDP	Left ventricular end-diastolic pressure
LVF	Left ventricular failure
LVH	Left ventricular hypertrophy
MAC	Minimum alveolar concentration
MAP	Mean arterial pressure
MBC	Maximum breathing capacity
MH	Malignant hyperthermia
MHRA	Medicines and Healthcare Products Regulatory Agency
MI	Myocardial infarction
MODS	Multiple organ dysfunction syndrome
MRSA	Methicillin-resistant staphylococcus aureus

MSSA	Methicillin-sensitive staphylococcus aureus
NMB	Neuromuscular blocking drug
NIBP	Non-invasive blood pressure
NICE	National Institute for Health and Clinical Excellence
NO	Nitric oxide
NSAID	Non-steroidal anti-inflammatory drug
OPCAB	Off-pump coronary artery bypass surgery
PA	Pulmonary artery
PAP	Pulmonary artery pressure
PCA	Patient-controlled analgesia
PCI	Percutaneous coronary intervention (angioplasty)
PCWP	Pulmonary capillary wedge pressure
PDA	Patent ductus arteriosus
PEA	Pulseless electrical activity
PEEP	Positive end-expiratory pressure
PEFR	Peak expiratory flow rate
$P_{ET}CO_2$	End-tidal carbon dioxide
PIP_2	Phosphoinositol 4,5-bisphosphate
PNS	Parasympathetic nervous system
PVC	Premature ventricular contraction
PVP	Pulmonary vascular pressure
PVR	Pulmonary vascular resistance
RA	Right atrium
ROC	Receiver operator curve
RPA	Right pulmonary artery
RPV	Right pulmonary vein
RSD	Reflex sympathetic dystrophy
RV	Right ventricle
RVP	Rendezvous point
SSEP	Somatosensory evoked potential
SIRS	Systemic inflammatory response syndrome
SNS	Sympathetic nervous system
STP	Standard temperature and pressure
SVC	Superior vena cava
SVR	Systemic vascular resistance
TBI	Traumatic brain injury
TCA	Tricarboxylic acid
TIA	Transient ischaemic attack
TOE	Transoesophageal echocardiography
TOF	Train of four
V_D	Volume of distribution
VF	Ventricular fibrillation
V_{O_2}	Oxygen consumption
VOC	Vaporizer outside the circle
VIC	Vaporizer inside the circle
VT	Ventricular tachycardia
VTE	Venous thromboembolism

Cardiovascular system 1

ANAESTHESIA AND CARDIAC DISEASE

New York Heart Association classification of cardiovascular disease

- I   Normal cardiac output. Asymptomatic on heavy exertion
- II   Normal cardiac output. Symptomatic on exertion
- III Normal cardiac output. Symptomatic on mild exercise
- IV   Cardiac output reduced at rest. Symptomatic at rest

ASSESSMENT OF RISK – Predictors in non-cardiac surgery

Cardiac complications are a major cause of perioperative morbidity and mortality, particularly vascular patients where mortality is 3–4% for open procedures. Perioperative MI accounts for 10–40% of all postoperative deaths. Risk stratification of patients with known, or at risk of, coronary artery disease is based on (1) the patient risk factors; (2) physiological status of the patient; (3) the risk factors of surgery.

Current thought is that if preoperative assessment reveals possible coronary artery disease, then patients booked for elective surgery should be referred to a cardiologist. Angioplasty in the lead up to elective surgery may increase overall 30-day mortality. CABG, however, may improve long-term outcomes in vascular surgical patients.

Previous ischaemia

Previous guidelines recommended waiting 6 months after an MI before non-cardiac surgery. It is now known that risk after an MI is related more to functional status of the ventricles and the amount of ischaemic myocardium. A small MI without residual angina, and good myocardial function, enables non-cardiac surgery 6 weeks post-MI. A large infarct, residual symptoms and LVEF <0.35 results in high risk even at 6 months post-MI.

- High risk: <6 weeks post-MI because myocardial healing is still ongoing
- Intermediate risk: 6 weeks to 3 months (longer if arrhythmias, ventricular dysfunction, or continued medical therapy)
- Low risk: >3 months post-MI with good myocardial function.

Box 1.1   Classification of cardiac risk factors for non-cardiac surgery

Major factors (unstable coronary artery disease):

- Congestive heart failure
- Malignant arrhythmias
- MI <6 weeks
- Angina class III/IV
- CABG/PCI <6 weeks

Intermediate factors (stable coronary disease):

- MI >6 weeks but <3 months
- Angina class I/II
- CABG or PCI within 3 months
- Diabetes mellitus
- Age >70 years
- Heart failure/ejection fraction <0.35

Minor factors (risk factors for coronary artery disease):

- Family history of ischaemic heart disease
- Uncontrolled hypertension
- Smoking
- ECG abnormalities (LVH, left bundle branch block)
- CABG or PCI >3 months but <6 years (symptom free and no therapy).

Previous cardiac surgery/angioplasty

There is increased risk with non-cardiac surgery if the patient is <3 months post-CABG. Asymptomatic patients >6 months post-CABG are low risk.

Non-cardiac surgery performed within 6 weeks of PCI results in a high risk of stent thrombosis and infarction if the antiplatelet medication is stopped, or of major bleeding if the treatment is maintained throughout the operation.

Important risk studies

- Mahar et al (1978): Patients with IHD who undergo coronary artery bypass grafting (CABG) subsequently have a normal risk of perioperative MI.
- Mangano et al (1990): Postoperative myocardial ischaemia is the most important predictor of adverse outcome. Risk increase ×9.2 (83% of ischaemic events are silent).

Hypertension

Diastolic blood pressure (DBP) is a good indicator of the severity of vascular disease. DBP >110 mmHg is associated with exaggerated swings in BP and an increased risk of perioperative complications. Severe (DBP >115 mmHg) or malignant (DBP >140 mmHg) hypertension should be treated before surgery. LV hypertrophy is associated with reduced ventricular compliance and these patients may benefit from perioperative monitoring of PCWP.

Perioperative hypertension doubles the risk of complications and is associated with increased silent ischaemia.

Investigations

Ambulatory ECG using 24 h Holter monitor. Ischaemic events are a highly significant predictor of adverse postoperative cardiac events. Silent preoperative ischaemia has a positive predictive value of 38% for postoperative cardiac events, whereas its absence precludes perioperative problems in non-vascular surgery in 99% of patients.

Exercise ECG (Bruce protocol). Aim for the target heart rate by stage 4. This is a good predictor of risk in patients with angina. Severe peripheral vascular disease limits exercising and may mask exercise-induced angina (consider the dobutamine stress test in these patients). ST-segment depression ≥ 0.1 mV during exercise is an independent predictor of perioperative ischaemic events.

ECHO. Ejection fraction, wall motion and valve abnormalities.

Thallium-201 scan. K^+ analogue injected i.v. and taken up by well-perfused myocardium, showing underperfused areas as cold spots. Cold spots resolving by 4 h are areas of ischaemia; those persisting are infarcted tissue.

Technetium-99m scan. Similar to thallium scan but underperfused areas show as hot spots.

Dipyridamole–thallium scan. Dipyridamole causes coronary vasodilation to assess coronary stenosis. Similar effect with dobutamine, which also increases myocardial work, i.e. pharmacological stress test. Good predictor of postoperative cardiac complications.

Angiography. Definitive investigation. (Right coronary artery supplies sinoatrial node in 60% of patients and atrioventricular node in 50%). Indicated for unstable angina, or when there is a possible indication for coronary revascularization.

General anaesthesia for non-cardiac surgery

Choice of anaesthetic technique or volatile agent has no proven effect on cardiac outcome. Aim to optimize myocardial oxygen balance (Table 1.1).

Laplace's law

Wall tension (preload and afterload) determined by Laplace's law:

$$\text{Wall tension} \propto \frac{\text{pressure} \times \text{internal radius}}{\text{wall thickness}}$$

Table 1.1 Factors affecting oxygen supply and demand

Supply	Demand
Coronary perfusion	Preload (LVEDP)
O_2 content	Afterload (SVR)
Heart rate	Heart rate
	Contractility

Premedication

Continue all cardiac medication until the day of surgery. Heavy premedication reduces anxiety, which may otherwise cause tachycardia, hypertension and myocardial ischaemia. Consider O_2 after morphine premedication to avoid hypoxaemia from respiratory depression; the prevention of tachycardia results in less myocardial ischaemia overall.

β-blockade. Not all studies have shown benefit from perioperative β-blockade. The Peri-Operative Ischemic Evaluation (POISE) trial showed a beneficial effect of high-dose metoprolol on reducing the risk of perioperative MI, but at the risk of increased stroke and overall mortality. AHA 2007 guidelines recommend continuing β-blocker therapy in patients already on this medication, and giving β-blockers only to high risk vascular surgery patients.

Aspirin. Although aspirin increases the risk of bleeding complications, it does not increase the severity level of the bleeding complication. A meta-analysis has shown that aspirin withdrawal was associated with a three-fold higher risk of major cardiac events (Biondi-Zoccai et al 2006).

Monitoring

ECG. Leads II and V_5 together detect 95% of myocardial ischaemic events. Leads II, V_5 and V4R together detect 100% of events. ST segment monitoring may be a more sensitive indicator.

BP (invasive/non-invasive). Invasive BP monitoring enables blood gases/acid–base and K^+ measurements.

CVP. Use the right atrium (RA) as zero reference point (midaxillary line, 4th costal cartilage). Normal range with spontaneous respiration is 0–6 cmH_2O. The manubriosternal junction is 5–10 cm above the RA when the patient is supine. Ischaemia causes abnormal 'v' waves.

Pulmonary artery catheter. Good monitor of LV function but low sensitivity for detection of myocardial ischaemia (ischaemia causes ↑PCWP and ↑PAP). Rao et al (1983) showed increased reinfarction risk if preoperative PCWP was >25 mmHg. Thus, monitoring of PCWP and aggressive treatment with inotropes/vasodilators may reduce the risk of reinfarction. If ejection fraction >0.50 and there is no dyssynergy, CVP is an accurate correlate of PCWP, and PAP monitoring may be unnecessary.

Transoesophageal ECHO (TOE). Developed in the 1950s by Edler and Hertz. Ultrasound waves are formed when a voltage is applied across a substance with piezoelectric properties (usually lead-zirconate-titanate-5, PZT-5). Ultrasound waves are reflected back to the PZT-5 transducer, and converted back into electrical energy. This signal is then processed and displayed on a monitor. TOE requires less penetration than transthoracic ECHO and therefore uses a higher frequency (3.5–7 MHz) to produces higher resolution images.

Useful to assess perioperative:

• Abnormal ventricular filling/function
• Extensive myocardial ischaemia
• Large air embolism
• Severe valvular dysfunction
• Large cardiac masses/thrombi
• Pericardial effusion
• Major lesions of great vessels (e.g. aortic dissection).

Myocardial wall motion abnormalities detected by TOE are a much more sensitive method than ECG in detecting myocardial ischaemia. Post-bypass TOE is a sensitive predictor of outcome (MI, LVF, cardiac death).

Induction

Aimed at limiting hypotensive response to induction agent and hypertensive pressor response to intubation. High-dose opioid is a popular technique.

Anaesthetic

Avoid CVS changes that precipitate ischaemia. Tachycardia and hypertension increase myocardial O_2 consumption and reduce diastolic coronary filling time. Hypotension reduces coronary perfusion pressure.

N_2O is a sympathetic stimulant, but will decrease sympathetic outflow if the SNS is already stimulated, e.g. LVF. In the presence of an opioid, it may cause CVS instability.

Volatiles. Enflurane and halothane both decrease coronary blood flow, but isoflurane, sevoflurane and desflurane increase coronary blood flow and maintain LV function in normotensive patients. Tachycardia with isoflurane increases myocardial work, but this is minimal with balanced anaesthesia. There is some concern that isoflurane may cause coronary steal (Fig 1.1) but it is thought not to do so as long as coronary perfusion pressure is maintained. There is growing evidence that isoflurane has myocardial protective properties, limiting infarct size and improving functional recovery. This mechanism mimics ischaemic pre-conditioning and involves the opening of ATP-dependent K^+ channels causing vasodilation and preservation of cellular ATP supplies. Desflurane and sevoflurane probably have similar but less marked cardioprotective effects.

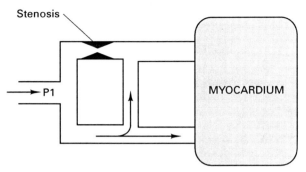

(A) P1 = perfusing pressure. Stenosis reduces
flow to myocardium but adequate perfusion is
achieved through collateral flow.

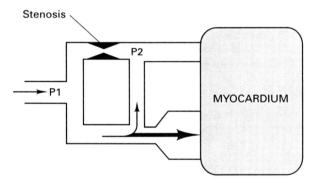

(B) Vasodilator increases run off, reducing
pressure at P2 and therefore reducing perfusion
pressure of myocardium

Figure 1.1 (A) Myocardial perfusion pressure (P1) reduced by stenosis. Adequate perfusion is achieved through collateral flow. (B) Vasodilator increases run-off, reducing pressure at (P2) and therefore reducing myocardial perfusion pressure distal to the stenosis.

Relaxants. Vecuronium combined with high-dose opioids tends towards bradycardia. Use of pancuronium avoids bradycardia.

Epidural/spinal

This decreases afterload and may improve LV function. General anaesthetic combined with epidural may cause severe hypotension because of vasodilation of vessels that have constricted above the block. In animals, redistribution of blood from epicardial to endocardial vessels reduces MI size. Angina following spinal anaesthesia tends to occur at cessation of the block, probably due to increased pre- and afterload aggravated by volume loading. Blocks below L_3 have no effect on the SNS. Blocks above T_{10} block sympathetic afferents to the adrenals and reduce catecholamine release. Blocks to T_1-T_4 interrupt cardioaccelerator fibres, preventing the coronary vasoconstrictive response to surgery, cause coronary vasodilation, decrease coronary perfusion pressure and decrease contractility and heart rate. Central hypovolaemia due to vasodilation causes a vagally mediated bradycardia which responds to fluid challenge.

Pacemakers

There are 200000 patients with implanted pacemakers in the UK.

Nomenclature

The type of permanent pacemaker is denoted by three or four letters (Fig. 1.2).

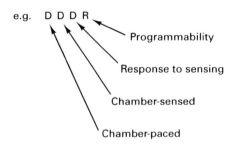

e.g. D D D R

— Programmability

— Response to sensing

— Chamber-sensed

— Chamber-paced

First and second letters
O = None
A = Atrium
V = Ventricle
D = Dual (atrium and ventricle)

Third letter
I = Inhibited
T = Triggered
D = Dual response

Fourth letter
O = None
P = Simple
M = Multi-programmable
R = Adaptive rate pacing

Figure 1.2 Pacemaker nomenclature. For example: DDDR = atrial and ventricular sensing and pacing with adaptive rate response; VVI = pacing wire triggers ventricular contraction. Any spontaneous electrical activity is sensed in the ventricle and inhibits pacemaker firing.

Indications for perioperative pacing

- Acute anterior MI
- First-degree heart block combined with bifascicular block or left bundle branch block
- Acute MI with Mobitz type II
- Third-degree heart block
- Sick sinus syndrome
- Faulty permanent pacemaker.

Intraoperative risks

Rate responsive pacemakers sense electrical activity or vibration around the pacing box and cause a tachycardia in response. Thus, shivering may cause a tachycardia. Fasciculations from suxamethonium are too transient to cause a tachycardia, but there is a case report of a pacemaker that stopped firing following administration of suxamethonium.

Pacemakers that sense blood temperature to control rate may trigger a tachycardia as a hypothermic patient is rewarmed. Those that measure respiratory rate by sensing thoracic impedance and adjust heart rate accordingly can also trigger a tachycardia if the ventilator is set at a high respiratory rate.

Risks associated with K⁺ are:

- hypokalaemia – risk of loss of pacing capture
- hyperkalaemia – risk of VT or VF.

Diathermy

Diathermy current risks reprogramming the pacemaker (not AOO, VOO), causing microshock and inducing VF. Bipolar diathermy is the safest. If unipolar, mount the diathermy plate away from the pacemaker and use short bursts of minimum current. Do not use within 15 cm of the pacing box.

Application of a magnet over a non-programmable ventricular-inhibited pacemaker (VVI) reverts it to asynchronous mode (VOO). Application of a magnet over a programmable pacemaker increases the risk of reprogramming, but it will remain in an asynchronous mode until the magnet is removed, when the reprogrammed mode will take over. Do not use any magnets unless the pacemaker reprogrammes during surgery.

Automatic implantable cardioverter defibrillators (AICDs)

There are 4000 patients with implanted pacemakers in the UK, usually for drug-resistant malignant ventricular arrhythmias. This has reduced 1-year mortality from 66% to 9%. AICDs consist of a lead electrode system for sensing, pacing and delivery of shocks for cardioversion/defibrillation and a control unit consisting of a pulse generator, microprocessor and battery. Modern devices also act as DDD pacemakers.

- In general, all AICDs should be deactivated with a programming device before surgery. In modern AICDs, the anti-bradycardia function can be left activated. Effects of magnets are not consistent between devices, but newer AICDs are inhibited by a magnet.
- Electromagnetic interference, e.g. diathermy, can inhibit the AICD or cause shock discharge. If used, place the diathermy plate as far as possible from the generator. Bipolar diathermy generates less current and is therefore preferential.

- External defibrillation pads should be placed prior to surgery, avoiding current pathways through the device. External defibrillation does not damage an AICD. If an AICD discharges, only a mild electric shock will be felt by anyone touching the patient.

Where the precise time since the onset of acute AF is uncertain, use oral antico-agulation for acute AF, as for persistent AF.

ATRIAL FIBRILLATION: THE MANAGEMENT OF ATRIAL FIBRILLATION
National Institute for Health and Clinical Excellence, June 2006

Guidance

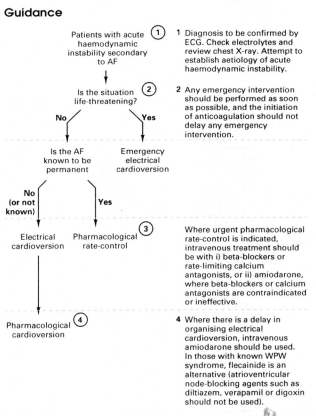

Patients with acute ① haemodynamic instability secondary to AF

1 Diagnosis to be confirmed by ECG. Check electrolytes and review chest X-ray. Attempt to establish aetiology of acute haemodynamic instability.

Is the situation ② life-threatening?

2 Any emergency intervention should be performed as soon as possible, and the initiation of anticoagulation should not delay any emergency intervention.

No / Yes

Is the AF known to be permanent

Emergency electrical cardioversion

No (or not known) / Yes

Electrical cardioversion

Pharmacological ③ rate-control

Where urgent pharmacological rate-control is indicated, intravenous treatment should be with i) beta-blockers or rate-limiting calcium antagonists, or ii) amiodarone, where beta-blockers or calcium antagonists are contraindicated or ineffective.

Pharmacological ④ cardioversion

4 Where there is a delay in organising electrical cardioversion, intravenous amiodarone should be used. In those with known WPW syndrome, flecainide is an alternative (atrioventricular node-blocking agents such as diltiazem, verapamil or digoxin should not be used).

Figure 1.3 Haemodynamically unstable and acute-onset AF. *NICE.*

Antithrombotic therapy for acute-onset atrial fibrillation (AF)

For patients with acute AF who are receiving no, or only sub-therapeutic anticoagulation therapy:

- start heparin at initial presentation, unless contraindicated
- continue heparin until a full risk assessment has been made and appropriate antithrombotic therapy started, based on risk stratification.

For patients with a confirmed diagnosis of acute AF (<48 h since onset), use oral anticoagulation if:

- stable sinus rhythm is not restored within the 48-h period following onset
- there are other risk factors for AF recurrence
- it is recommended by the stroke risk stratification algorithm.

Where a patient with acute AF is haemodynamically unstable, begin emergency treatment as soon as possible. Do not delay emergency intervention in order to begin anticoagulation treatment first.

Anaesthetic considerations for heart surgery

Aortic stenosis

Aortic stenosis becomes symptomatic when the normal valve area of 3 cm² is reduced by >25%. Gradient >70 mmHg is severe (= 0.6 cm²); low cardiac output, dependent upon rate. Bradycardia reduces cardiac output and therefore BP. Tachycardia is poorly tolerated because reduced time for LV filling reduces ejection time and diastolic time during which coronary perfusion occurs. Aortic diastolic pressure must be maintained to preserve coronary blood flow. Ischaemia occurs even with normal coronaries. Atrial contraction is important to fill a poorly compliant LV. A fall in SVR is poorly tolerated. Therefore, maintain both pre- and afterload and avoid regional techniques.

Aortic regurgitation

This causes a dilated, overloaded and failing LV. Low aortic diastolic pressure impairs coronary perfusion. Slight tachycardia reduces regurgitant time and keeps LV small (Laplace's law), thereby improving LV efficiency. A slight reduction in SVR reduces regurgitation but may reduce coronary perfusion pressure.

Mitral stenosis

A value area <1 cm² is severe. There is poor LV filling and a fixed output, dependent upon rate. Low CO is worsened by tachydysrhythmia. Rapid heart rate reduces diastolic time for ventricular filling and thus reduces cardiac output, so bradycardia is beneficial. A high PVP risks pulmonary oedema with overtransfusion, but it is important to maintain adequate filling. A fall in SVR is poorly tolerated. Consider inotropes and pulmonary vasodilators.

Mitral regurgitation

Often well tolerated; PVP remains low. There is slight tachycardia and reduction in SVR which reduce regurgitation. Ischaemia is not usually a problem. General anaesthesia is normally well tolerated, unless pulmonary hypertension has developed, when inotropic support may also be indicated.

Hypertrophic obstructive cardiomyopathy (HOCM)

HOCM is autosomal dominant with variable penetrance. There is variable subaortic obstruction and impaired diastolic function. Try to avoid drugs that depress LV function. Increase pre- and afterload, maintain sinus rhythm and avoid excessive tachy/bradycardia. There is usually good LV function. Ventricular arrhythmias are common. Depression of myocardial contractility reduces outflow obstruction. β-agonists increase outflow obstruction.

Ischaemic heart disease

Rate pressure product (RPP) = heart rate × systolic pressure. Aim to maintain value at below 12 000.

Decrease preload (wall tension) and maintain afterload. A slight decrease in both contractility and rate can be beneficial by reducing work if there is good LV function. Myocardial depression may improve oxygenation unless there is severe IHD or aortic stenosis. If ischaemia occurs, decrease heart rate (β-blockers, calcium-channel blockers), increase ventricular volume (GTN) and increase afterload.

Pulmonary hypertension

Defined as mean pulmonary artery pressure (MPAP) >25 mmHg at rest. Overall, those with severe disease have a 5-year survival of only 27% from time of diagnosis, increasing to 54% with treatment.

Classification of pulmonary artery hypertension

- Idiopathic pulmonary hypertension:
  - Sporadic
  - Familial
- Secondary:
  - Collagen vascular disease (e.g. systemic sclerosis)
  - Portal hypertension (e.g. pulmonary thromboembolism)
  - Congenital heart disease
  - HIV infection
  - Drugs/toxins
  - Persistent pulmonary hypertension of the newborn
  - Congenital heart disease.

Causes increased pulmonary vascular resistance (PVR) with increased load on the right heart causing right heart failure. Treatment aims to reduce PVR. Correct reversible causes (e.g. pulmonary thromboembolectomy, congenital heart disease, etc.). Pulmonary vasodilators include epoprostenol (prostacyclin) with its analogues (iloprost and treprostinil), endothelin receptor antagonists (bosentan), phosphodiesterase inhibitors (sildenafil) and inhaled nitric oxide.

Shunts

- *Right-to-left shunt* (Fallot's tetralogy, Eisenmenger's syndrome). Risk from microemboli, LVF and cyanosis. Shunt worsens with ↑ PVR or ↓ SVR. Keep lung inflation pressures low.
- *Left-to-right shunt* (ASD, VSD, PDA). Shunt worsens with ↓ PVR or ↑ SVR. IPPV increases PVR.

Endocarditis prophylaxis

ANTIMICROBIAL PROPHYLAXIS AGAINST INFECTIVE ENDOCARDITIS IN ADULTS AND CHILDREN UNDERGOING INTERVENTIONAL PROCEDURES
National Institute for Health and Clinical Excellence, March 2008 (http://www.nice.org.uk/nicemedia/pdf/CG64PIEQRG.pdf)

Summary

Antibacterial prophylaxis is not recommended for the prevention of infective endocarditis (IE) in patients undergoing procedures of the:

- upper and lower respiratory tract (including ENT procedures and bronchoscopy)
- genito-urinary tract (including urological, gynaecological and obstetric procedures)
- upper and lower gastrointestinal tract
- dental procedures.

While these procedures can cause bacteraemia, there is no clear association with the development of infective endocarditis.

If patients at risk of endocarditis are undergoing a gastrointestinal or genito-urinary tract procedure at a site where infection is suspected, they should receive appropriate antibacterial therapy that includes cover against organisms that cause endocarditis.

Risk factors for the development of infective endocarditis

- acquired valvular heart disease with stenosis or regurgitation
- valve replacement
- structural congenital heart disease, including surgically corrected or palliated structural conditions, but excluding isolated atrial septal defect, fully repaired ventricular septal or fully repaired patent ductus arteriosus, and closure devices that are judged to be endothelialised.
- hypertrophic cardiomyopathy
- previous infective endocarditis
- (atrial septal defect, repaired ventricular septal defect/patent ductus arteriosus not at risk).

GUIDELINES FOR THE PREVENTION OF ENDOCARDITIS

Report of the Working Party of the British Society for Antimicrobial Chemotherapy, 2006

High-risk patients:
- Previous infective endocarditis
- Cardiac valve replacement surgery (mechanical or tissue)
- Surgically constructed shunts or conduits.

Dental procedures

Prophylaxis is only recommended for high-risk patients
Amoxicillin: p.o. – 3 g 1 h preoperatively;
i.v. – 1 g at induction.

If allergic to penicillin

Clindamycin: p.o. 600 mg p.o. 1 h preoperatively;
i.v. – 300 mg immediately preoperatively.

Endocarditis prophylaxis for non-dental procedures

All patients at risk of endocarditis should receive prophylactic antibiotics for invasive genito-urinary, gastrointestinal, respiratory or obstetric/gynaecological procedures as follows:
Amoxicillin 1 g i.v. + gentamicin 1.5 mg.kg^{-1} i.v. immediately preoperatively.

If allergic to penicillin

Teicoplanin 400 mg i.v. + gentamicin 1.5 mg.kg^{-1} i.v. immediately preoperatively.

Bibliography

ACC/AHA: Guideline Update for Perioperative Cardiovascular Evaluation for Noncardiac Surgery – Executive Summary, *Anesth Analg* 94:1052–1064, 2002.

Agnew NM, Pennefather SH, Russell GN: Isoflurane and coronary heart disease, *Anaesthesia* 57:338–347, 2002.

Allen M: Pacemakers and implantable cardioverter defibrillators, *Anaesthesia* 61:883–890, 2006.

Biccard BM: Peri-operative β-blockade and haemodynamic optimization in patients with coronary artery disease and decreasing exercise tolerance, *Anaesthesia* 59:60–68, 2004.

Biondi-Zoccai GG, Lotrionte M, Agostoni P, et al: A systematic review and meta-analysis on the hazards of discontinuing or not adhering to aspiring among 50,279 patients at risk for coronary artery disease, *Eur Heart J* 27:2667–2674, 2006.

British Society for Antimicrobial Chemotherapy: *Guidelines for the Prevention of Endocarditis. Report of a Working Party*, 2006. http://jac.oxfordjournals.org/cgi/reprint/dkl121v1.

Chassot PG, Delabays A, Spahn DR: Preoperative evaluation of patients with, or at risk of, coronary artery disease undergoing non-cardiac surgery, *Br J Anaesth* 89:747–759, 2002. National Institute of Health and Clinical Excellence http://www.nice.org.uk/nicemedia/pdf/CG036niceguideline.pdf.

De Hert SG: Preoperative cardiovascular assessment in noncardiac surgery: an update, *Eur J Anaesthesiol* 26:449–457, 2009.

Fleisher LA, Beckman JA, Brown KA, et al: ACC/AHA Guidelines on perioperative cardiovascular evaluation and care for noncardiac surgery, *Circulation* 116:1971–1996, 2007.

Gould FK, Elliott TSJ, Foweraker J, et al: Guidelines for the prevention of endocarditis: report of the Working Party of the British Society for Antimicrobial Chemotherapy, *J Antimicrob Chemother* 57:1035–1042, 2006.

Howell SJ: Peri-operative β-blockade, *Br J Anaesth* 86:161–164, 2001.

Howell SJ, Sear JW, Foëx P: Hypertension, hypertensive heart disease and perioperative cardiac risk, *Br J Anaesth* 92:570–583, 2004.

Mahar LJ, Steen PA, Tinker JH, et al: Perioperative myocardial infarction in patients with coronary artery disease with and without aorta-coronary bypass grafts, *J Thorac Cardiovasc Surg* 76:533–537, 1978.

Mangano DT, Browner WS, Hollenberg M, et al: Association of perioperative myocardial ischaemia with cardiac morbidity and mortality in men undergoing non-cardiac surgery. The study of the Perioperative Ischaemia Research Group, *N Engl J Med* 323:1781–1788, 1990.

Mythen M: Pre-operative coronary revascularization before non-cardiac surgery: think long and hard before making a pre-operative referral, *Anaesthesia* 64: 1045–1050, 2009.

Newby DE, Nimmo AF: Prevention of cardiac complications of non-cardiac surgery: stenosis and thrombosis, *Br J Anaesth* 92:628–632, 2004.

NICE: *Atrial Fibrillation: the Management of Atrial Fibrillation*, 2006. June www.nice.org.uk/CG036NICEguideline.

NICE: *Antimicrobial Prophylaxis against Infective Endocarditis in Adults and Children Undergoing Interventional Procedures*, 2008. March www.nice.org.uk/nicemedia/pdf/CG64PIEQRG.pdf.

Moppett I, Sharjar M: Transoesophageal echocardiography, *Br J Anaesth CEPD Reviews* 1:72–75, 2001.

Ng A, Swanevelder J: Perioperative echocardiography for non-cardiac surgery: what is its role in routine haemodynamic monitoring? *Br J Anaesth* 102:731–733, 2009.

POISE study group, Devereaux PJ, Yang H, Yusuf S, et al: Effects of extended-release metoprolol succinate in patients undergoing noncardiac surgery (POISE trial): a randomized controlled trial, *Lancet* 371:1839–1847, 2008.

Roscoe A, Strang T: Echocardiography in intensive care, *Cont Edu Anaesth, Crit Care Pain* 8:46–49, 2008.

Salukhe TV, Dob D, Sutton R: Pacemakers and defibrillators: anaesthetic implications, *Br J Anaesth* 93:95–104, 2004.

CARDIAC SURGERY

General

There are 20000 cardiac operations per annum in the UK. Surgical mortality is only 1–2% for low-risk patients. In uncomplicated cases, patients are generally rewarmed and extubated within 3–4h of the completion of surgery (fast-tracking).

More than 90% of cases are performed using cardiopulmonary bypass (CPB), but off-pump coronary artery bypass grafting (OPCAB) may be performed while the heart is still beating. This avoids costs of CPB circuit, reduces micro-emboli (may lessen postoperative cognitive dysfunction) and reduces inflammatory response to bypass. However, it results in limited surgical access to more posterior coronary arteries and is associated with increased haemodynamic instability. Analysis of the National Adult Cardiac Surgery Database of 3396 off-pump procedures showed a reduction in risk adjusted mortality from 2.9% in CABG to 2.3% for OPCAB. The complication rate was also reduced from 12% (CABG) to 8% (OPCAB). Other studies have not demonstrated a difference in mortality or morbidity.

Risk factors for major postoperative complications

- Previous heart surgery
- Low cardiac output
- Reduced LV ejection fraction
- Peripheral vascular disease
- Renal failure
- Preoperative IPPV
- Age.

New ischaemia occurring prior to cardiopulmonary bypass (CPB) increases the risk of perioperative MI in patients undergoing CABG (Slogoff 1985).

Cardiopulmonary bypass

Drug pharmacokinetics

- Haemodilution on bypass decreases plasma drug concentration but is counterbalanced by reduced total protein binding, due to decreased plasma protein concentration.
- Decreased flow into peripheral vascular beds results in decreased drug uptake by peripheral tissues and decreased mobilization of previously stored drugs out of peripheral tissues.
- Decreased liver perfusion and decreased hepatic metabolism.

Therefore, there is little change in most drug concentrations during bypass. Neuromuscular blockers have a small V_D and therefore are greatly diluted on bypass and additional perioperative doses may be needed. Plasma levels of fentanyl rise on rewarming and after separation from CPB due to reperfusion of peripheral compartments and washout of drug bound in lung.

Bypass circuit

A cardiopulmonary bypass circuit is illustrated in Figure 1.4.

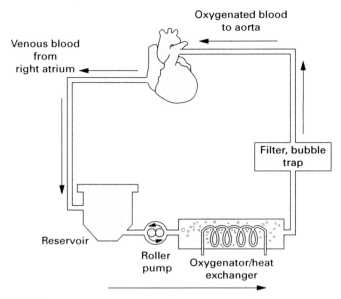

Figure 1.4 Membrane oxygenator circuit.

Advantages of membrane over bubble oxygenators

- Less blood trauma and complement activation
- Fewer microemboli
- Ability to regulate O_2 and CO_2 separately
- Less neuroendocrine stress response.

Pump

Most centres now use non-pulsatile flow. However, pulsatile pumps cause less neuroendocrine stress response.

Lower bypass pressure results in less mechanical damage to blood, reduces aortic trauma at the clamp site and allows use of smaller arterial and venous catheters. However, higher pressures (60–90 mmHg) avoid loss of CNS autoregulation (occurs at <50 mmHg) with less postoperative neurological dysfunction.

Pump flow rate is set at 2.4 L/m², pressure at 40–80 mmHg; 99% O_2 ± 1–5% CO_2. Priming volume approx. 2000 mL, usually with crystalloid but blood is used for paediatric bypass. Priming without blood decreases haematocrit to 20–25%, which offsets the increase in viscosity caused by hypothermia.

Cardioplegia solution

This solution, used to arrest and protect the myocardium, contains 15–30 mEq.L⁻¹ K⁺. It may also contain:

- citrate (to bind Ca^{2+})
- GTN (improves distribution)

- glucose and insulin (energy for cells)
- mannitol (decreases cellular swelling)
- bicarbonate (increases intracellular shift of K$^+$).

Anaesthesia for cardiac surgery

Preoperative assessment

Assess risk factors: age >60 year, arterial and/or pulmonary hypertension, BMI <20 or >35 kg.m^{-2}, congestive cardiac failure, peripheral vascular disease, aortic atheroma, diabetes mellitus, renal insufficiency, acute coronary syndromes, chronic pulmonary disease, neurological disease and previous cardiac surgery. Assess for drugs that interfere with coagulation (aspirin, NSAIDs, clopidogrel, glycoprotein IIb/IIIa antagonists, thrombolytics, heparin, warfarin). Assess for drugs affecting the cardiovascular system (β-blockers, ACE inhibitors).

Premedication

Benzodiazepines and opiates. (Anxiety increases endogenous catecholamines and causes coronary vasospasm.) Heavy premedication may cause hypoventilation and hypoxaemia so consider starting oxygen at time of premedication.

Monitoring

ECG. Either CM5 or combinations including lead II (inferolateral wall) or posterior wall (oesophageal lead).

BP. Radial arterial line. Internal mammary artery dissection can dampen ipsilateral arterial line trace.

CVP. Monitoring through multi-lumen line.

Pulmonary artery catheter. Controversial but may improve outcome in selected patients.

Other. Urinary catheter and core temperature (nasopharyngeal, oesophageal, or tympanic thermocouple).

TOE. Detects wall motion abnormalities and is a more sensitive indicator of myocardial ischaemia than ECG or invasive pressure monitoring.

Induction

Aim is to obtund sympathetic response to surgical stimulation in order to avoid tachycardia and hypertension which worsens myocardial ischaemia. Achieved using anaesthesia based on a high-dose opiate technique (50–100 μg.kg^{-1} fentanyl), which requires postoperative IPPV but improves perioperative cardiovascular stability. Thiopentone, propofol, midazolam and etomidate have all been used as induction agents. Propofol and thiopentone may cause more hypotension on induction, especially in the presence of poor LV function.

Use of thoracic epidural in patients undergoing coronary artery bypass surgery is associated with fewer pulmonary complications but does not decrease the incidence of myocardial infarction or overall mortality.

Intubation

Minimize the pressor response (which worsens ischaemia) by the use of opiates. Use of β-blockers, clonidine or lidocaine also described. Non-depolarizing relaxants reduce chest wall rigidity caused by high-dose opioids.

Maintenance

All volatiles decrease myocardial oxygen demand but also decrease coronary perfusion pressure. Isoflurane/desflurane cause least myocardial depression. There is some evidence that volatile agents have cardioprotective properties, with better preservation of postoperative myocardial function and reduced postoperative myocardial damage. Cessation of pulmonary blood flow during CPB requires maintenance of anaesthesia during this period with propofol infusion or alternatively, volatile agent given directly into the bypass circuit.

Vecuronium avoids CVS side-effects present in other neuromuscular blockers, but mild tachycardia induced by pancuronium may be useful to offset the bradycardia seen with high-dose opioids.

Sternotomy and aortic manipulation cause intense sympathetic stimulation. Further increments of fentanyl may be needed. If there is no CNS disease, a MAP of 35–40 mmHg is adequate when a patient is hypothermic.

Avoid N_2O because of risk of air bubble emboli expanding, especially dangerous with right-to-left shunt. Aim for a haematocrit of 20–30%.

Anticoagulation

Use 3 mg/kg heparin (= 300 U/kg), which accelerates antithrombin III to neutralize clotting factors II, X, XI, XII and XIII. Aim for activated clotting time (ACT) >400. (Celite in test tube at 37°C triggers clotting.) Normal ACT = 120–150 s. Half-life of heparin = 100 min.

Reverse heparin with protamine at 1 mg/100 U heparin. Protamine may increase PVR causing right ventricular failure and also causes hypotension by binding to Ca^{2+}.

Acid–base management

- *pH-stat approach* – arterial blood gases corrected for temperature (pH kept constant)
- *Alpha-stat approach* – arterial blood gases not corrected for temperature.

pH-stat results in relative hypercarbia and acidaemia which increases cerebral blood flow and may increase the risk of cerebral emboli. Cerebral autoregulation, which keeps blood flow constant at arterial pressures of 50–150 mmHg, is lost during pH-stat and cerebral blood flow becomes pressure-dependent. pH-stat management may be optimal for children undergoing deep hypothermic circulatory arrest, because it increases the rate of brain cooling and results in slower exhaustion of brain O_2 stores, providing better CNS protection.

Alpha-stat management maintains cerebral autoregulation, offers better control of cerebral blood flow and demand, and limits cerebral microemboli load. However, the pressure-dependent characteristics of pH-stat may improve cooling and oxygen delivery to the brain.

CABG patients

Good LV function. The main problem is hyperdynamic circulation. Avoid tachycardia and hypertension. Aim to decrease myocardial work, e.g. with volatiles, β-blockers.

Poor LV function. The main problem is cardiac failure. Minimize use of drugs causing myocardial depression, i.e. use high-dose opioids. Use volatiles sparingly. May require inotrope infusion to wean from bypass which is continued in the immediate postoperative period.

Sequence of events in CABG surgery

Anaesthesia. Invasive monitoring and induction of general anaesthesia.

Pre-bypass. Surgical incision and sternal splitting. Disconnect the ventilator during sternal splitting, allowing lungs to deflate, reducing risk of damage from the sternal saw.

Heparin is administered into a central vein and ACT checked prior to commencing CPB.

Pericardial stretching during cardiac manipulation may impair venous return and lower BP.

Nitrous oxide is discontinued to avoid enlargement of any air emboli (or not used at all).

Establishment of bypass. The aortic cannula is first inserted through a purse string suture into the ascending aorta to allow infusion of volume from the bypass reservoir if the BP drops. The venous cannula is then inserted into the right atrium or superior and inferior venae cavae.

CPB is then initiated. Ventilation is stopped when full bypass is established. The aorta is clamped proximal to the cannula and cardioplegia solution infused into the aortic root where it perfuses the coronary arteries causing asystole (Fig. 1.5).

Hypothermia is achieved by cooling the blood through a heat exchanger to reduce myocardial and cerebral oxygen requirements. Core temperature ≈ 32°C is adequate for most cases.

Coronary artery surgery. The vein grafts are anastomosed to the diseased coronary arteries, the distal anastomosis being performed first to enable administration of cardioplegia solution distal to the stenosis.

Rewarming is begun once the final distal anastomosis is complete. The aorta is unclamped, which results in washout of cardioplegia solution from the myocardium. The proximal vein graft anastomoses are completed.

Weaning from bypass. Once the heart is rewarmed, it begins to contract. Internal paddles (10J) are used to defibrillate the heart if VF/VT occurs. Lungs are re-expanded to peak pressure of 30–40 cmH$_2$O with 100% O$_2$ and IPPV is started. Flow through the venous cannulae is reduced to allow the heart to refill and spontaneous cardiac output subsequently increases. Once adequate filling and output are established, the venous and then arterial cannulae are clamped.

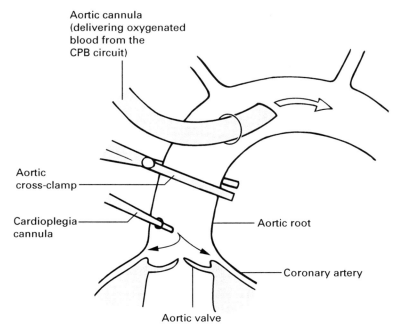

Aortic cannula
(delivering oxygenated
blood from the
CPB circuit)

Aortic
cross-clamp

Cardioplegia
cannula

Aortic root

Coronary artery

Aortic valve

Figure 1.5 Diagram of aortic root showing arrangement of cannulae and cross-clamp for administration of cardioplegia.

Post-bypass management. If the patient remains hypotensive, give fluid challenge in 50–100 mL increments from venous reservoir. Further fluid continues to be needed because of continued rewarming of vascular beds causing vasodilation, changing ventricular diastolic compliance and continued bleeding before heparin reversal. If hypotension persists despite adequate filling, inotropes and/or vasoconstrictors may be required.

Once adequate output is established, venous and arterial cannulae are removed and the effects of heparin are reversed with protamine.

Weaning from bypass

Difficulty occurs usually due to ischaemia following aortic cross-clamping or myocardial stunning.

Causes of failure to wean from cardiopulmonary bypass are:

- Ischaemia
  - graft failure: clot, air bubble, kink
  - inadequate coronary blood flow: coronary spasm, inadequate coronary perfusion pressure or flow
- Valve failure

- Inadequate gas exchange
  - low F_iO_2, bronchospasm, pulmonary oedema
- Hypovolaemia
- Reperfusion injury
- Electrolyte or acid–base imbalance
- Negatively inotropic drugs
- Pre-existing LV failure.

Intra-aortic balloon-pump counterpulsation

This is used as a mechanical assist device for the failing myocardium. The intra-aortic balloon is placed in the aortic arch/early descending thoracic aorta via the femoral artery so that the tip lies distal to left subclavian artery, but is not occluding renal arteries (Fig. 1.6).

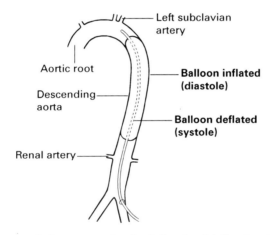

Figure 1.6 Intra-aortic balloon pump showing inflated and deflated position.

- *Diastolic effects.* Expands during diastole, increasing aortic diastolic pressure and therefore coronary perfusion pressure.
- *Systolic effects.* Sudden decrease in balloon volume prior to systole decreases systemic vascular resistance, afterload and myocardial work, and increases cardiac output, cerebral and renal perfusion (Fig. 1.7).

Perioperative placement is considered in high-risk patients, e.g. severe LV dysfunction, congestive heart failure, cardiomyopathy, prolonged bypass. The IABP decreases afterload, increases cardiac output and increases coronary and systemic perfusion, facilitating the patient's weaning from CPB.

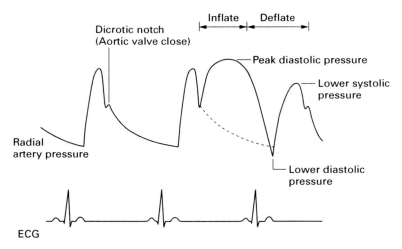

Figure 1.7 Arterial pressure changes using an intra-aortic balloon pump.

Postoperative complications

Cardiac. Avoid postoperative hypertension, common in fit young patients with good LV function, post-aortic valve replacement for aortic stenosis or those with pre-existing hypertension. Worsened by inadequate analgesia/sedation and hypothermia. Often due to neuroendocrine responses to CPB (renin–angiotensin activation).

Low-output syndrome is associated with poor preoperative LV function, intraoperative damage and effects of bypass.

Respiratory. Infection and sputum retention are relatively common. Cardiogenic and non-cardiogenic pulmonary oedema may develop at any time in the postoperative period.

Neurological. 2–6% of patients have neurological damage following CPB. Usually slight (neuropsychiatric) rather than gross. Cause of subtle damage may be unknown but may include micro/macroemboli (particularly common at insertion of aortic cannula and initiation of bypass), air bubbles, effect of non-pulsatile flow, inadequate cerebral perfusion or hyperglycaemia during neuroischaemia. Known risk factors include age, prolonged bypass, severe atherosclerosis and hypertension.

Renal. Risk of prerenal failure and failure from direct tubular damage, e.g. myoglobin, antibiotics.

Haematology. Haemorrhage is a major complication, usually due to platelet dysfunction. Worsened by preoperative aspirin and/or clopidogrel. Antifibrinolytic agents (e.g. aprotinin, tranexamic acid, aminocaproic acid) preserve the adhesive capacity of platelets, which are altered by circulation through the CPB circuit, and may reduce postoperative blood loss. Platelet transfusions and FFP may be needed if bleeding persists. Thromboelastography is useful to identify causes of coagulopathy (inadequate protamine, lack of clotting factors, poor platelet function, fibrinolysis).

Neurological monitoring and protection

Monitoring

Unmodified EEG. Some evidence for correlation with outcome.
Processed EEG. Easier to interpret.
Transcranial Doppler. Research tool. Correlates with neuroinsults.
Jugular bulb O_2 saturation. Desaturation is common but significance is not known.
Regional cerebral blood flow. Research tool.
Cerebral oximetry. Non-invasive and only monitors small regions.

Protection

Physiological. Pulsatile flow, hypothermia, alpha-stat management, euglycaemia, filtration of arterial blood to remove microemboli.
Pharmacological.
Barbiturates: may protect in high doses (>30 mg/kg) but conflicting studies.
Steroids: no evidence for benefit.

DEATH FOLLOWING A FIRST TIME, ISOLATED CORONARY ARTERY BYPASS GRAFT
A report of the National Confidential Enquiry into Patient Outcome and Death, 2008

Recommendations

Multidisciplinary case planning

- Each unit undertaking coronary artery bypass grafting should hold regular preoperative MDT meetings to discuss appropriate cases. Core membership should be agreed and a regular audit of attendance should be performed.

Patient investigations

- There must be a system in place to ensure that preoperative investigations are reviewed by a senior clinician and acted upon.

Medical management

- NCEPOD supports the guidance of the American College of Cardiology and the American Heart Association that clopidogrel should be stopped prior to surgery wherever practicable.

Non-elective, urgent, in-hospital cases

- There should be a protocol to ensure a timely and appropriate review of unstable cases that involves both cardiologists and cardiac surgeons.
- A 'track and trigger' system should be used to provide early recognition of clinical deterioration and early involvement of consultant staff.

Comorbidities

- Where preoperative comorbidity exists, there should be a clear written management plan, which is followed in order to optimize the physical status of the patient prior to surgery, and identify the need for specific postoperative support to be available.

Perioperative management and postoperative care

- Cardiac recovery areas/critical care units are best suited to managing the majority of patients who recover uneventfully.
- Patients who are developing critical illness and additional organ failure should be managed in an environment with sufficient throughput of such patients to have the resources and experience to provide optimum outcomes.
- Senior clinicians should be readily available throughout the perioperative period in order to ensure that complications are recognized without delay and managed appropriately.

Communication, continuity of care and consent

- Protocols must exist for handover between clinical teams and patient locations to ensure effective communication and continuity of care.
- A consultant should obtain consent for coronary artery bypass grafting.

Multidisciplinary review and audit

- Morbidity and mortality audit meetings should be held in all cardiothoracic units. The majority of units should hold meetings at least monthly. If the numbers of cases performed in a unit are small, alternative arrangements should be made to incorporate these cases in other surgical audit meetings.
- A common system for grading of quality of care of patients should be employed for all patients discussed in morbidity and mortality audit meetings. The peer review scale used by NCEPOD provides such a system.

Free radical scavengers (e.g. superoxide dysmutase) and calcium channel blockers remain experimental.

Bibliography

Cornelissen H, Arrowsmith JE: Preoperative assessment for cardiac surgery, *Contin Edu Anaesth, Crit Care & Pain* 6:109–113, 2006.

Feneck RO: Cardiac anaesthesia: the last 10 years, *Anaesthesia* 58:1171–1177, 2003.

Hett DA: Anaesthesia for off-pump coronary artery surgery, *Contin Edu Anaesth, Crit Care & Pain* 6:60–62, 2006.

Krishna M, Zacharowski K: Principles of intra-aortic balloon pump counterpulsation, *Contin Edu Anaesth, Crit Care & Pain* 9:24–28, 2009.

Machin D, Allsager C: Principles of cardiopulmonary bypass, *Contin Edu Anaesth, Crit Care & Pain* 6:176–181, 2006.

National Confidential Enquiry into Patient Outcome and Death: *Death Following a First Time, Isolated Coronary Artery Bypass Graft*, 2008. www.ncepod.org.uk/2008report2/Downloads/CABG_summary.pdf.

Royse CF: High thoracic epidural anaesthesia for cardiac surgery, *Curr Opin Anaesthesiol* 22:84–87, 2009.

Russell IA, Rouine-Rapp K, Stratmann G, et al: Congenital heart disease in the adult: a review, *Anesth Analg* 102–694, 102–723, 2006.

Scott T, Swanevelder J: Perioperative myocardial protection, *Contin Edu Anaesth, Crit Care & Pain* 9:97–101, 2009.

Shaaban Ali M, Harmer M, Kirkham F: Cardiopulmonary bypass and brain function, *Anaesthesia* 60:365–372, 2005.

MAJOR VASCULAR SURGERY

Abdominal aortic aneurysm

Pathogenesis

Destruction of elastin in the media results in abnormal widening of all three layers of the vessel wall. Genetic predisposition, acquired risk factors (smoking, hypertension, atherosclerosis), defective and decreased elastin. If >6 cm, 50% rupture in 10 years.

Associated common pathology:

- hypertension (50%)
- COPD (30%)
- diabetes (10%)
- chronic renal failure (10%).

Mortality

- elective: 6%
- emergency: 65% if ruptured.

Anaesthetic aims

- maintain cardiovascular stability
- blood replacement
- maintain renal function
- temperature control.

Anaesthetic management

Preoperative. Mostly elderly patients. Full cardiac work-up for elective patients. Assess severity and treat other co-existing diseases. Systolic BP at presentation is the most important predictor of survival.

Fluid resuscitation. There is some evidence that aggressive preoperative fluid resuscitation may increase mortality by accelerating bleeding, increasing the risk of clot dislodgement and causing a dilutional coagulopathy. Bleeding makes surgery more difficult and distended veins (IVC and left renal vein) are at greater risk of rupture. It is suggested that the MAP should be maintained at ≈ 65 mmHg until the aorta has been clamped, after which blood, FFP and platelets should be given to restore haemodynamic parameters. All fluids should be warmed.

Preparation. Prepare and drape the patient in the operating theatre. Induction may result in cardiovascular collapse as the tamponading effect of abdominal muscle tone is lost and surgeons must therefore be ready to start immediately.

Adequate analgesia with small doses of i.v. opioids prevents hyperventilation, hypertension, increased endocrine stress response and increased oxygen consumption.

Induction. Ketamine may be of benefit with severe haemorrhagic shock but increases cardiac work, possibly precipitating ischaemia. Induction with combined opioid (e.g. fentanyl) and hypnotic (e.g. midazolam) provides the best CVS stability. Thiopentone and propofol may cause CVS collapse if the patient is haemodynamically unstable. Commence GTN infusion if known IHD or ischaemic ECG changes.

Maintenance of anaesthesia

General anaesthesia. Nitrous oxide–oxygen–relaxant technique and nitrous oxide–oxygen–relaxant–volatile technique alone are associated with depressed ventricular performance and hyperdynamic circulation. Addition of high-dose fentanyl/remifentanil maintains cardiac function and is not associated with hyperdynamic changes. Isoflurane is relatively stable on the cardiovascular system and has been shown to maintain a higher GFR than halothane during aneurysm surgery.

Combined regional and general anaesthesia. Regional anaesthesia combined with a light GA may reduce operative mortality and postoperative morbidity. Epidural followed by heparinization does not increase the risk of epidural haematoma. Regional techniques may improve regional blood flow and maintain GFR although there is no evidence for improved postoperative creatinine clearance. Increases perioperative fluid requirements in elective surgery by 25–50%.

Haemodynamic changes

Mesenteric traction syndrome. Causes flushing, hypotension and tachycardia due to prostacyclin and $PGF_1\alpha$ release. Treat with fluids and vasoconstrictors. Abolish if patient on NSAIDs.

Aortic cross-clamping. Location of clamp determines degree of cardiovascular stress and increase in MAP. Increased afterload increases myocardial wall tension and may worsen LV function. Infrarenal clamping reduces stroke volume by 15–35%, increases SVR by 40% and reduces renal cortical blood flow. Results in increased perfusion proximal to the clamp and anaerobic metabolism distal to the clamp.

Decrease afterload with vasodilators. Nitroglycerine infusion at 0.25–5 µg. $kg^{-1}.min^{-1}$ reduces myocardial wall tension by reducing pre- and afterload, and may maintain normal myocardial blood flow, decrease arterial blood pressure, lower SVR and reduce myocardial oxygen consumption. Lumbar epidurals attenuate the increased SVR that occurs with cross-clamping.

Declamping. Hypoxic vasodilation, sequestration of blood in pelvic and lower limb capacitance vessels, hypovolaemia and release of vasoactive and myocardial depressant metabolites (lactate, K^+) cause hypotension. Severity of hypotension is related to cross-clamp time and the speed at which the clamp is released. Fluid loading until PCWP is 3–5 mmHg above preoperative value prior to declamping reduces hypotension. Severe hypotension may necessitate vasoconstrictor/inotrope support and partial reclamping. Epidurals may exaggerate hypotension after declamping but tend to produce greater CVS stability.

Postoperative. Ventilate until warm, well-filled and cardiovascularly stable. Correct any clotting abnormalities. Monitor renal function closely. Good analgesia is important. Postoperative complications are common and include MI (40%), respiratory failure (40%), renal failure (35%), bleeding (15%) and stroke (5%).

Arterial supply to the spinal cord

The major arterial supply to the spinal cord is a single anterior spinal artery lying in the anterior median fissure of the cord and two posterior spinal arteries located just medial to the dorsal roots. The anterior spinal artery is fed from several sources (Figs 1.8, 1.9):

- C_1–T_4: vertebral, thyrocervical and costocervical arteries
- T_4–T_9: intercostal arterial branches
- below T_9: artery of Adamkiewicz which arises from the aorta between T_9 and L_2.

The anterior spinal artery supplies the anterior two-thirds of the cord and anastomoses with both posterior spinal arteries.

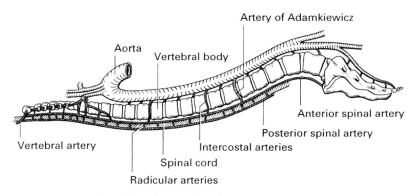

Figure 1.8 Arterial supply to the spinal cord.

Spinal cord injury

Impaired flow in the artery of Adamkiewicz during cross-clamping results in cord ischaemia and paraplegia. There is a 40% incidence of paraplegia following emergency repair of a dissecting aneurysm compared with 0.1% for elective infrarenal procedures. Motor damage–sensory damage. Poor recovery. Attempts to protect cord function include:

- avoiding glucose-containing solutions
- monitoring of cord function with SSEPs

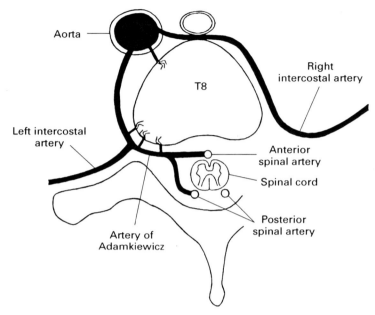

Figure 1.9 Cross-section of the spine showing the relationship between the artery of Adamkiewicz and the anterior spinal artery. (Reproduced from Djurberg & Haddad 1995.)

- maintaining distal aortic pressure with shunts
- 3 mL 1% preservative-free epidural papaverine has been shown to protect the cord during prolonged aortic cross-clamping by dilating anterior spinal arteries
- cross-clamping causes increased CSF pressure, further decreasing cord perfusion. Lumbar drain insertion in an attempt to decrease CSF pressure has shown variable results in reducing cord damage
- steroids, barbiturates and superoxide dismutase
- regional lumbar spinal cord cooling.

Renal function

There is a high risk of renal failure due to hypovolaemia, renal atherosclerosis, changes in renal perfusion with cross-clamping and nephrotoxic drugs.

Optimize fluid and electrolyte balance and consider mannitol, furosemide and renal-dose dopamine. Prophylactic administration of mannitol (25–50 mL 25% solution) prior to cross-clamping may protect against renal cortical ischaemia by several mechanisms:

- osmotic diuresis
- volume expansion, increasing renal blood flow and GFR
- haemodilution

- free radical scavenger activity
- atrial expansion, suppressing renin release
- reducing endothelial cell swelling.

Postoperative

Patients are prone to developing abdominal compartment syndrome (ACS), defined as intra-abdominal pressure >20 mmHg. Risk factors for ACS are anaemia, prolonged ↓ BP, CPR, hypothermia, severe acidosis (base deficit >14 mEq) and massive blood transfusion.

Carotid artery surgery

Patients with severe carotid artery stenosis (>70%) have a better outcome with surgery. Benefits for moderate stenosis (30–69%) are unclear. Surgery for carotid artery obstruction may be carried out if patient is having transient ischaemic attacks:

- 80% TIAs from carotid territory
- 20% TIAs from vertebrobasilar territory.

Vessels distal to a stenosis are maximally dilated and further flow can only come via collaterals from the circle of Willis. Thus, these patients are extremely sensitive to hypotension. If non-diseased areas vasodilate, a 'reverse steal' may occur, reducing collateral flow to post-stenotic areas.

Preoperative

A detailed preoperative neurological examination is needed to enable assessment of the postoperative neurological state. Also, examine the cardiovascular system to assess the degree of atherosclerosis. Diabetes and hypertension are common. Stop smoking.

Anaesthetic techniques

Recent GALA trial (Lancet 2008) failed to show a difference in outcome between local and general anaesthetic techniques.

Premedication. Short-acting only to prevent prolonged postoperative somnolence and allow early assessment of neurological function. Short-acting benzodiazepine is suitable.

Monitoring

CVS. Potential for large swings in heart rate and BP due to manipulation of carotid baroreceptors. Consider invasive BP monitoring.

Neurological. The awake patient allows continuous assessment of multiple levels of neurological function, but this is less sensitive if the patient is sedated. Also consider EEG, SSEPs, transcranial Doppler or intracarotid xenon wash-out curve to measure cerebral blood flow (CBF), and internal carotid artery distal stump pressure >50 mmHg (but poor correlation with regional CBF).

Regional technique (C_2–C_4). Deep and superficial cervical plexus block or cervical extradural anaesthesia. Provides excellent haemodynamic stability resulting in a very low incidence of perioperative MI. However, oxygenation and ventilation are poorly controlled and hypoxaemia/hypercarbia may necessitate intubation during surgery.

General anaesthesia. No specific technique has been shown to be of any advantage. Pre-oxygenate. Induction with thiopentone followed by vecuronium/rocuronium. Avoid pressor response to intubation (topical/i.v. lidocaine, opioids, esmolol, nitroprusside, etc.). Oxygen–air mixture + isoflurane may provide more EEG depression than halothane or enflurane for a given blood flow. Animals pretreated with barbiturates show protection from ischaemia, but there is no evidence suggesting thiopentone protects in humans.

Swings in BP are best treated with changes in volatile concentration, because use of short-acting haemodynamic drugs (nitroprusside, nitroglycerine, adrenaline, etc.) is associated with greater myocardial ischaemia.

Hyperglycaemia during ischaemia may worsen the neurological outcome by increasing anaerobic metabolism. Patients with poorly controlled blood glucose following a stroke have a worse outcome. Therefore, although no outcome studies have proven the risks of hyperglycaemia in carotid artery surgery, maintain tight control of perioperative glucose in diabetic patients.

Postoperative

Avoid postoperative hypertension and hypercapnia, which increase the risk of cerebral oedema and haemorrhage, because maximally vasodilated areas are unable to autoregulate. Hypocapnia may cause cerebral ischaemia.

Wound haematoma may cause airway obstruction. Laryngeal and hypoglossal nerve injury has been documented. Myocardial infarction is the commonest cause of perioperative mortality.

Bibliography

Augoustides JG: The year in cardiothoracic and vascular anesthesia: selected highlights from 2008, *J Cardiothorac Vasc Anesth* 23:1–7, 2009.

Djurberg H, Haddad M: Anterior spinal artery syndrome, *Anaethesia* 50:345–348, 1995.

GALA Trial Collaborative Group: General anaesthesia versus local anaesthesia for carotid surgery (GALA): a multicentre, randomised controlled trial, *Lancet* 372:2132–2142, 2008.

Hebballi R, Swanevelder J: Diagnosis and management of aortic dissection, *Contin Edu Anaesth, Criti Care & Pain* 8:14–18, 2009.

Leonard A, Thompson J: Anaesthesia for ruptured abdominal aortic aneurysm, *Contin Edu Anaesth, Criti Care & Pain* 8:11–15, 2008.

Sloan TB: Advancing the multidisciplinary approach to spinal cord injury risk reduction in thoracoabdominal aortic aneurysm repair, *Anesthesiology* 108:555–556, 2008.

Spargo JR, Thomas D: Local anaesthesia for carotid endarterectomy, *Contin Edu Anaesth, Criti Care & Pain* 4:62–65, 2004.

Tuman KJ: Anesthetic considerations for carotid artery surgery, *Anesth Analg* 2000 Review Course Lectures (Suppl).

HYPOTENSIVE ANAESTHESIA

First described by Gardner in 1946 who used controlled haemorrhage to induce hypotension. (Introduced clinically by Griffiths & Gillie in 1948.) There was initial concern over high morbidity and mortality, but recent studies suggest that when carefully performed, the technique is reasonably safe. East Grinstead reported a mortality rate of 1 in 4128 cases.

Benefits

- Improves surgical field, e.g. ENT, maxillofacial and plastic surgery
- Reduces blood loss
- Reduces risk of cerebral aneurysm rupture during clipping.

Contraindications

- Hypertension: BP may be extremely labile
- Ischaemic heart disease: hypotension reduces myocardial perfusion
- Severe cerebrovascular disease
- Respiratory disease: vasodilating drugs abolish hypoxic pulmonary vasoconstriction, making shunting worse. Reversible airways obstruction may be made worse by the use of β-blockers or ganglion-blocking drugs
- Diabetes: ganglion blockade impairs stress-induced gluconeogenesis. β-blockers potentiate hypoglycaemia
- Hypovolaemia, anaemia
- Renal and hepatic disease
- Pregnancy.

Effects of hypotension

CVS. Reduced diastolic pressure reduces coronary perfusion pressure.

Respiratory. Greatly increased physiological dead space, $\uparrow$ V/Q (ventilation/perfusion) mismatch and $\downarrow$ FRC. Volatile agents may further impair hypoxic pulmonary vasoconstriction. May need F_iO_2 >0.3 to maintain arterial saturation.

CNS. Loss of cerebral autoregulation <50 mmHg. Risk of ischaemia in the presence of hypocapnia.

Renal. Poor GFR below 50 mmHg with risk of renal failure.

Techniques of induced hypotension

Premedication

Avoid atropine. Ensure patient is well sedated. Consider droperidol/ chlorpromazine.

Induction

Spray cords. Thiopentone, fentanyl and neuromuscular blocker (not pancuronium which causes tachycardia – tubocurare was used because of its hypotensive effects). Maintenance with isoflurane/N_2O and a high F_iO_2.

Posture

Head-up tilt reduces arterial and venous pressure in tissues higher than the heart.

IPPV

Positive intrathoracic pressure reduces venous return and thus cardiac output. Reflex vasoconstriction then normally maintains the BP but ganglion blockade or β-blockers may abolish this compensatory reflex. Positive end-expiratory pressure (PEEP) produces a further reduction in venous return and BP. Hyperventilation augments hypotension.

Volatiles

Halothane > enflurane causes peripheral vasodilation and myocardial depression. Isoflurane/sevoflurane/desflurane have little effect on myocardial contractility and hypotension is a result of peripheral vasodilation. Increasing doses cause CNS depression, which limits any reflex tachycardia. Isoflurane/sevoflurane/desflurane have the advantage that their cardiovascular effects can be altered with a change in inspired concentration faster than enflurane or halothane and they have less effect on intracranial pressure.

Sympathetic ganglion blockade

Trimetaphan (3–4 mg.min^{-1}) blocks nicotinic receptors at PNS and SNS ganglia. The SNS block reduces myocardial contractility but the PNS block results in tachycardia which may impair the degree of hypotension. Tachyphylaxis is marked.

Non-depolarizing neuromuscular blockers

Alcuronium and d-tubocurarine induce hypotension through histamine release. Mild ganglionic blockade also contributes to the hypotensive effect.

Alpha-adrenoceptor blockade

Phentolamine (5–10 mg i.v.), phenoxybenzamine, chlorpromazine and droperidol all produce competitive blockade of sympathetic postsynaptic noradrenergic receptors. Phentolamine is short-acting whereas phenoxybenzamine is usually used preoperatively for chronic vascular expansion. Droperidol and chlorpromazine are useful additions to the premedication.

Beta-adrenoceptor blockade

Reduces cardiac output and heart rate. Labetalol (50 mg i.v. over 1 min; max. 200 mg) is short-acting and also has some α-blocking action. Esmolol (100–300 μg.min⁻¹) is a short-acting drug which may be suitable for intraoperative i.v. use. Preoperative oral administration of β-blockers, e.g. propanolol, may prevent wide fluctuations in BP.

Direct-acting vasodilators

The very short half-life of sodium nitroprusside (SNP) enables rapid reduction in BP and equally rapid restoration (2–4 min). It dilates resistance and capacitance vessels. Vasodilation causes raised intracranial pressure and SNP should not be used in neurosurgery until the cranium has been opened. SNP increases aortic flow, increasing shearing pressure; therefore β-blockers may need to be used in addition. Start at $0.3 \mu g.kg^{-1}.min^{-1}$ to limit cyanide toxicity (max. 8 μg. $kg^{-1}.min^{-1}$). Base deficit >–7 mmol.L⁻¹ is suggestive of CN^- toxicity. Sodium thiosulphate reduces CN^- levels by providing sulphydryl groups at the rate-limiting step (Fig. 1.10).

Glyceryl trinitrate (0.25–$5.0 \mu g.kg^{-1}.min^{-1}$) causes a slower reduction and recovery in BP (10–20 min) than SNP, with a greater effect on the systolic than on the diastolic BP. Dilates capacitance vessels with little effect on resistance vessels. Maintains coronary perfusion pressure more effectively than SNP but may raise intracranial pressure even more. Degree of hypotension achievable may be limited. Hydralazine (5–10 mg i.v. slowly) is also suitable for rapid control of BP.

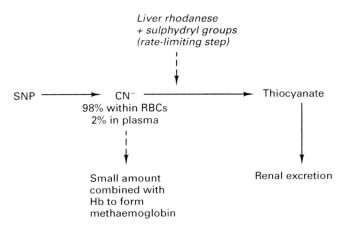

Figure 1.10 Metabolism of nitroprusside.

Regional anaesthesia

Spinal and epidural anaesthesia with blocks extending to thoracic levels will produce hypotension by arterial and venous dilatation. Blocks extending to cardioaccelerator fibres (T2–T4) augment the hypotension further by preventing a compensatory tachycardia.

Bibliography

Degoute CS: Controlled hypotension: a guide to drug choice, *Drugs* 67:1053–1076, 2007.

Simpson PJ: Hypotensive anaesthesia, *Curr Anaesth Crit Care* 3:90–97, 1992.

ASSESSING THE AIRWAY

During routine anaesthesia, the incidence of difficult tracheal intubation (≥3 attempts at intubation or >10 min to accomplish it) has been estimated as 3–15%. Tracheal intubation is best achieved with the neck flexed and the atlantoaxial joint extended ('sniffing the morning air'). Factors affecting this position may result in difficult intubation.

History and examination

Remember to check anaesthetic notes for previous difficulties and ask the patient if he or she is aware of any anaesthetic problems.

Visual inspection

The following features suggest a difficult intubation: obesity, pregnancy, large breasts, short muscular neck, full dentition, limited neck flexion or head extension, receding jaw, prominent upper incisors, limited mouth opening, high arched palate.

Cormack and Lehane grading (1984)

Used to grade the view at laryngoscopy (Fig. 2.1):

- Grade I – visualization of the entire laryngeal aperture
- Grade II – visualization of the posterior part of the laryngeal aperture
- Grade III – visualization of epiglottis only
- Grade IV – not even the epiglottis is visible.

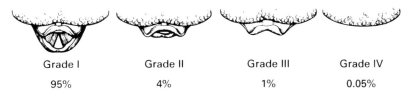

Grade I	Grade II	Grade III	Grade IV
95%	4%	1%	0.05%

Figure 2.1 Cormack & Lehane grading. (Adapted from Cormack & Lehane 1984.)

Recent reclassification has subdivided grade II view further:

- Grade IIa – only part of the glottis is visible
- Grade IIb – only the arytenoids or the very posterior origin of the cords are visible.

Predictive tests
Mallampati classification (Mallampati et al 1985)

The patient sits upright with the head in the neutral position and the mouth open as wide as possible, with the tongue extended to maximum. The following structures are visible (Fig. 2.2):

- Class I – hard palate, soft palate, uvula, tonsillar pillars
- Class II – hard palate, soft palate, uvula
- Class III – hard palate, soft palate
- Class IV – hard palate.

Class I view is grade I intubation >99% of the time. Class IV view is grade III or IV intubation 100% of the time.

This classification may fail to predict >50% of difficult intubations.

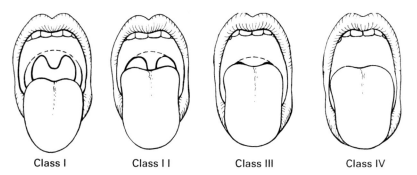

Class I   Class I I   Class III   Class IV

Figure 2.2 Mallampati classification. (Reproduced from Mallampati et al 1985.)

Thyromental distance (Patil et al 1983)

Measure from the upper edge of the thyroid cartilage to tip of the jaw with the head fully extended (Fig. 2.3). A short thyromental distance equates with an anterior larynx which is at a more acute angle and also results in less space for the tongue to be compressed into by the laryngoscope blade. This is a relatively unreliable test unless combined with other tests:

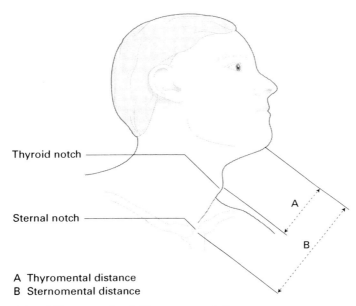

Thyroid notch

Sternal notch

A
B

A Thyromental distance
B Sternomental distance

Figure 2.3 (A) Thyromental and (B) sternomental distance.

- Thyromental distance >6.5 cm = easy intubation
- Thyromental distance <6.0 cm = difficult intubation.

Sternomental distance (Savva 1994)

Measure from the sternum to the tip of the mandible with the head extended (Fig. 2.3). A sternomental distance of ≤12.5 cm predicts difficult intubation.

Horizontal length of mandible

Horizontal mandibular length >9 cm is suggestive of a good laryngoscopic view.

Cervical spine movements

The effect of mobility of the atlanto-occipital and atlantoaxial joints on ease of intubation is probably underestimated. It may be best assessed by asking patients to extend their head while their neck is in full flexion. Extension of the head with atlantoaxial joint immobility results in greater cervical spine convexity which pushes the larynx anteriorly and impairs the laryngoscopic view.

Prayer sign

The inability to place both palms flat together suggests difficult intubation. It is probably a reflection of generalized joint and cartilage immobility limiting atlantoaxial and cervical extension. It may be particularly common in diabetics.

Wilson risk score (Wilson 1993; see Table 2.1)

A total of 3 predicts 75% of difficult intubations, while a total of 4 predicts 90%. However, the test has a poor specificity and may fail to predict >50% of difficult intubations. Many of the measurements are subjective.

Table 2.1 Wilson risk score

Parameter	Risk level
Weight	0–2 (e.g. >90 kg = 1; >110 kg = 2)
Head and neck movement	0–2
Jaw movement	0–2
Receding mandible	0–2
Buck teeth	0–2
Maximum	10 points

Radiographic predictors of difficult intubation

These have the disadvantage of X-ray exposure and thus cannot be performed as routine tests.

Mandibulohyoid distance (Chou and Wu 1993)

This is the vertical distance between the anterior edge of the hyoid and the mandible vertically above measured by lateral X-ray. A distance >6 cm is suggestive of difficult intubation. A longer distance results in more of the tongue being present in the hypopharynx, which must be displaced to view the vocal cords.

Cass et al (1956) (absolute measurements not given)

- Incisor tooth to posterior border of ramus
- Alveolar margin to lower border of the mandible
- Angle of the mandible.

White and Kander (1975)

- Increased length of mandible
- Increased depth of mandible
- Reduced distance between occiput and spinous process of C_1 or reduced distance between C_1–C_2 interspinous gap.

Nichol and Zuck (1983)

These authors stressed the importance of a reduced atlanto-occipital distance as a predictor of ability to extend the head during laryngoscopy.

Combined indicators

By combining prognostic indicators, a greater specificity for predicting difficult intubation may be achieved.

- Freck (1991) found that a thyromental distance of 7 cm in patients with Mallampati class III/IV predicts a grade IV intubation. The test has high sensitivity and specificity.
- Benumof (1991) suggested that a combination of relative tongue/pharyngeal size, atlantoaxial joint extension and anterior mandibular space provides a good predictor of difficult intubation and that the tests are quick and easy to perform.
- Best multifactorial index scores the following criteria to give sensitivity and specificity >90% in prediction of difficult intubation (Arné et al 1998):
  - Previous history of difficult intubation
  - Pathologies associated with difficult intubation
  - Clinical symptoms of a pathological airway
  - Inter-incisor gap
  - Thyromental distance
  - Head and neck movement
  - Mallampati's modified test.

Bibliography

Arné J, Descoins P, Ingrand P, et al: Preoperative assessment for difficult intubation in general and ENT surgery: predictive value of a clinical multivariate risk index, *Br J Anaesth* 80:140–146, 1998.

Benumof JL: Management of the difficult airway, *Anesthesiology* 75:1087–1110, 1991.

Cass NM, James NR, Lines V: Difficult laryngoscopy complicating intubation for anaesthesia, *BMJ* 1:488–489, 1956.

Charters P: What future is there for predicting difficult intubation? *Br J Anaesth* 77:309–311, 1996.

DIFFICULT AIRWAY SOCIETY GUIDELINES FOR MANAGEMENT OF THE UNANTICIPATED DIFFICULT INTUBATION 2004

Problems with tracheal intubation are the most frequent cause of anaesthetic death in the analyses of records of the UK medical defence societies. The Difficult Airway Society (DAS) has developed guidelines for management of the unanticipated difficult intubation in an adult non-obstetric patient, see http://www.das.uk.com/home

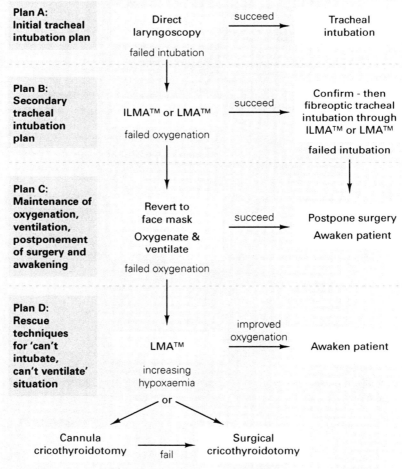

Figure 2.4 Simple composite chart. (*Difficult Airway Society, 2004*)

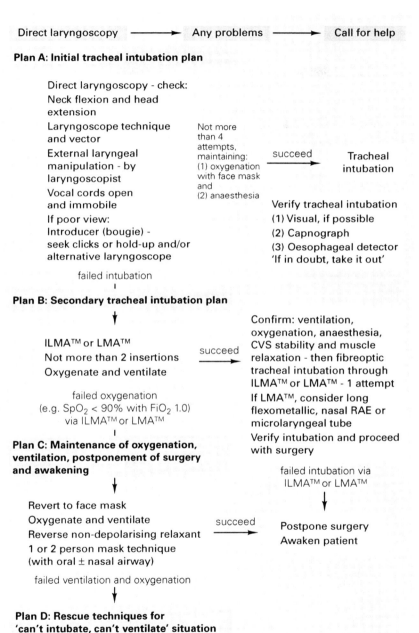

Figure 2.5 Unanticipated difficult tracheal intubation. *(Difficult Airway Society, 2004)*

failed intubation and difficult ventilation (other than laryngospasm)

Face mask
Oxygenate and ventilate patient
Maximum head extension
Maximum jaw thrust
Assistance with mask seal
Oral ± 6 mm nasal airway
Reduce cricoid force - if necessary

failed oxygenation with face mask (e.g. SpO_2 < 90% with FiO_2 1.0)

call for help

↓

LMA™ Oxygenate and ventilate patient
Maximum 2 attempts at insertion
Reduce any cricoid force during insertion

succeed → Oxygenation satisfactory and stable: maintain oxygenation and awaken patient

↓

'can't intubate, can't ventilate' situation with increasing hypoxaemia

Plan D: Rescue techniques for 'can't intubate, can't ventilate' situation

or

Cannula cricothyroidotomy

Equipment: Kink-resistant cannula, e.g. Patil (Cook) or Ravussin (VBM)
High-pressure ventilation system, e.g. Manujet III (VBM)
Technique:
1. Insert cannula through cricothyroid membrane
2. Maintain position of cannula - assistant's hand
3. Confirm tracheal position by air aspiration -20 mL syringe
4. Attach ventilation system to cannula
5. Commence cautious ventilation
6. Confirm ventilation of lungs, and exhalation through upper airway
7. If ventilation fails, or surgical emphysema or any other complication develops - convert immediately to surgical cricothyroidotomy

fail →

Surgical cricothyroidotomy

Equipment: scalpel - short and rounded (no. 20 or Minitrach scalpel)
Small (e.g. 6 or 7 mm) cuffed tracheal or tracheostomy tube
4-step technique:
1. Identify cricothyroid membrane
2. Stab incision through skin and membrane. Enlarge incision with blunt dissection (e.g. scalpel handle, forceps or dilator)
3. Caudal traction on cricoid cartilage with tracheal hook
4. Insert tube and inflate cuff

Ventilate with low-pressure source
Verify tube position and pulmonary ventilation

Notes:
1. These techniques can have serious complications - use only in life-threatening situations
2. Convert to definitive airway as soon as possible
3. Postoperative management - see other difficult airway guidelines and flow-charts
4. 4 mm cannula with low-pressure ventilation may be successful in patient breathing spontaneously

Difficult Airway Society guidelines Flow-chart 2004 (use with DAS guidelines paper)

Figure 2.6 Failed intubation. *(Difficult Airway Society, 2004)*

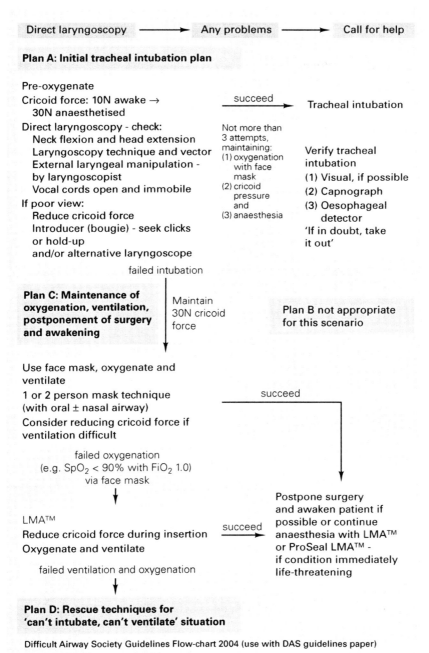

Direct laryngoscopy ⟶ Any problems ⟶ Call for help

Plan A: Initial tracheal intubation plan

Pre-oxygenate
Cricoid force: 10N awake →
   30N anaesthetised

succeed → Tracheal intubation

Direct laryngoscopy - check:
   Neck flexion and head extension
   Laryngoscopy technique and vector
   External laryngeal manipulation -
    by laryngoscopist
   Vocal cords open and immobile
If poor view:
   Reduce cricoid force
   Introducer (bougie) - seek clicks
    or hold-up
   and/or alternative laryngoscope

Not more than
3 attempts,
maintaining:
(1) oxygenation
   with face
   mask
(2) cricoid
   pressure
   and
(3) anaesthesia

Verify tracheal
intubation
(1) Visual, if possible
(2) Capnograph
(3) Oesophageal
   detector
'If in doubt, take
it out'

failed intubation

**Plan C: Maintenance of
oxygenation, ventilation,
postponement of surgery
and awakening**

Maintain
30N cricoid
force

Plan B not appropriate
for this scenario

Use face mask, oxygenate and
ventilate
1 or 2 person mask technique
(with oral ± nasal airway)
Consider reducing cricoid force if
ventilation difficult

succeed

failed oxygenation
(e.g. SpO_2 < 90% with FiO_2 1.0)
via face mask

LMA™
Reduce cricoid force during insertion
Oxygenate and ventilate

succeed

Postpone surgery
and awaken patient if
possible or continue
anaesthesia with LMA™
or ProSeal LMA™ -
if condition immediately
life-threatening

failed ventilation and oxygenation

**Plan D: Rescue techniques for
'can't intubate, can't ventilate' situation**

Difficult Airway Society Guidelines Flow-chart 2004 (use with DAS guidelines paper)

Figure 2.7 Management of unanticipated difficult tracheal intubation. *(Difficult Airway Society, 2004)*

Chou HC, Wu TL: Mandibulohyoid distance in difficult laryngoscopy, *Br J Anaesth* 71:335–339, 1993.

Cormack RS, Lehane: Difficult tracheal intubation in obstetrics, *Anaesthesia* 39:1105–1111, 1984.

Difficult Airway Society, 2004, British Airway Society Guidelines Flow-chart 2004, http://www.das.uk.com/files/rsi-Jul04-A4.pdf.

Freck CM: Predicting difficult intubation, *Anaesthesia* 46:1005–1008, 1991.

Henderson JJ, Popat MT, Latto IP, et al: Difficult Airway Society guidelines for management of the unanticipated difficult intubation, *Anaesthesia* 59:675–694, 2004.

Lavery GG, McCloskey BV: The difficult airway in adult critical care, *Crit Care Med* 36:2163a–2173a, 2008.

Lee A, Fan LTY, Gin T, et al: A systematic review (meta-analysis) of the accuracy of the Mallampati tests to predict the difficult airway, *Anesth Analg* 102:1867–1878, 2006.

Mallampati SR, Gatt SP, Gugino LD, et al: A clinical sign to predict difficult intubation: a prospective study, *Can J Anaesth* 32:429–434, 1985.

Nichol HL, Zuck D: Difficult laryngoscopy – the 'anterior' larynx and the atlanto-occipital gap, *Br J Anaesth* 55:141–143, 1983.

Patil VU, Stehling LC, Zaunder HL: *Fibreoptic endoscopy in anaesthesia*, Chicago, 1983, Year Book Medical Publishers.

Popat M: The airway, *Anaesthesia* 58:1166–1170, 2003.

Savva D: Prediction of difficult tracheal intubation, *Br J Anaesth* 73:149–153, 1994.

Vaughan RS: Predicting difficult airways, *BJA CEPD Reviews* 1:44–47, 2001.

White A, Kander PL: Anatomical factors in difficult direct laryngoscopy, *Br J Anaesth* 47:468–474, 1975.

Wilson ME: Predicting difficult intubation, *Br J Anaesth* 71:333–334, 1993.

ANAESTHESIA AND RESPIRATORY DISEASE

Smoking

Postoperative pulmonary complications occur in 22% of current smokers but only 5% of those who have never smoked.

Effects of smoking

- Increased oxygen demand through nicotine activation of the sympatho-adrenergic system ($\uparrow$HR, $\uparrow$BP and $\uparrow$SVR)
- Decreased oxygen supply via carboxyhaemoglobinaemia (HbCO) and raised coronary vascular resistance
- Increased airway reactivity with greater risk of laryngospasm
- Increased mucus production
- Decreased ciliary motility

- Increased closing capacity
- Impaired humoral and cell-mediated immunity ($\downarrow$ immunoglobulins and $\downarrow$ leucocyte activity)
- Increased risk of chest infection
- Impaired wound healing
- Cor pulmonale
- Lung cancer.

Preoperative cessation of smoking (Box 2.1)

A study in patients undergoing CABG (Warner 2006) showed that in those stopping smoking, the incidence of postoperative pulmonary complications did not fall until at least 8 weeks had elapsed:

- current smokers – 33% incidence
- ex-smokers <8 weeks – 57% incidence
- ex-smokers >8 weeks – 15% incidence.

Box 2.1   Effects of cessation of smoking

12–24 h	Clearance of carbon monoxide
2–10 days	Decreased upper airway reactivity
1–2 months	Increase in postoperative pulmonary complications (Bluman et al 1998)
6 months	Decrease in postoperative pulmonary complications
Years	Reduced risk of COPD, ischaemic heart disease, lung cancer and cerebrovascular disease

---

Chronic bronchitis

Chronic bronchitis is defined as productive cough >3 months of the year for ≥ 2 years.

Postoperative pneumonia

Predisposed by:

- decreased ciliary activity
- sputum retention
- poor cough
- lack of humidification.

Viral upper respiratory tract infection (URTI)

Common in paediatric ENT patients. Causes worsening of asthma and ↑ bronchial reactivity for up to 6 weeks following resolution of symptoms. May be due to viral-mediated damage to vagus releasing acetylcholine and potentiating bronchoconstriction.

In children, there is a 2–7-fold increase in respiratory related adverse events, if intubated, an 11-fold increase in adverse events, and an increased risk of transient hypoxaemia in the postoperative period. In adults with URTI, upper airway reactivity is also increased by an amount related to severity of symptoms.

Therefore, postpone routine surgery for at least 2–3 weeks. If anaesthesia is given during this period, consider topical anaesthesia to larynx to reduce vagally mediated reflexes and consider the use of atropine to block hyperreactivity. Monitor O_2 saturation postoperatively.

Effects of general anaesthesia

- Central respiratory depression
- Reduced compliance
- Cranial shift of diaphragm, atelectasis, reduced tone of chest wall and reduced thoracic blood volume cause ↓ FRC (17%, 500 mL)
- FRC approaches and may exceed closing capacity (CC)
- Impaired O_2 and CO_2 exchange
- Increased spread of V/Q ratios. Increased shunting (shunt fraction during GA: 11% during spontaneous breathing, 14% during IPPV)
- Hypoxic pulmonary vasoconstriction inhibited by up to 25% with volatiles but not by i.v. agents.

All these factors result in an increased $A-aO_2$ (difference in alveolar and arterial oxygen tensions), which persists for at least 1–2 h postoperatively. Diaphragm may recover from neuromuscular blockade prior to muscles involved in coughing and swallowing. Postoperative wound pain, abdominal distension, pulmonary venous congestion and a supine posture all increase CC–FRC and result in further alveolar collapse.

Anaesthesia for chronic respiratory disease
Risk factors for postoperative pulmonary complications

American Society of Anesthesiologists (ASA) classification:

- Extremes of age
- Obesity ($\downarrow$ compliance, $\downarrow$ FRC)
- Suboptimal respiratory therapy
- Smoking (need to stop >8 weeks to be of benefit)
- Severe dyspnoea at rest
- Copious sputum production
- Respiratory failure ($P_a co_2$ >6.7 kPa)
- Pulmonary hypertension
- Surgery >4 h duration
- Thoracic, upper > lower abdominal surgery (decreases postoperative FEV_1 and FVC by 50%)
- Midline > transverse incisions
- Bowel distension.

Respiratory function tests predicting increased postoperative morbidity with chronic respiratory disease

- $\dfrac{FEV_1}{FVC}$ <50% = high risk (obstructive pattern)

    (FEV_1 = forced expiratory volume in 1 s, FVC = forced vital capacity)

- $\dfrac{RV}{TLC}$ <50% = high risk (restrictive pattern)

    (RV = residual volume, TLC = total lung capacity)

    FEV_1 <1000 mL or <50% predicted

    FVC <1500 mL or <50% predicted

- Maximum breathing capacity (MBC) <50% predicted

    (MBC = PEFR × 0.25 or FEV_1 × 35)

- Forced expiratory time : >4 s is abnormal

    >10 s indicates severe obstruction.

    Morbidity of high-risk patients can be reduced by:

- Pre- and postoperative physiotherapy
- Humidified oxygen
- Optimization of medication (antibiotics, bronchodilators, steroids, etc.)
- Optimization of nutritional status.

Anaesthetic techniques

Aims

- Avoid bronchospasm (which causes autoPEEP)
- Avoid hypoxia or hypercapnia
- Minimize postoperative complications (e.g. pain relief reduces atelectasis)
- Avoid postoperative ventilation (reduces ciliary motility, acts as route for infection, causes bronchospasm).

Use either regional/local technique or maximal support approach with GA. Plan elective surgery for summer.

Regional technique

Requires the patient to be able to lie flat for the duration of surgery and not cough. Avoid sedation which may precipitate respiratory failure. Can be combined with a light GA and spontaneous ventilation, but reactive airways are irritated by an endotracheal tube which may cause severe bronchospasm. Avoided by using local/regional technique.

General anaesthetic

The technique of choice for patients with respiratory failure or upper abdominal/thoracic surgery. Light/no premedication. Use a heat and moisture exchanger or humidifier. Use drugs allowing rapid recovery. IPPV allows control of O_2 and CO_2 and enables airway suctioning and may need to be continued postoperatively. Use slow inspiratory flow to allow equilibration of fast and slow alveoli. A long expiratory time reduces air trapping. Avoid PEEP in patients with COPD. If there are high-frequency bullae, avoid N_2O and consider double-lumen tube. Spontaneous respiration or jet ventilation (HFJV) may be appropriate with bullae.

At the end of surgery, ensure bowel is decompressed and drain any peritoneal air. Sit patient up postoperatively, which increases FRC. Epidurals also increase FRC (bupivacaine > morphine). Prior to extubation, ensure cardiovascular stability and fluid balance and ensure no residual effects of anaesthetic or neuromuscular blockade.

Anaesthesia for asthmatics

Asthma affects 4–5% of the population. There are 1400 deaths p.a. in the UK. Prevalence and mortality are increasing. Avoid factors precipitating bronchospasm (differential diagnosis = aspiration, pulmonary oedema, endobronchial intubation, patient too light, mechanical obstruction of the tube).

Preoperative

Assess severity: severe if patient unable to speak sentences, pulse >120/min, pulsus paradoxus >20 mmHg, FEV_1 <25%, $\uparrow P_a co_2$. Consider bronchodilators, hydration, antibiotics and steroids. Measure baseline arterial blood gases (ABGs). Percussive physiotherapy is contraindicated because it exhausts the patient further.

Premedication

Atropine limits vagal reflexes that cause bronchospasm. The small doses used for premedication do not cause bronchodilation but increase the viscosity of sputum. Consider nebulized salbutamol.

Anaesthetic

Use of a regional or local technique avoids most precipitating factors. Induction with ketamine ($\uparrow$ secretions but is the best bronchodilator), propofol, etomidate or benzodiazepines. Thiopentone causes histamine release and may cause bronchoconstriction.

Although suxamethonium causes histamine release, there is no evidence that it precipitates bronchospasm. Intubate deep to avoid stimulating reflexes which cause bronchospasm and avoid excessively light anaesthesia which may also cause endotracheal tube irritation and bronchoconstriction. Consider topical lidocaine or lidocaine 1.5 mg.kg^{-1} i.v. pre-intubation.

Isoflurane and sevoflurane, but not desflurane cause moderate bronchodilation. Desflurane causes bronchoconstriction in patients who currently smoke. If theophylline infusion is running (6 mg.kg^{-1} loading dose, 0.5 mg.kg^{-1}.h^{-1} maintenance), halve the rate because general anaesthesia decreases liver blood flow. If the patient is ventilated, aim for slow inflation for optimal alveolar gas distribution. Slow exhalation reduces air trapping. There is little work on the effects of neuromuscular blockers on asthma. Avoid those that cause histamine release. Remember to give steroid supplements if the patient is taking steroids.

Perioperative complications (bronchospasm, laryngospasm) are more common in older patients (>50 years) and those with active asthma.

Reversal

Anticholinesterases cause bronchospasm, prevented by the addition of an anticholinergic.

INITIAL ASSESSMENT

MODERATE EXACERBATION

SpO_2 <92% PEF 33-50%
- increasing symptoms
- PEF >50-75% best or predicted
- no features of acute severe asthma

ACUTE SEVERE

Any one of:
- PEF 33-50% best or predicted
- respiratory rate ≥25/min heart rate ≥ 110/min
- inability to complete sentences in one breath

LIFE THREATENING

In a patient with severe asthma any one of:
- PEF <33% best or predicted
- SpO_2 <92%
- PaO_2 <8 kPa
- normal $PaCO_2$ (4.6-6.0 kPa)
- silent chest
- cyanosis
- poor respiratory effort
- arrhythmia
- exhaustion, altered conscious level

NEAR FATAL

Raised $PaCO_2$ and/or requiring mechanical ventilation with raised inflation pressures

Clinical features	Severe breathlessness (including too breathless to complete sentences in one breath), tachypnea, tachycardia, silent chest, cyanosis or collapse *None of these singly or together is specific and their absence does not exclude a severe attack*
PEF or FEV_1	PEF or FEV_1 are useful and valid measures of airway calibre. PEF expressed as a % of the patient's previous best value is most useful clinically. In the absence of this, PEF as a % of predicted is a rough guide.
Pulse oximetry	Oxygen saturation (SpO_2) measured by pulse oximetry determines the adequacy of oxygen therapy and the need for arterial blood gas (ABG). The aim of oxygen therapy is to maintain SpO_2 94-98%
Blood gases (ABG)	Patients with SpO_2 <92% or other features of life threatening asthma require ABG measurement
Chest X-Ray	Chest X-ray is not routinely recommended of in the absence of: - suspected pneumomediastinum or pneumothorax - suspected consolidation - life threatening asthma failure to respond to treatment satisfactorily - requirement for ventilation

Figure 2.8 (A) British Guideline on the Management of Asthma. Management of Acute Asthma in Adults. (British Thoracic Society & Scottish Intercollegiate Guidelines Network 2009.)

MANAGEMENT OF ACUTE ASTHMA IN ADULTS

CRITERIA FOR ADMISSION

B Admit patients with any feature of a life threatening or near fatal attack.

B Admit patients with any feature of a severe attack persisting after initial treatment.

C Patients whose peak flow is greater than 75% best or predicted one hour after initial treatment may be discharged from ED, unless there are other reasons why admission may be appropriate.

TREATMENT OF ACUTE ASTHMA

OXYGEN

C • Give supplementary oxygen to all hypoxaemic patients with acute asthma to maintain an SpO_2 level of 94-98%. Lack of pulse oximetry should not prevent the use of oxygen

A • In hospital, ambulance and primary care, nebulized β_2 agonist broncho-dilators should be driven by oxygen

C • The absence of supplemental oxygen should not prevent nebulized therapy being given if indicated.

STEROID THERAPY

A Give steroids in adequate doses in all cases of acute asthma.

☑ Continue prednisolone 40-50mg daily for at least five days or until recovery.

OTHER THERAPIES

B Consider giving a single dose of IV magnesium sulphate for patients with:
• acute severe asthma who have not had a good initial response to inhaled bronchodilator therapy
• life threatening or near fatal asthma.

☑ IV magnesium sulphate (1.2–2 g IV infusion over 20 minutes) should only be used following consultation with medical staff.

B Routine prescription of antibiotics is not indication for patients with acute asthma

β_2 AGONIST BRONCHODILATORS

A Use high dose inhaled β_2 agonists as first line agents in acute asthma and administer as early as possible. Reserve intravenous β_2 agonists for those patients in whom inhaled therapy cannot be used reliably.

☑ In acute asthma with life threatening features the nebulized route (oxygen-driven) is recommended.

A In patients with severe asthma that is poorly responsive to an initial bolus dose of β_2 agonist, consider continuous nebulization with an appropriate nebulizer.

IPRATROPIUM BROMIDE

B Add nebulized ipratropium bromide (0.5 mg 4-6 hourly) to $\beta2$ agonist treatment for patients with acute severe or life threatening asthma or those with a poor initial response to β_2 agonist therapy.

REFERRAL TO INTENSIVE CARE

Refer any patient:
• requiring ventilatory support
• with acute severe or life threatening asthma, failing to respond to therapy, evidenced by:
  - deteriorating PEF
  - persisting or worsening hypoxia
  - hypercapnea
  - ABG analysis showing ↓ph or ↑H+
  - exhaustion, feeble respiration
  - drowsiness, confusion, altered conscious state
  - respiratory arrest

Figure 2.8, cont'd (B) British Guideline on the Management of Asthma. Management of Acute Asthma in Children aged over 2 years. (British Thoracic Society & Scottish Intercollegiate Guidelines Network 2009.)

Continued

MANAGEMENT OF ACUTE ASTHMA IN CHILDREN AGED OVER 2 YEARS

ACUTE SEVERE

SpO_2 <92% PEF 33-50%
- Can't complete sentences in one breath or too breathless to talk or feed
- Pulse >125 (>5 years) or >140 (2 to 5 years)
- Respiration >30 breaths/min (>5 years) or >40 (2 to 5 years)

LIFE THREATENING

SpO_2 <92% PEF <33-50% best or predicted
- Hypertension
- Exhaustion
- Confusion
- Coma
- Silent chest
- Cyanosis
- Poor respiratory effort

CRITERIA FOR ADMISSION

☑ β_2 agonists should be given as first line treatment. Increase β_2 agonist dose by two puffs every two minutes according to response up to ten puffs.

☑ • Children with acute asthma in primary care who have not improved after receiving up to 10 puffs of β_2 agonist should be referred to hospital. Further doses of bronchodilator should be given as necessary whilst awaiting transfer.
- Treat children transported to hospital by ambulance with oxygen and nebulized β_2 agonists during the journey.

☑ Paramedics attending to children with acute asthma should administer nebulized salbutamol driven by oxygen if symptoms are severe whilst transferring the child to the emergency department.

☑ Children with severe or life threatening asthma should be transferred to hospital urgently.

B **Consider intensive inpatient treatment for children with SpO_2 <92% on air after initial bronchodilator treatment.**

The following clinical signs should be recorded:
- **Pulse rate** - increasing tachycardia generally denotes worsening asthma; a fall in heart rate in life threatening asthma is a pre-terminal event
- **Respiratory rate and degree of breathlessness** - i.e. too breathless to complete sentences in one breath of to feed
- **Use of accessory muscles of respiration** - best noted by palpation of neck muscles
- **Amount of wheezing** - which might become biphasic or less apparent with increasing airways obstruction
- **Degree of agitation and conscious level** - always give calm reassurance

NB Clinical signs correlate poorly with the severity of airways obstruction. Some children with acute asthma do not appear distressed.

Figure 2.8, cont'd (C) British Guideline on the Management of Asthma. Management of Acute Asthma in Children aged under 2 years. (British Thoracic Society & Scottish Intercollegiate Guidelines Network 2009.)

TREATMENT OF ACUTE ASTHMA

OXYGEN

☑ Children with life threatening asthma or SpO_2 <94% should receive high flow oxygen via a tight fitting face mask or nasal cannula at sufficient flow rates to achieve normal saturations.

β_2 AGONIST BRONCHODILATORS

A • **Inhaled β_2 agonists are the first line treatment for acute asthma**
   • **A pMDI + spacer is the preferred option in mild to moderate asthma.**

B individualize drug dosing according to severity and adjust according to the patient's response.

B Consider early addition of a single bolus dose of IV salbutamol (15 mcg/kg over 10 minutes) in severe cases where the patient has not responded to initial inhaled therapy.

☑ Discontinue long-acting β_2 agonists when short-acting β_2 agonists are requires more often than four-hourly.

MANAGEMENT OF ACUTE ASTHMA IN CHILDREN AGED OVER 2 YEARS

STEROID THERAPY

A **Give prednisolone early in the treatment of acute asthma attacks.**

☑ • Use a dose of 20 mg prednisolone for children aged 2 to 5 years and a dose of 30-40 mg for children >5 years. Those already receiving maintenance steroid tablets should receive 2 mg/kg prednisolone up to a maximum dose of 60 mg
   • Repeat the dose of prednisolone in children in children who vomit and consider IV steroids.
   • Treatment for up to three days is usually sufficient, but the length of course should be tailored to the number of days necessary to bring about recover. Weaning is unnecessary unless the course of steroids exceeds 14 days.

OTHER THERAPIES

A **If symptoms are refractory to initial β_2 agonist treatment, add ipratropium bromide (250 mcg/dose mixed with the nebulized β_2 agonist solution)**

☑ Repeated doses of ipratropium bromide should be given clearly to treat children poorly responsive to β_2 agonists.

A • **Aminophylline is not recommended in children with mild to moderate acute asthma**

C • **Consider aminophylline in an HDU or PICU setting for children with severe or life threatening bronchspasm unresponsive to maximal doses of bronchodilators plus steroids.**

☑ Do not give antibiotics routinely in the management of acute childhood asthma.

Figure 2.8, cont'd

Continued

MANAGEMENT OF ACUTE ASTHMA IN CHILDREN AGED UNDER 2 YEARS

- The assessment of acute asthma in early childhood can be difficult
- Intermittent wheezing attacks are usually due to viral infection and the response to asthma medication is inconsistent
- The differential diagnosis of symptoms includes:
  - aspiration pneumonitis
  - pneumonia
  - bronchiolitis
  - tracheomalacia
  - complications of underlying conditions such as congenital anomalies and cystic fibrosis
- Prematurity and low birth weight are risk factors for recurrent wheezing

TREATMENT OF ACUTE ASTHMA

β_2 AGONIST BRONCHODILATORS

B Oral β_2 agonists are not recommended for acute asthma in infants.

A For mild to moderate acute asthma a pDMI + spacer is the optimal drug delivery device.

STEROID THERAPY

B Consider steroid tablets in infants early in the management of moderate to severe episodes of acute asthma in the hospital setting.

☑ Steroid tablet therapy (10 mg of soluble prednisolone for up to three days) is the preferred steroid preparation for use in this age group.

B Consider inhaled ipratropium bromide in combination with an inhaled β_2 agonist for more severe symptoms.

Figure 2.8, cont'd

Anaesthesia for cystic fibrosis

Cystic fibrosis is caused by an autosomal recessive gene localized to chromosome 7, occurring in 1:2000 births. It is the commonest fatal inherited disease. The prognosis is improving, with median life expectancy of 40 years. Gene encodes for cystic fibrosis transmembrane inductance regulator, which is involved in chloride transport on epithelial cell membranes. Results in impaired chloride and sodium transport with increased electrolyte content of secretions.

Presents as meconium ileus, recurrent respiratory infections, steatorrhoea and failure to thrive. Diagnosed by sweat test with sweat sodium and chloride >60 mmol.L^{-1}.

Pathophysiology

Cardiovascular. Chronic hypoxaemia and pulmonary disease result in cor pulmonale. Left ventricular abnormalities and cardiomyopathy.

Respiratory. Chronic sinusitis, nasal polyps, turbinate hypertrophy, mucous plugging of airways, hyperinflation, bronchial hyperreactivity, bronchiectasis, chronic infection (*Staphylococcus aureus*, *Haemophilus influenzae*, *Pseudomonas*), obstructive and restrictive defects.

Gastrointestinal. Gastro-oesophageal reflux, impaired liver function, biliary cirrhosis causing portal hypertension, insulin-dependent diabetes and malabsorption secondary to pancreatic insufficiency causing malnutrition.

Other. Anaemia of chronic disease, renal impairment secondary to aminoglycosides, diabetes and amyloidosis.

Anaesthesia

Preoperative. Urea and electrolytes, liver function tests, glucose, full blood count, chest X-ray. Pulmonary function tests (FEV_1 <30% = poor prognosis), arterial blood gases, exclusion of active infection, vigorous physiotherapy, good diabetic control.

Premedication. Sedatives and narcotics best avoided. Anticholinergics probably of little benefit. Give H_2 antagonists if reflux.

Induction. Gas induction slow due to V/Q mismatch but may be unavoidable, particularly in children with poor venous access. Coughing and laryngospasm are common. Pre-oxygenate to avoid desaturation. Ketamine increases secretions and is relatively contraindicated. Aim to intubate for most procedures to allow tracheobronchial suctioning and control of ventilation. Ensure adequate depth of anaesthesia prior to intubation in view of bronchial hyperreactivity. Low airway pressures reduce the risk of pneumothorax.

Maintenance. Humidify inspiratory gases. Sevoflurane/desflurane allows rapid recovery permitting early physiotherapy. Long-acting muscle relaxants risk incomplete postoperative reversal. Aminoglycoside antibiotics may prolong neuromuscular blockade. Aim for early extubation.

Postoperative. Effective analgesia is essential to allow good coughing and regular physiotherapy. Maintain adequate hydration.

Pulmonary hypertension

Tachycardia reduces filling time, causing ischaemia. Hypoxia causes pulmonary vasoconstriction and precipitates right heart failure. Pulmonary hypertension results in coronary filling during diastole rather than systole.

Obstructive sleep apnoea

Defined as absence of airflow for >10 s, occurring >30 times in 7 h sleep. Either obstructive or central (no respiratory movements). Associated with obesity, hypertension and diabetes. Patients are at even greater risk with i.v. sedation.

Common symptoms are snoring, daytime somnolence, restless sleep.

Reduced activity of genioglossus muscle combined with negative pressure from the diaphragm causes pharyngeal obstruction, just posterior to the soft palate. Also impaired contractility of respiratory muscles.

Nasal CPAP abolishes sleep apnoea in most patients and improves the clinical symptoms. It improves daytime oxygenation by increasing FRC and hence alveolar ventilation and improves chronic CCF and LV function. Nocturnal O_2 may also be of benefit.

Postoperative hypoxia

Severity and incidence of arterial desaturation are closely related to the surgical site and are greatest for thoracoabdominal surgery, less for upper abdominal surgery and least for peripheral surgery.

Early hypoxaemia. One-third of patients being transferred from theatre to recovery room developed O_2 saturation <90%, despite being given 100% O_2 for 5 min at the end of surgery. This early phase hypoxaemia is mostly due to upper airway obstruction, increased oxygen consumption, alveolar hypoventilation, atelectasis, V/Q mismatch, diffusion hypoxia, aspiration or central or obstructive apnoea.

Late hypoxaemia is due to impaired gas exchange (atelectasis), impaired control of breathing (sleep, analgesia), impaired diaphragmatic contractility and collapse of pharynx with negative inspiratory pressures and reduced muscle tone. Persists for up to 5 days. Related temporally to hypertension, tachycardia, myocardial ischaemia and arrhythmias. Some episodes of postoperative LVF and myocardial infarction are probably related to this ischaemia. Hypoxaemia may impair wound healing and promote bacterial infection.

Nasal oxygen delivery is more comfortable than a mask and does not require additional humidification, but 35% patients fail to keep O_2 on overnight. Intratracheal and nasopharyngeal catheters may be more effective.

Recommendations (Powell et al 1996) include:

- Use of pulse oximetry to monitor all postoperative patients in the recovery room
- Patients at risk of prolonged postoperative hypoxaemia need prolonged monitoring and oxygen supplementation (obese patients with BMI >27–35 kg/m², upper abdominal surgery or thoracotomy, patients receiving opioids and those with respiratory disease)
- Patients with impaired O_2 delivery (hypovolaemia, anaemia, myocardial/cerebral ischaemia, sickle cell disease) all require postoperative oxygen therapy
- Oxygen should be continued until S_aO_2 exceeds 93% or reaches preoperative value.

Bibliography

Bluman LG, Mosca L, Newman N, et al: Preoperative smoking habits and postoperative pulmonary complications, *Chest* 113:883–889, 1998.

British Thoracic Society & Scottish Intercollegiate Guidelines Network: *British Guideline on the Management of Asthma*, 2009. www.brit-thoracic.org.uk/ClinicalInformation/Asthma/AsthmaGuidelines/tabid/83/Default.aspx.

Edrich T, Sadovnikoff N: Anesthesia for patients with severe chronic obstructive pulmonary disease, *Curr Opin Anaesthesiol* 2009. E-pub doi: 10.1097/ACO.0b013e328331ea5b.

Mills GH: Respiratory physiology and anaesthesia, *BJA CEPD Rev* 1:35–39, 2001.

Powell JF, Menon DK, Jones JG: The effects of hypoxaemia and recommendations for postoperative oxygen therapy, *Anaesthesia* 51:769–772, 1996.

Stanley D, Tunnicliffe W: Management of life-threatening asthma in adults, *Continuing Education in Anaesthesia, Critical Care & Pain* 8:95–99, 2008.

Stather DR, Stewart TE: Clinical review: mechanical ventilation in severe asthma, *Crit Care* 9:581–587, 2005.

Sweeney BP, Grayling M: Smoking and anaesthesia: the pharmacological implications, *Anaesthesia* 64:179–186, 2009.

Tonnesen H, Nielsen PR, Lauritzen JB, et al: Smoking and alcohol intervention before surgery: evidence for best practice, *Br J Anaesth* 102:297–306, 2009.

Vaschetto R, Bellotti E, Turucz E, et al: Inhalational anesthetics in acute severe asthma, *Curr Drug Targets* 10:826–832, 2009.

Walsh TS, Young CH: Anaesthesia and cystic fibrosis, *Anaesthesia* 50:614–622, 1995.

Warner DO: Perioperative Abstinence from Cigarettes: Physiologic and Clinical Consequences, *Anesthesiology* 104:356–367, 2006.

THORACIC ANAESTHESIA

Anaesthesia for thoracotomy

Preoperative

Full cardiovascular and respiratory work-up, including room air ABGs and pulmonary function tests. Patient is often arteriopathic with end-organ damage.

Lung function tests

1. Predicted postoperative FEV_1 and FVC as a percentage of preoperative values:
   - One lobe resection – 80%
   - Left lung – 60%
   - Right lung – 40%.
2. Predicted postoperative FEV_1:
   - <0.8 L – ventilator-dependent; therefore resection is contraindicated
   - <1.0 L – sputum retention.
3. $\% \dfrac{\text{preop. FVC}}{\text{postop. FVC}} + \% \dfrac{\text{preop. }FEV_1}{\text{postop. }FEV_1} < 100 \Rightarrow$ postoperative IPPV necessary.

4. Postoperative maximum breathing capacity (MBC):
   - <25 L/min – respiratory cripple
   - 25–50 L/min – severe respiratory impairment
   - >60 L/min – normal (60–200).
5. Preoperative FEV_1 >1.5 L is needed for pneumonectomy.

Pulmonary artery pressure (PAP)

High risk if mean PAP >25 mmHg at rest. Hypoxic pulmonary vasoconstriction (HPV) increases shunt by diverting blood to non-ventilated lung. Worsened by most sympathomimetics, although least with dopamine.

Operative

Monitoring. ECG, good venous access, CVP line on side of thoracotomy for easier access, chest drain positioned on same side postoperatively avoids risks of pneumothorax on opposite side to surgery. Arterial line placed in contralateral radial artery. Wright's respirometer to measure expired air volumes, pulse oximeter and capnograph.

Positioning. Take care with positioning because of risk of nerve injury (axillary rolls cause brachial plexus compression). Dependent pooling in head and legs reduces cardiac output. Worse with hypovolaemia.

Intubation and ventilation. Use bronchial blockers if patient is too small for a double-lumen tube. Intubate with double-lumen tube and use fibreoptic scope if necessary to check position. Usually intubate left main bronchus unless this would interfere with surgery. IPPV with muscle relaxation prevents coughing and high-volume IPPV ensures more even ventilation.

Maintenance. Use volatiles and high F_iO_2. Intravenous anaesthetic agents may suppress hypoxic pulmonary vasoconstriction less than volatiles.

Reversal. Inflate lungs to 40 cmH$_2$O for 40 s to reverse atelectasis and check for leaks. Ensure complete reversal and return of protective reflexes before extubation.

Postoperative analgesia

Pain pathways are:
- Visceral
  - PNS: vagus
  - SNS: T_2–T_5
- Somatic
  - diaphragm: C_2–C_5 (phrenic)
  - chest wall: T_2–T_{12}.

Pneumonectomy removes most of the visceral input.

Use thoracic epidural or intrathecal analgesia (avoids vagus and phrenic nerves), intercostal nerve blocks, interpleural local anaesthetic or paravertebral blocks. Use systemic opioids sparingly. Epidurals improve postoperative pulmonary outcome.

Anaesthesia for one-lung ventilation

Predictors of risk for one-lung surgery

- Pulmonary hypertension
- FEV_1 <50% predicted
- FVC <50% predicted
- MBC <50% predicted.

Physiology of spontaneous ventilation in lateral decubitus position

GA reduces compliance of both upper and lower lungs, which is returned to normal values by the application of PEEP.

Weight of mediastinum and pressure of abdominal contents on diaphragm impair lower lung expansion and cause decreased FRC. However, greater curvature of the diaphragm results in more efficient contraction with greater expansion matching increased blood flow to dependent lung, i.e. V/Q remains balanced.

During spontaneous ventilation, dependent diaphragm moves cephalad on expiration, pushing the mediastinum upwards, resulting in inefficient ventilation. This mediastinal shift causes sympathetic activation, reduces venous return and reduces cardiac output.

When the upper chest is opened during spontaneous ventilation, paradoxical respiration results. During inspiration, gases are drawn from upper lung, which collapses. During expiration, gases pass from lower into upper lung causing upper lung inflation. Mediastinal shift as a result of paradoxical respiration also generates more work.

Physiology of two-lung IPPV in lateral decubitus position

IPPV results in most ventilation being directed to the upper rather than the lower lung, with perfusion remaining greatest in the lower lung, thus increasing the V/Q mismatch.

- High F_IO_2 (0.8–1.0) causes vasodilation and increases flow in the dependent lung
- Aim for 10 mL/kg IPPV once single-lung ventilation established
- Aim for P_aCO_2 of 6 kPa. Since the overall tidal volume is decreased by about 20%, respiratory rate may need to be increased by a similar amount to maintain minute volume
- PEEP to dependent lung may improve oxygenation by recruiting closed alveoli and restoring compliance to normal, but may worsen oxygenation by compressing pulmonary vasculature and diverting more blood to the upper unventilated lung. Countered by upper lung CPAP
- Blood flow through unventilated lung is the main determinant of PO_2.

Maintain two-lung ventilation until pleura is opened.

Hypoxia during single-lung IPPV

If this occurs:

- Check position of double-lumen tube. Suction down ETT
- Non-dependent lung CPAP (5–10 cmH$_2$O)
- Dependent lung PEEP
- Operative lung HFJV
- Intermittent IPPV to operative lung
- Clamp pulmonary artery.

Postoperative

Any V/Q̇ mismatch is improved by nursing the patient in a lateral position with the healthy lung lowermost if breathing spontaneously, or the healthy side uppermost if IPPV.

Double-lumen tubes

Because of the wide variation in anatomical position of the right upper lobe bronchus, a left-sided tube is usually chosen unless surgery is to the left main bronchus (carina to left upper lobe = 5.0 cm; carina to right upper lobe = 2.5 cm). The presence of a carinal hook increases the stability of the tube but makes insertion more difficult.

The following are types of double-lumen tube:

- *Carlens* (left-sided) and *White* (right-sided): carinal hook; four sizes
- *Robertshaw*: left/right; no carinal hook; small/medium/large
- *Gordon–Green*: single-lumen right-sided tube; carinal hook
- *Bryce–Smith*: left/right; no carinal hook.

Carlens and White tubes have lumens of a smaller diameter than the Robertshaw tubes.

Indications

- Soiling below cuff (empyema, bronchiectasis, haemoptysis, tracheo-oesophageal fistula, TOF)
- Gas leak below cuff (TOF, bronchopleural fistula, ruptured cyst).

Insertion of tube with carinal hook

1. Advance tip of tube through cords and then turn 180° so that hook is anterior.
2. Once hook is through cords, rotate to correct position and advance until resistance is felt.
3. Ventilate both lungs first; then inflate tracheal cuff and listen at the mouth for any air leak. Inflate endobronchial cuff and inflate single lung through endobronchial port. Check there are no air leaks via tracheal port. Inflate opposite lung via tracheal port and check there are no air leaks via endobronchial port. Measure expired air volumes to check for leaks.

Complications

- Trauma to laryngeal cartilage and trachea during insertion
- Tube malposition resulting in hypoxia
- Surgical compression can displace tube and disrupt isolation of operative lung
- Tube displacement may result in ball valve effect with hypercapnia and prolonged expiratory flow.

Anaesthesia for bronchopleural fistula

Fistula usually occurs after lung resection; also with abscess, tumour, or bullae. Results in sudden onset of productive cough, worse at night.

Diagnosed by fall in fluid level on CXR, failure of hemithorax to opacify, return of mediastinum to midline, and consolidation of healthy lung from overspill from infected lung.

Sit patient up, with the affected side lowermost and the fistula clear of pleural fluid. Give oxygen, resuscitate preoperatively. Carry out early endo-bronchial intubation to isolate fistula. Induction by:

- awake intubation, but risk of coughing and contamination
- rapid sequence induction, but trachea may be distorted following pneumonectomy
- deep volatile induction, but marked CVS depression in shocked patient.

Aim for early extubation to avoid pressure from IPPV on stump sutures.

Anaesthesia for lung cysts/bullae

Lung cysts are often compliant and therefore preferentially ventilated. IPPV may deliver large volumes to the cyst, resulting in its rupture. Therefore aim for small tidal volumes, low inflation pressure, no PEEP and long expiratory phase. Spontaneous respiration until chest opening may avoid hyperinflation. A ball-valve effect may occur with mucous plugs, causing tensioning of the cyst. Avoid N_2O which may rupture the cyst. Consider spontaneous respiration or HFJV.

Good postoperative pain relief (e.g. epidural) allows quicker return of normal lung function.

Anaesthesia for tracheal resection

A partially obstructed airway is at risk of complete obstruction. Therefore avoid sedative premedication and use gas induction in case a paralysed apnoeic patient cannot be ventilated. Airway obstruction will slow induction. Since ventilation may be dependent upon a patient's spontaneous respiratory effort, avoid neuromuscular blockers until obstruction resected.

When the trachea is divided, the surgeon places a Tovell endotracheal tube in distal trachea to continue ventilation and the original tube is then withdrawn.

When the trachea is reanastomosed, the neck is kept flexed to prevent strain on sutures. Aim to extubate as soon as possible to avoid high airway pressures on anastomosis.

Anaesthesia for bronchoscopy

Methods of anaesthesia for bronchoscopy include:

- *Apnoeic oxygenation.* Apnoea with insufflation of O_2 via catheter placed at carina. Arterial CO_2 rises by 0.26–0.66 kPa.min^{-1}, therefore use for short periods only
- *Flexible fibreoptic bronchoscope*
- *Ventilating (rigid) bronchoscope with sidearm.* Glass window opened for passage of instruments prevents effective ventilation
- *Sanders injector.* Injection of O_2 at 4 bar through 16 G cannula with entrainment of air by Venturi effect. F_iO_2 uncertain.

Complications include dental and laryngeal damage, tracheal rupture, haemorrhage and pneumothorax.

Laser surgery

Carbon dioxide or Nd-Yag laser used for surgery to thoracic neoplasms. Associated with a risk of fire and explosion in the airway, risk of ignition of the endotracheal tube and risk to eyesight from laser beam.

Endotracheal tube must be shielded from the laser by coating of aluminium foil or use of a stainless steel tube. Use double cuff in case laser bursts upper cuff. Fill cuffs with water, which absorbs stray energy better than air. Both O_2 and N_2O support combustion. Reduce risk of fire by keeping F_iO_2 <0.40, adding helium and using laser for as short a burst as possible. Use saline-soaked swabs to protect surrounding tissue from laser. Everyone in theatre should wear protective goggles.

Bibliography

Eastwood J, Mahajan R: One-lung anaesthesia, *Br J Anaesth CEPD Rev* 2:83–87, 2002.

Grichnik KP, Shaw A: Update on one-lung ventilation: the use of continuous positive airway pressure ventilation and positive end-expiratory pressure ventilation – clinical application, *Curr Opin Anaesthesiol* 22:23–30, 2009.

Hillier J, Gillbe C: Anesthesia for lung volume reduction surgery, *Anaesthesia* 58:1210–1219, 2003.

Karzai W, Schwarzkopf K: Hypoxemia during one-lung ventilation: prediction, prevention, and treatment, *Anesthesiology* 110:1402–1411, 2009.

Slinger P: Update on anesthetic management for pneumonectomy, *Curr Opin Anaesth* 22:31–37, 2009.

Tschernko EM, Kritzinger M, Gruber EM, et al: Lung volume reduction surgery: preoperative functional predictors for post-operative outcome, *Anesth Analges* 88:28–33, 1999.
Vaughan RS: Pain relief after thoracotomy, *Br J Anaesth* 87:681–683, 2001.

MECHANICAL VENTILATION

History

Mechanical ventilation was first described in the sixteenth century by Vesalius, who used bellows to ventilate a donkey. Advances in mechanical ventilation were encouraged by the 1952 polio epidemic in Copenhagen during which Lassen organized relays of medical students to ventilate hundreds of patients by hand for many weeks.

Aims of intubation

- Establish and maintain an upper airway
- Protect the lower airway
- Facilitate IPPV ± hyperventilation
- Reduce dead space
- Facilitate airway suctioning.

Respiratory failure
Definition

- $P_a o_2 < 8.0\,\text{kPa}$
- $P_a co_2 > 6.7\,\text{kPa}$.

Causes
Ventilatory failure

- Hypoventilation (lesion in medulla $\rightarrow$ spinal cord $\rightarrow$ lungs)
- $\uparrow$ dead space.

Intrapulmonary shunt

- True shunt (collapse, consolidation, pulmonary oedema etc.)

$$\text{Shunt equation} = \frac{Q_S}{Q_t} = \frac{C_c o_2 - C_a o_2}{C_c o_2 - C_v o_2}$$

- $\uparrow$ V/$\dot{Q}$ scatter

$$(\text{normal } V/\dot{Q} = \frac{4000\,\text{mL / min}}{5000\,\text{mL / min}} = 0.8)$$

Indications for ventilation

Subjective. Clinical grounds, trends in condition, response to treatment, ability to cough, etc.

Objective

- Respiratory rate >40/min
- V_t <5 mL/kg
- Vital capacity <10–15 mL/kg
- ABGs: $P_a o_2$ <8 kPa, $P_a co_2$ >8 kPa.

Time constants

- Time constant = resistance (cmH_2O) × compliance (L/cmH_2O) = time for 63% of change in pressure to be distributed through lungs
- Five time constants = complete equalization of pressure
- Short inspiratory time favours fast units (short time constant) with incomplete filling of slower units.

Mechanical ventilation

Ventilators

There are four main groups of ventilator:

1. Minute volume dividers, e.g. Manley Pulmovent, Blease Brompton
2. Bag squeezers, e.g. Cape Waine ventilator, Manley Servovent
3. Thumb occluders, e.g. occlusion of T-piece outlet by thumb
4. Intermittent blowers, e.g. Pneupac ventilator, Nuffield Penlon 200.

Initiation of inspiration

- Time initiated – inspiratory mode begins after a set time
- Pressure initiated – inspiratory mode begins when pressure falls below the baseline pressure.

Termination of inspiration

- Volume cycle: ends inspiration after a preset volume is delivered
- Pressure cycle: ends inspiration when circuit pressure reaches predetermined level
- Time cycle: ends inspiration after a set time. Commonest used trigger
- Flow cycle: ends inspiration when circuit flow diminishes to a predetermined level.

Infant ventilators are usually pressure-limited, time-cycled flow generators. Adult ventilators are usually volume-limited ventilators.

Ventilatory modes
Intermittent positive pressure ventilation (IPPV)
Effects of IPPV
- $\uparrow V_D : V_T$, $\downarrow$ FRC
- $\uparrow$ Spread V/Q ratios, $\uparrow$ venous admixture
- Increased pulmonary vascular resistance due to compression and stretching of vessels
- Impaired venous return.

Large tidal volume (V_T)
- Compensates for $\uparrow$ dead space that occurs with IPPV
- Reduces basal atelectasis
- Better tolerated by conscious patients.

Therefore, in the absence of lung pathology, use 12–15mL/kg at 10–12 breaths/min.

IMV, SIMV and MMV

Intermittent mandatory ventilation (IMV). Patient able to breathe spontaneously on CPAP between mandatory tidal volumes.

Synchronized intermittent mandatory ventilation (SIMV). As above, but synchronized with patient's respiratory efforts.

Mandatory minute ventilation (MMV). Spontaneous ventilation but if minute ventilation falls below set level, IPPV takes over.

Advantages of IMV, SIMV and MMV
- Lowers mean airway pressure (improves myocardial and renal blood flow)
- More physiological gas distribution
- Reduces sedation requirements
- Avoids hyperventilation causing respiratory alkalosis
- Easier and earlier weaning, exercises respiratory muscles.

Disadvantages of IMV, SIMV and MMV
- Increases work of breathing if resistance is present in spontaneous breathing circuits
- Respiratory muscle fatigue
- Prolongs weaning if decrease in IMV is too slow
- Hypoventilation may cause respiratory acidosis
- Added dead space.

High-frequency ventilation

High-frequency positive pressure ventilation (HFPPV) (1–2 Hz). Jet injector delivers gas into normal ventilator tubing. Low-velocity wavefront acts as a piston within the tracheal tube. Expiration is passive.

High-frequency jet ventilation (HFJV) (2–6 Hz). High-pressure (5 bar) pulses of gas delivered into tracheal tube, entraining air in the flow. Expiration is passive.

High-frequency oscillatory ventilation (HFOV) (3–20 Hz). Loudspeaker cone used to produce a sinusoidal pattern of gas flow superimposed on a continuous oxygen flow. Expiration is also active. Not shown to be of any benefit for preterm infants where the mortality and incidence of chronic lung disease are not improved in comparison with conventional ventilation. Associated with higher incidence of intraventricular haemorrhage (possibly from interference with cerebral vascular autoregulation) and inotropic support (possibly from interference with baroreflex).

Advantages

- ↓ mean airway pressure, thereby reducing pulmonary barotrauma
- Provides PEEP (↑ as frequency increases)
- Less depression of cardiac output
- Reduction in pulmonary shunting
- Allows patient to breathe spontaneously
- Reduced sedation requirements
- Reduced air leak with pneumothorax.

Disadvantages

- Humidification difficult
- Atelectasis in dependent areas of lung
- Inefficient CO_2 removal at >3 Hz
- Difficult to monitor lung volumes and pressures.

Oxygenation of alveoli occurs by several proposed mechanisms:

- Direct alveolar ventilation of proximal alveoli
- Central core of oxygen
- Convective streaming – peripheral flow to alveoli
- Turbulent dispersion
- Resonance enhances spread of oxygen
- Pendelluft – exchange of gas between alveoli with different time constants at end of inspiration.

Continuous positive airway pressure (CPAP)

Advantages

- Increased airway pressure
- Increased FRC
- Recruitment of collapsed alveoli
- Decreased airway resistance
- Reduced V/$\dot{Q}$ mismatch
- Improved distribution of inspired gas
- Reduced work of breathing.

Disadvantages

- Impaired CO_2 elimination
- Reduced cardiac output
- Reduced GFR.

Positive end expiratory pressure (PEEP)

Effects of PEEP

- $\uparrow$ pulmonary vascular resistance. $\downarrow$ flow in West's zone 1 causes increased dead space
- $\uparrow$ work of breathing if patient breathing spontaneously because patient must generate a negative inspiratory pressure greater than the PEEP pressure to inspire
- $\uparrow P_aO_2$ due to $\uparrow$ FRC >CC
- Prevents surfactant aggregation, reducing alveolar collapse
- Worsens right-to-left shunt and may worsen shunt if applied just to lower lung in one-lung ventilation.

Optimum PEEP/CPAP

- Reduces physiological shunt to <15%
- Restores FRC to normal
- Corresponds to optimal compliance
- Minimizes work of breathing.

CPAP may be uncomfortable for the awake patient and cause gastric distension. Therefore, the patient must be cooperative, able to protect the airway, cough and have the energy to breathe spontaneously.

Other ventilatory modes

Pressure support ventilation (also known as assisted spontaneous breathing, ASB)

Ventilator senses inspiratory flow, pressure or volume and then increases airway pressure to a set level. This inspiratory pressure is then maintained until expiration is triggered by low inspiratory gas flow or increasing airway pressure. Limits peak airway pressure and may improve distribution of alveolar gas in poorly compliant lungs. Encourages respiratory muscle effort to accelerate the weaning process.

Biphasic positive airway pressure (BiPAP)

Similar to APRV, except that inspiration:expiration ratios are normal, not inversed, and it is partially synchronized with the patient's ventilation. The ventilator time-cycles between two set pressure levels (P_{Insp} and PEEP), with the ability of the patient to breathe spontaneously at both levels while the airway pressure is automatically adjusted to remain at preset levels. As weaning continues, P_{Insp} can be reduced to zero until the patient is effectively on CPAP.

Airway pressure release ventilation (APRV)

Forerunner of BiPAP. Differs in that the time held in inspiration is much longer than the expiratory phase. Aims to maximize alveolar recruitment by maintaining a higher mean airway pressure than that achieved by BiPAP.

Inverse ratio ventilation

Allows reduction in airway pressures and may improve expansion and thus gas exchange across slow alveolar units. Causes an abnormal breathing pattern and discomfort, requiring patient sedation.

Permissive hypoxaemia. A P_aO_2 of 8 kPa is not thought to be detrimental in critically ill patients if it allows avoidance of high PEEP, high airway pressures or F_iO_2 >0.6.

Permissive hypercapnia. In diseased lungs, the large minute volume needed to achieve normocapnia may cause overdistension of the lungs and further alveolar damage. P_aCO_2 >6.7 kPa is acceptable if pH >7.25 with adequate cardiovascular function.

Weaning from ventilation

The following criteria must first be met:

- Adequate oxygenation (P_aO_2 >8 kPa with F_iO_2 <0.6)
- Adequate CO_2 clearance
- Able to protect airway
- Control of pain, agitation and depression
- Control of precipitating illness, fever and infection
- Optimization of electrolytes and haemoglobin
- Optimization of nutritional state.

Prognostic variables for failure to wean

- Tidal volume <5 mL/kg
- Vital capacity <10 mL/kg
- Minute volume <10 L/min
- Max. inspiratory pressure <−20 cmH$_2$O
- A–ao$_2$ difference >300 mmHg
- Dead space/tidal volume >0.6
- Respiratory rate:tidal volume >100.

CROP index

Calculated from:

- thoracic compliance (C_{dyn})
- respiratory rate
- arterial oxygenation – P_aO_2 >8.0 kPa on F_iO_2 <0.35
- maximum inspiratory pressure (P_imax) > –30 cmH_2O is a good predictor.

$$CROP = C_{dyn} \times P_imax \times [P_aO_2 / P_aO_2] / rate$$

The threshold value predicting successful weaning was 13 mL/breath per min, giving a sensitivity of 0.81 and a specificity of 0.57.

All variables are of limited value in predicting the success of weaning because it generally requires maximum effort from the patient and there are difficulties in obtaining accurate measurements.

Other factors to be considered:

- Cuff deflation improves laryngeal and pharyngeal muscle function and coordination pre-extubation
- Normalizing arterial P_aCO_2 pre-extubation increases the ventilatory response to hypercapnia
- Respiratory muscle strength, endurance and coordination are maximized by ventilation strategies that increase respiratory muscle work during weaning
- Psychological state is difficult to measure quantitatively but is a major factor in success of weaning.

Overlooked factors contributing to failure to wean include:

- Acute left ventricular failure
- Sleep deprivation
- Excessive CO_2 production from overfeeding.

Bibliography

Bouchut J-C, Godard J, Claris O: High frequency oscillatory ventilation, *Anesthesiology* 100:1007–1012, 2004.

Edwards SM, Matthews PC: Current modes of conventional ventilation in intensive care, *Br J Anaesth CEPD Rev* 2:41–44, 2002.

Hawker FF: PEEP and CPAP, *Curr Anaesth Crit Care* 7:236–242, 1996.

Lia Graciano A, Freid EB: High-frequency oscillatory ventilation in infants and children, *Curr Opin Anesth* 15:161–166, 2002.

Shelly MP, Nightingale P: ABC of intensive care: respiratory support, *BMJ* 318:1674–1677, 1999.

Soni N, Williams P: Positive pressure ventilation: what is the real cost? *Br J Anaesth* 101:446–457, 2008.

Stocker R, Biro P: Airway management and artificial ventilation in intensive care, *Curr Opin Anesth* 18:35–45, 2005.

Sydow M, Burchardi H: Inverse ratio ventilation and airway pressure release ventilation, *Curr Opin Anaesth* 9:523–528, 1997.

Neurology

NEUROLOGY AND NEUROMUSCULAR DISORDERS

Epilepsy

Affects 1/200 of the general population. Continue anticonvulsants peri-operatively.

Anaesthetic problems

- *Enzyme induction.* Chronic medication induces hepatic enzymes with resistance to i.v. induction agents and volatiles.
- *Risk of seizures.* Particularly with enflurane in a hypocapnic patient, methohexitone, ketamine and etomidate. Although propofol has not been demonstrated to cause significant EEG changes, excitatory phenomena are more common. Because patients risk losing their driving licence after an epileptiform event, it is recommended to avoid propofol in patients who are driving. Several case reports document successful use of propofol for the treatment of status epilepticus.
- *Underlying pathology causing epilepsy.*

Cerebrovascular disease

A cerebrovascular accident (CVA) is defined as a rapidly evolving episode of loss of cerebral function with symptoms lasting more than 24 h (<24 h = transient ischaemic attack) or leading to death. Annual incidence is 1–2/1000 in the UK, with a mortality of 15–30%.

Risk of perioperative stroke following general surgery is 0.2–0.7% in patients without a history of cerebrovascular disease. Most CVAs occur 2–10 days post-operatively, with an average of 7 days, and have an associated mortality of 26%. In those with a history of cerebrovascular disease, the risk is 2.9% with a mortality of 60%.

Risk factors include age, systolic hypertension, atrial fibrillation (AF), peripheral vascular disease and diabetes. Hyperextension or rotation of the patients neck during head surgery may reduce flow in vertebral and internal carotid arteries.

Preventative measures

Preoperative measures include treating risk factors and anticoagulation for patients in AF. The European Carotid Surgery Trial (ECST) and the North American Symptomatic Carotid Endarterectomy Trial (NACEST) suggest that carotid endarterectomy would benefit symptomatic patients with >70% carotid stenosis. Surgery should be deferred for 4–6 weeks after an acute event.

Intraoperative measures. Avoid hypocapnia (steal syndrome) or hypercapnia (inverse steal syndrome), avoid hypo- or hyperglycaemia, and avoid extreme cervical spine rotation or extension. Maintain BP within normal range.

Postoperative measures. Avoid hypotension, dehydration and hypoxia.

Parkinsons disease

Disorder of the extrapyramidal system with degeneration of dopaminergic neurones in the substantia nigra of the basal ganglia, giving rise to intention tremor, 'cogwheel' rigidity, akinesia and postural changes. Dysautonomia also common (orthostatic hypotension, urinary dysfunction, sleep disorders). Prevalence 1% in those >65 years age. First described as 'the shaking palsy' by James Parkinson in 1817.

Patients are already confused in a strange environment, which is worsened by GA. Patients are often difficult to assess preoperatively, with reduced pulmonary function, upper airway obstruction, weakness and incoordination of inspiratory and expiratory muscles. The usual drug regimen should be continued preoperatively. If patient is well controlled on L-DOPA, both general and regional anaesthesia is usually well tolerated. Avoid drugs that exacerbate Parkinson's (phenothiazines, droperidol, metoclopramide).

Continue anti-Parkinsonian medication immediately postoperatively, via nasogastric (NG) tube if necessary. Delayed mobilization postoperatively increases risk of respiratory complications and deep vein thrombosis (DVT). Avoid antiemetics that are dopamine antagonists (e.g. prochlorperazine), although all may cause extrapyramidal and movement disorders.

Multiple sclerosis (MS)

Chronic progressive demyelinating disease characterized by repeated exacerbations and partial remissions. Affects 1:2000; equal incidence in both sexes. Upper motor neurone lesions, cerebellar lesions and sensory deficits are common.

General anaesthesia does not exacerbate MS. Use normal doses of muscle relaxants.

Regional blockade. New lesions may develop coincidentally at the time of regional blockade and subsequent symptoms may be difficult to differentiate from nerve injury or may be blamed on the block. Therefore regional blockade is relatively contraindicated.

Motor neurone disease

Progressive degeneration of motor function with sparing of higher mental function and sensory function. Involves both upper and lower motor neurones. Progressive muscle atrophy, spasticity, pseudobulbar palsy. Affects smooth, striated and cardiac muscle.

General anaesthesia. Risk of aspiration from delayed gastric emptying and bulbar weakness. Weak respiratory muscles. Suxamethonium may cause hyperkalaemia. Increased sensitivity to non-depolarizing relaxants and induction agents.

Regional anaesthesia. Avoid impairment of respiratory muscles but otherwise safe.

Autoimmune disease
Myasthenia gravis

Affects 1:20 000. A result of autoantibodies directed against the neuromuscular junction. Ocular, facial, bulbar and limb weakness in 85% of patients.

Preoperative. Continue anticholinesterases and steroids. Intubate if vital capacity falls below 1000 mL. Consider β-blockers and atropine to stabilize the autonomic nervous system.

GA. Greatly increased sensitivity to non-depolarizers; decreased sensitivity to depolarizing blockers. Give conventional anticholinesterase dose at end of surgery and then restart anticholinesterases at a decreased dose. Extubate when inspiratory pressure $>-30\,cmH_2O$ or FVC $>15\,mL.kg^{-1}$.

Postoperative. Risk factors for postoperative ventilation are:

- disease for >6 years
- chronic respiratory disease
- pyridostigmine $>750\,mg.day^{-1}$
- FVC <2.9 L.

Eaton–Lambert syndrome

Severe muscle weakness found in association with 1% of patients with bronchial carcinoma, thyroid disease and connective tissue disorders (systemic lupus erythematosus, polyarteritis nodosa). Unlike myasthenia gravis, causes proximal rather than bulbar weakness, muscle power increases with exercise and no fade occurs on tetanic stimulation.

Increased sensitivity to both non-depolarizing and depolarizing blockers.

Associated with ↑ ACTH (hypertension, diabetes) and ↑ PTH (↑ Ca^{2+}, dehydration).

Myotonia
Myotonic dystrophy

Affects 1:25000. Autosomal dominant. Myotonia with difficulty releasing hand grip, muscle weakness, cataracts, 'inverted smile', bilateral ptosis, frontal balding, masseter and sternomastoid wasting, and bulbar weakness (aspiration and chest infections); also cardiac conduction defects, cardiomyopathy, valve defects, obstructive sleep apnoea, dysphagia and reduced gastric emptying.

Sensitivity to sedatives, induction agents (barbiturates, propofol), opioids and non-depolarizing neuromuscular blockers. Anticholinesterases, cold and shivering may worsen myotonia. Suxamethonium may produce a generalized myotonic response. Non-depolarizing relaxants are safe. Myotonic contraction with surgical diathermy may be a major problem. Postoperative complications are usually related to cardiac pathology or muscle weakness leading to aspiration. Postoperative shivering may induce a myotonic crisis.

Pregnancy may exacerbate myotonia and muscle weakness.

Myotonia congenita (Thomsen's disease)

Affects 1:25000. Autosomal dominant. Generalized muscular hypertrophy, stiffness on initiating movement, relieved by exercise. Myotonia may be severe but no muscle weakness. Anaesthetic problems are as for myotonic dystrophy. Association with malignant hyperthermia.

Familial periodic paralysis
Hyperkalaemic periodic paralysis

Episodes of flaccid paralysis associated with hyperkalaemia. Paralysis may occur with potassium levels no greater than 4.0 mmol, possibly due to a defect in the sarcolemma causing spontaneous depolarization. Triggered by stress, cold, hunger and exercise. Vital to avoid hyperkalaemia perioperatively, using insulin/dextrose and loop diuretics. Suxamethonium may cause sufficient hyperkalaemia to precipitate an attack.

Hypokalaemic periodic paralysis

Unrelated to hyperkalaemic periodic paralysis. Asymmetric paralysis involving arms, legs, trunk and neck. Usually spares diaphragm and facial muscles. Associated with reduced cell membrane potential, making muscle more excitable. Precipitated by heavy carbohydrate meals, diuretics, alkalosis and hypothermia. The effect of muscle relaxants may be clinically similar to the paralysis itself.

Bibliography

Berrouschot J, Baumann I, Kalischewski P, et al: Therapy of myasthenic crisis, *Crit Care Med* 25:1228–1235, 1997.

Eriksson LI: Neuromuscular disorders and anaesthesia, *Curr Opin Anaesth* 8:275–281, 1995.

Errington DR, Severn AM, Meara J: Parkinson's disease, *BJA CEPD Rev* 2:69–73, 2002.

Kam PCA, Calcroft RM: Perioperative stroke in general surgical patients, *Anaesthesia* 52:879–883, 1997.

Le Corre F, Plaud B: Neuromuscular disorders, *Curr Opin Anaesth* 11:333–337, 1998.

Nicholson G, Pereira AC, Hall GM: Parkinson's disease and anaesthesia, *Br J Anaesth* 89:904–916, 2002.

Sneyd JR: Propofol and epilepsy, *Br J Anaesth* 82:168–169, 1999.

Thavasothy M, Hirsch N: Myasthenia gravis, *BJA CEPD Rev* 2:88–90, 2002.

NEUROANAESTHESIA

Physiology

Cerebrospinal fluid (CSF)

Secreted by the choroid plexus in the lateral, III and IV ventricles. Flows through foramen of Magendie and Lushka and is absorbed by arachnoid villi: 720 mL. day^{-1}. Contents are:

- pH 7.3
- CSF >plasma: Na^+, Cl^-, Mg^{2+}
- CSF <plasma: K^+, HCO_3^-, glucose, protein.

Intracranial pressure (ICP)

Munro–Kelly hypothesis (1852) stated that the contents of cranium are not compressible (60% water, 40% solid). Therefore, increasing the volume within the cranium causes a rapid increase in pressure (Fig. 3.1).

However, compression of veins and communication of CSF with spinal column result in a small range of compensation before pressure increases (Fig. 3.2).

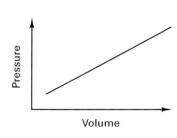

Figure 3.1 Theoretical intracranial pressure–volume relationship.

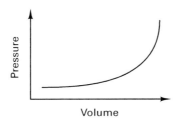

Figure 3.2 Actual intracranial pressure–volume relationship.

Normal CSF pressure = 0–10 mmHg. Neurosurgical patients often have raised ICP and so are already on the steep part of curve. Active treatment is needed if ICP >25–30 mmHg. CSF pressure oscillates with arterial pulse and swings with respiration.

Cushing reflex. Increased ICP causes hypertension and bradycardia.

Coning

All coning causes an autonomic storm. High pulmonary artery pressures may then result in neurogenic pulmonary oedema. ECG changes are now thought to be indicative of myocardial ischaemia. Reduced ADH secretion causes diabetes insipidus. Metabolic response is similar to that of the stress response following surgery.

- *Temporal (tentorial) coning.* Ipsilateral III nerve palsy, ↓ consciousness, Cushing reflex, decerebrate rigidity
- *Cerebellar (medullary) coning.* Cheyne–Stokes breathing, sudden apnoea, neck stiffness.

Pressure waves in CSF (described by Lundberg in 1960)

- *A-waves* – large amplitude waves lasting 5–20 min. Indicate failure of vasomotor compensation for raised ICP
- *B-waves* – 1/min. Associated with brainstem disorders
- *C-waves* – 6/min. Indicative of cerebral disorders.

Cerebral circulation

$$CPP = MAP - (ICP + CVP)$$

where CPP = cerebral perfusion pressure, MAP = mean arterial pressure, ICP = intracranial pressure, CVP = central venous pressure at jugular bulb (usually zero).

Raised intrathoracic pressure increases CVP and reduces CPP further.

- *Normal flow* = 50 mL.100 g^{-1}.min^{-1} 15–20% of cardiac output.
- *Critical flow* occurs if MAP <50 mmHg, i.e. <20 mL.100 g^{-1}.min^{-1}.

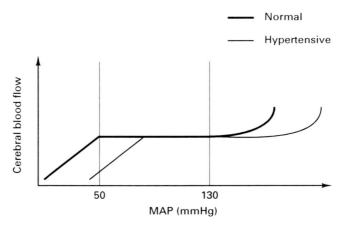

Figure 3.3 Autoregulatory limits of cerebral blood flow.

Local metabolites are the main regulator of cerebral blood flow (CBF) by effects on extracellular H^+ concentration. Lactic acid metabolites maximally vasodilate diseased tissues, e.g. infarct, tumour, head injury, subarachnoid haemorrhage. Subsequently, any cerebral vasodilator will increase flow to normal tissue and may reduce flow in diseased tissue. Known as 'reverse steal'.

Normal brain autoregulates over a range of 50–130 mmHg (Fig. 3.3). Hypertension shifts the curve to the right. Autoregulation is lost with volatile anaesthetic agents, tumour, trauma, infarction, intracranial bleed, hypoxia, hypercarbia, seizure disorders, hypotension and hypertension. In these conditions, CBF $\propto$ MAP.

CO_2

Affects CBF through vasodilation by changing the pH of extracellular fluid (ECF) (Fig. 3.4). Aim for a $P_a\text{co}_2$ of 3.5 kPa to lower ICP without excessive vasoconstriction and prevent 'reverse steal'. Volatile agents increase effects of CO_2 on vasodilation. A 3% change in CBF occurs for each 0.1 kPa change in $P_a\text{co}_2$.

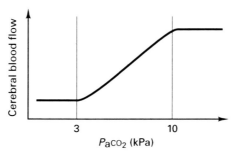

Figure 3.4 Effect of $P_a\text{co}_2$ on cerebral blood flow.

Acute changes of hyperventilation return to normal values after 48 h due to normalization of CSF pH and a compensatory increase in CSF volume.

O_2

Has less influence on CBF until P_aO_2 <8 kPa (Fig. 3.5). Hyperoxia causes mild cerebral vasoconstriction of 5–10% at 60 kPa.

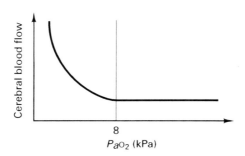

Figure 3.5 Effect of P_aO_2 on cerebral blood flow.

Monitoring

Table 3.1 Glasgow Coma Scale

Eye opening		Motor response		Verbal response	
Spontaneous	4	Obeys commands	6	Orientated	5
To speech	3	Localizes pain	5	Confused	4
To pain	2	Normal flexion	4	Inappropriate words	3
Nil	1	Abnormal flexion	3	Sounds	2
		Extension	2	Nil	1
		Nil	1		

EEG

- Unmodified EEG
- Cerebral function monitor – EEG filtered to derive mean amplitude
- Fourier analysis – displays frequency versus amplitude.

Waves

- alpha (α): 8–13 Hz; awake, eyes closed
- beta (β): >13 Hz; alert, eyes open
- theta (θ): 4–7 Hz; abnormal in elderly patients
- delta (δ): 0.5–1 Hz; abnormal in all patients.

Sudden reduction in CBF reduces amplitude of all waves and increases β and δ activity.

Evoked potentials

Measure latency and amplitude.

- Somatosensory: e.g. median or posterior tibial nerve. Record over sensory cortex. Used for spinal cord and posterior fossa surgery
- Auditory: auditory clicks. Record over mastoid to assess brainstem function, e.g. acoustic neuroma surgery
- Visual: flashes of light over eyes. Record over visual cortex, e.g. for pituitary surgery.

Measurement of intracranial pressure

- Intraventricular catheter: attached to transducer. Most accurate but risk of infection
- Subdural bolt: tends to under-read at high pressures
- Subdural catheter
- Extradural catheter: either pressure transducer at tip of catheter or fibreoptic light shining onto mirror at tip which is displaced as ICP increases and alters amount of light reflected back onto the catheter.

Anaesthetic drugs

Alter CBF by effects on vascular smooth muscle, cerebral metabolism and alveolar ventilation (P_aCO_2).

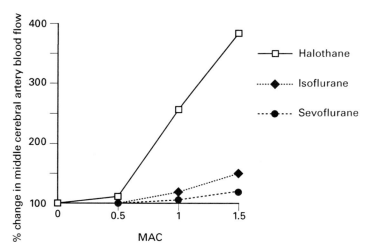

Figure 3.6 Percentage change in middle cerebral artery blood flow with increasing minimum alveolar concentration (MAC).

Volatile agents

All volatiles with the exception of desflurane reduce cerebral metabolism and oxygen demand. Effect is most marked with isoflurane. All increase ICP and abolish autoregulation in sufficient doses. Halothane causes most cerebral vasodilation (Table 3.2). At 1 MAC (minimum alveolar concentration), isoflurane has minimal effect on ICP, autoregulation or EEG depression. At 2.5 MAC, the EEG becomes isoelectric. Isoflurane reduces cerebral O_2 demand more than any other volatile and reduces cerebral blood flow without evidence of ischaemia. Sevoflurane and desflurane appear similar to isoflurane in their CNS and CVS effects.

N_2O is a weak vasodilator causing moderate increases in CBF and cerebral metabolic rate (CMR). Changes in CBF are variable and may be more related to changes in F_iO_2.

Table 3.2 Cerebral effects of anaesthetic drugs

	Autoregulation	Cerebral blood flow	Intracranial pressure	Cerebral metabolic rate ($CMRO_2$)
Inhaled agents				
Nitrous oxide	N	↑	↑	↑
Halothane	↓	↑	↑	↓
Isoflurane	↓	↑	↑	↓
Sevoflurane	↓	↑	↑	↓
Desflurane	↓	↑	↑	N
Intravenous agents				
Thiopentone	N	↓	↓	↓
Propofol	N	↓	↓	↓
Midazolam	N	↓	↓	↓
Ketamine	N	↑	↑	↑
Etomidate	N	↓	↓	↓
Opioids				
Morphine	N	N	N	N
Fentanyl	N	N	N	N
Alfentanil	N	↓	↓	↓
Remifentanil	N	↓	↓	↓
Muscle relaxants				
Depolarizing	N	↑	↑	N
Non-depolarizing	N	N	N	N

↑, Increase; ↓, Decrease; N, Normal

Intravenous agents

All i.v. induction agents, except ketamine, decrease ICP, and all have little effect on autoregulation. Both thiopentone and propofol cause dose-related decreases in CBF and O_2 demand and both are good attenuators of increased ICP during intubation. Propofol has nine Committee on Safety of Medicines reports (August 1987) warning of grand mal seizures.

Ketamine increases CBF, ICP and O_2 demand. Avoid in neuroanaesthesia.

Suxamethonium causes a transient rise in ICP through muscle fasciculations, increasing venous pressure and muscle spindle efferents activated by fasciculations.

Anaesthesia for neurosurgery

Aims

- Maintain safe airway
- Maximize O_2 delivery
- Minimize O_2 demand
- Avoid sudden hypertensive insults
- Maintain CPP ($\rightarrow$ MAP, $\downarrow$ ICP, $\downarrow$ CVP)
- Use agents allowing rapid postoperative recovery.

Preoperative

Assess gag reflex (?aspiration), $\downarrow$ cough reflex (?sputum retention), drowsiness (?drug-induced or CNS pathology), nausea and vomiting causing electrolyte disturbance and dehydration. Assess signs of raised ICP (headache, nausea and vomiting, Cushing reflex, downward gaze of eyes). Assess drug treatment: steroids decrease ICP, anticonvulsants induce liver enzymes. Assess pituitary dysfunction.

Premedication

Avoid drugs causing neurological or respiratory depression. Prescribe midazolam and glycopyrrolate if necessary.

Monitoring

Arterial line, CVP via long line (neck lines impair venous drainage of head and may require head-down position for insertion), ECG, temperature, end-tidal CO_2, S_aO_2, neuromuscular stimulator, regular blood gases and electrolytes.

Positioning

Avoid obstructing venous drainage of head. 15° head up. Protect eyes.

Induction

Thiopentone is often the drug of choice because of its anticonvulsant properties. Give slowly to avoid a decrease in BP reducing CPP. Propofol is also popular and appears not to cause postoperative seizures. Consider additional agent to attenuate pressor response to intubation, e.g. lidocaine, high-dose opioids, β-blockers, hydralazine. Topical anaesthesia to larynx. Etomidate causes coughing, hiccoughs and vomiting which raises ICP. Propofol may cause epileptiform EEG but lowers ICP and is suitable for induction and maintenance.

Suxamethonium causes hyperkalaemia in the presence of spastic paraplegia. Wait for full paralysis before intubation to avoid coughing and straining on endotracheal tube (ETT). Use armoured ETT to prevent kinking. Tape ETT, because a tie may cause venous obstruction of head and neck, increasing ICP. Consider NG tube.

Maintenance

Use a balanced technique with opioid in combination with O_2 and N_2O/air and muscle relaxants, which produces good cardiovascular stability. N_2O may increase ICP but detrimental affects of using this as part of balanced anaesthesia have not been demonstrated. Sevoflurane is the volatile of choice as it causes less vasodilation ($\uparrow$ ICP) and preserves autoregulation compared with isoflurane and desflurane. If greatly increased ICP, avoid volatiles until dura has been opened. Vecuronium/rocuronium are the relaxants of choice – use high dose to avoid coughing or straining. Ventilate to maintain $P_a\text{co}_2$ at 3.5 kPa. Fentanyl is a suitable opioid, but remifentanil may allow faster waking and neuroassessment. TIVA is gaining popularity using propofol/remifentanil infusion, but some concern that it increases cerebral oxygen demand.

Reversal

Avoid coughing. Early extubation allows CNS monitoring for signs of deterioration. Avoid sudden hypertension which causes cerebral oedema through loss of autoregulation.

Fluids

Maintain plasma osmolality at the upper end of normal. Avoid fluids with low osmolality which increase free brain water (Table 3.3). Avoid glucose-containing solutions which accelerate anaerobic metabolism and may worsen neurological morbidity.

Postoperative

Any change in Glasgow Coma Scale can be assumed to be due to surgical complications. Aim for a similar BP as the preoperative value. Codeine phosphate is usually sufficient for analgesia. Start anticonvulsants. Watch for diabetes insipidus, tension pneumocephalus and cranial nerve injury.

Table 3.3 Osmolality of intravenous fluids

Solution	Osmolality (mOsm.L⁻¹)
Normal saline	310
Mannitol	300
Hartmann's solution	272
Dextrose saline	262
5% dextrose	250

Anaesthesia for intracranial aneurysm

Nimodipine reduces the risk of re-bleeding in patients following a subarachnoid haemorrhage and may reduce the severity of vasospasm. Vasospasm is maximal between days 3 and 10. Generally, aim for early surgery (within 48 h) if no severe neurological deficit, or late surgery if patient is comatose (to assess potential degree of recovery over about 10 days). Hyperventilation may worsen vasospasm.

Opening the dura reduces ICP, resulting in increased transmural pressure across the aneurysm wall. Therefore, may need perioperative hypotensive anaesthesia. Vasodilation with sodium nitroprusside causes increased ICP unless dura is opened. Trimetaphan can be used with the dura closed but is of slower onset, causes dilated pupils (ganglion blockade), making CNS assessment difficult, and triggers histamine release. Both drugs may cause rebound hypertension on cessation.

If aneurysm ruptures, press on ipsilateral carotid artery, give 100% O_2 and consider transient hypotension with sodium nitroprusside.

Anaesthesia for posterior fossa surgery

The posterior fossa comprises midbrain, pons, medulla, cerebellum and cranial nerves V–XII. Patient position to be either:

- sitting – reduces blood loss but high risk of air embolus and hypotension
- park bench position – greatly reduces the risk of air embolus.

Complications of surgery

Air embolus. Usually gradual leak rather than sudden bolus. Occurs due to veins being prevented from collapsing by tethering to dura (dural sinuses) or periosteum (emissary sinuses). Reduce incidence with 10 cm PEEP, neck tourniquet and G-suit.

Spontaneous respiration provides further indicators of brainstem function but increased risk of air embolus (negative intrathoracic pressure) and hypercapnia.

Sensitivity of detection. Precordial Doppler $>P_aO_2 >P_{ET}CO_2 >PAP >P_aCO_2 >CVP$ $>CO >BP >ECG>$'mill-wheel' murmur using stethoscope.

Treatment. Occlude wound with wet swab, 100% O_2, raise CVP by levelling table and neck compression, aspirate CVP line (tip should be placed in RA preoperatively), position patient in left lateral position with head down if possible.

Other complications

- Stimulation of posterior fossa causing the Cushing reflex
- Vagal stimulation causes bradycardia
- Stimulation of V (trigeminal) cranial nerve causes hypertension
- Damage to dorsal group neurones causes postoperative apnoea
- Bulbar palsy
- Increased sensitivity to respiratory depressants.

Postoperative

Loss of gag (glossopharyngeal (IX) damage) increases risk of aspiration following extubation. Therefore assess prior to extubation. Watch for respiratory failure and hydrocephalus.

Treatment of raised ICP

- 15° head-up tilt. Ensure good venous drainage of head and neck
- Avoid hypoxia. Keep P_aCO_2 lower limit of normal. No PEEP
- Keep CVP low
- Avoid cerebral vasodilating drugs
- Adequate muscle relaxation
- Osmotic/loop diuretics (mannitol 1 g.kg^{-1}; effect prolonged by furosemide). Consider hypertonic saline as an alternative to mannitol.
- Consider CSF drainage.

RECOMMENDATIONS FOR THE SAFE TRANSFER OF PATIENTS WITH BRAIN INJURY
Association of Anaesthetists of Great Britain and Ireland 2006

Summary

1. High quality transfer of patients with brain injury improves outcome.
2. There should be designated consultants in the referring hospitals and the neuroscience units with overall responsibility for the transfer of patients with brain injuries.
3. Local guidelines on the transfer of patients with brain injuries should be drawn up between the referring hospital trusts, the neurosciences unit and the local ambulance service. These should be consistent with

established national guidelines. Details of the transfer of responsibility for patient care should also be agreed.

4. While it is understood that transfer is often urgent, thorough resuscitation and stabilization of the patient must be completed before transfer to avoid complications during the journey.

5. All patients with a Glasgow Coma Scale (GCS) ≤8 requiring transfer to a neurosciences unit should be intubated and ventilated.

6. Patients with brain injuries should be accompanied by a doctor with appropriate training and experience in the transfer of patients with acute brain injury. They must have a dedicated and adequately trained assistant. Arrangements for medical indemnity and personal accident insurance should be in place.

7. The standard of monitoring during transport should adhere to previously published standards.

8. The transfer team must be provided with a means of communication – a mobile telephone is suitable.

9. Education, training and audit are crucial to improving standards of transfer.

Bibliography

Association of Anaesthetists of Great Britain and Ireland, 2006. Recommedations for The Safe Transfer of Patients With brain injury. Reproduced with the kind permission of the Association of anaesthetists of Great Britain and Ireland.

Dinsmore J: Anaesthesia for elective neurosurgery, Br J Anaesth 99:68–74, 2007.

Hancock SM, Nathanson MH: Nitrous oxide or remifentanil for the 'at risk' brain, Anaesthesia 59:313–315, 2004.

Hirsch N: Advances in neuroanaesthesia, Anaesthesia 58:1162–1165, 2003.

Moss E: The cerebral circulation, BJA CEPD Rev 1:67–71, 2001.

Pasternak JJ, William LW: Neuroanesthesiology update, J Neurosurg Anesth 21:73–97, 2009.

AUTONOMIC NERVOUS SYSTEM

Sympathetic nervous system (Fig. 3.7)

Centres in the brainstem give rise to descending tracts which innervate SNS preganglionic neurones in intermediolateral columns in the spinal cord. They emerge at T_1–L_2, then either synapse in SNS chain or synapse at a distance, e.g. coeliac plexus (splanchnic) or hypogastric plexus (bladder). SNS fibres for skin and vessels re-enter the cord to re-emerge with skeletal nerves.

SNS

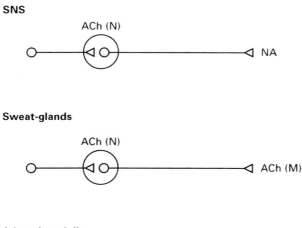

Sweat-glands

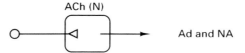

Adrenal medulla

Figure 3.7 SNS synapse. N, nicotinic receptor; M, muscarinic receptor; NA, noradrenaline; Ad, adrenaline; O, ganglia; □, adrenal medulla.

Parasympathetic nervous system (Fig. 3.8)

Parasympathetic nerve fibres run in cranial nerves II, V, VII, IX, X, S_2–S_4. 75% of PNS fibres run in the vagus to supply heart, lungs, upper GI tract and liver. Preganglionic fibres terminate in the end organ and postganglionic fibres are very short.

PNS

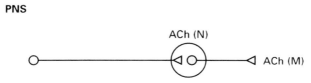

Figure 3.8 PNS synapse. N, nicotine receptor; M, muscarinic receptor; ACh, acetylcholine; O, ganglia.

Valsalva manoeuvre

- *Phase I*
  - forced expiration against resistance (or a closed glottis) to a pressure of 40 mmHg for 10 s
  - raised intrathoracic pressure transmitted to arteries causing initial hypertension and compensatory bradycardia
- *Phase II*
  - reduced venous return causes hypotension with compensatory tachycardia
- *Phase III*
  - release of Valsalva
  - reduced intrathoracic pressure causes hypotension and compensatory tachycardia
- *Phase IV*
  - hypertension due to vasoconstriction as venous return and thus cardiac output increases, causing a reflex bradycardia.

Autonomic neuropathy

Causes

- Elderly
- Diabetes (IDDM >NIDDM)
- CVA
- Guillain–Barré syndrome
- Parkinson's disease
- Shy–Drager syndrome
- AIDS.

Symptoms and signs

- Loss of diurnal BP variation
- Fixed heart rate (tachycardia) and loss of R–R variation
- Orthostatic hypotension
- Painless MI
- Failure of kidneys to concentrate urine at night, causing nocturia
- Increased gastric emptying time.

Assessment

Abnormal response to Valsalva manoeuvre with BP continuing to fall during phase II. No overshoot of BP on release of Valsalva. No tachy- or bradycardia.

- *SNS*
  - degree of postural hypotension (decrease systolic >30 mmHg)
  - thermoregulatory sweating test.
- *PNS*
  - degree of bradycardia with Valsalva manoeuvre (<5 beats.min^{-1} is abnormal)
  - degree of sinus arrhythmia during deep breathing (difference between maximum and minimum HR <15 beats.min^{-1} is abnormal).

Anaesthetic problems

- Blood pressure dependent upon ECF volume with subsequent hypotension on induction
- Arrhythmias common
- Reduced sensitivity to hypoxia and hypercapnia
- Ventilation not associated with the usual Valsalva-type response
- Reduced response to indirect-acting catecholamines (e.g. ephedrine) but exaggerated response to direct catecholamines (e.g. adrenaline) due to a denervation hypersensitivity.

Bibliography

Foëx P: The heart and autonomic nervous system. In Nimmo WS, Rowbotham DJ, Smith G, editors: *Anaesthesia*, ed 2, Oxford, 1994, Blackwell Scientific Publications, pp 195–242.

Keyl C, Lemberger P, Palitzsch KD, et al: Cardiovascular autonomic dysfunction and haemodynamic response to anesthetic induction in patients with coronary artery disease and diabetes mellitus, *Anesth Analg* 88:985–991, 1999.

Tusiewicz K: The autonomic nervous system. In Kaufman L, editor: *Anaesthesia Review 5*, Edinburgh, 1988, Churchill Livingstone, pp 54–66.

4 Other systems

DENTAL ANAESTHESIA

The first dental GA was given by Cotton and Wells in 1844. Currently, 300 000 dental GAs are given per annum (70% children) and, until recently, numbers have been declining owing to less tooth decay.

Mortality is 1:150 000 (2 deaths/year), compared with 1:250 000 non-dental day-case GAs, and is usually due to respiratory difficulties or sudden cardiovascular collapse.

Recent deaths in the dental chair have prompted moves to stop dental anaesthesia being carried out in dental surgeries.

POSWILLO REPORT
Department of Health 1990

This report discusses general anaesthesia, sedation and resuscitation in dental surgeries. Its main recommendations are:

- Same standards required for GA in dental surgeries as in hospitals.
- Minimum monitoring standards.
- Dental surgeries to be inspected and registered.
- Accredited anaesthetists only.

STANDARDS AND GUIDELINES FOR GENERAL ANAESTHESIA FOR DENTISTRY
The Royal College of Anaesthetists 1999

Introduction

- There are concerns over a recent increase in the number of dental anaesthetics administered in the community.
- Deaths (usually young, healthy patients) continue to occur. Criticism of anaesthetic standards has led to increase in public concern.
- The Royal College of Anaesthetists expects the same standards in dental anaesthesia as are widely accepted for anaesthesia in other clinical settings in the UK.

Background

- GAs are often used inappropriately as a method of anxiety control rather than pain relief.
- Risks of community GAs are often not appreciated, with frequent failings in standards of patient care, monitoring and resuscitation skills. Compromise in standards is almost inevitable because of economic pressure.
- The Poswillo Report and guidelines from the General Dental Council have not improved standards as intended.

Recommended standards

General anaesthesia should be limited to:

1. Control of pain that cannot be achieved with local anaesthesia ± sedation
2. Patients with problems related to age/maturity or physical/mental disability
3. Patients in whom dental phobia will be induced or prolonged.

Patient assessment

The final decision as to the benefit:risk of a dental GA can only be made after consultation between the patient, anaesthetist and dentist.

Clinical setting

Risks of death are greater should a complication occur. There must be written protocols for the management of patients requiring resuscitation or transfer.

Equipment and drugs

Equipment should be appropriate to the dental setting and anaesthetic technique. Routine maintenance must be performed and checks of equipment must be made before use. Back-up equipment and resuscitation drugs must be available.

Staffing standards

Dental anaesthesia should only be administered by:

1. Anaesthetists on the specialist register
2. Trainees working under supervision
3. Non-consultant-grade anaesthetists working under the supervision of a named consultant. Trained assistance must be provided by an operating department practitioner or dental nurse. Patients must be supervised in recovery until fully awake.

Aftercare

Patients must be discharged home according to the same criteria as day-case surgery.

Audit

This should examine all aspects of practice.

The way forward
- Greater patient education in the non-GA techniques that are available
- Better anaesthetic training in control of pain and anxiety
- Centralization of GA services in centres with adequate facilities.

Main anaesthetic problems

- Shared airway
- Day-case anaesthesia
- Paediatrics
- Mentally handicapped patients from institutions are at higher risk of hepatitis B
- Lack of premedication causing ↑ anxiety, ↑ arrhythmias and difficult i.v. access.

Techniques

Local anaesthetic

Sedation

A state of CNS depression during which *verbal contact with the patient is maintained*. Achieved with Entonox, oral/i.v. benzodiazepines, i.v. methohexitone.

General anaesthetic

Intubation. Avoid suxamethonium, which has high morbidity. High-dose alfentanil (30 µg/kg) together with propofol enables intubation without relaxant.

Indicated for mental handicap, prolonged or painful surgery and nasal airway obstruction. Use nasopharyngeal pack.

Cardiovascular side-effects

Dysrhythmias. These are common due to sympathetic and parasympathetic activity, high levels of endogenous catecholamines, halothane and airway obstruction with hypoxia and hypercarbia:

- nodal rhythms – 25%
- multifocal PVCs – 8%.

They mostly occur during surgery and are worse during trigeminal nerve stimulation. Atropine increases the incidence of dysrrhythmias.

Less common with i.v. induction than with gaseous induction. Less common with volatile agents other than halothane.

More common following recent Coxsackie B infection due to (?) viral myocarditis.

Arrhythmias may be the primary cause of high mortality seen with dental GAs.

Fainting. Only in conscious patients! May need large doses of atropine. Abandon procedure because CVS instability persists for up to 90 min.

High mortality in erect patients was attributed to unrecognized fainting, but mortality is the same in supine patients. Supine position is associated with more pharyngeal soiling. It is now recommended that all surgery should be performed in the supine position which gives better CVS stability.

Bibliography

Cartwright DP: Death in the dental chair, *Anaesthesia* 54:105–107, 1999.

Department of Health: *General anaesthesia, sedation and resuscitation in dentistry (Poswillo Report)*, London, 1990, HMSO.

Flynn PJ, Strunin L: General anaesthesia for dentistry, *Anaesth Intens Care Med* 6:263–265, 2005.

Royal College of Anaesthetists: *Standards and guidelines for general anaesthesia and dentistry*, London, 1999, RCA.

Worthington LM, Flynn PJ, Strunin L: Death in the dental chair: an avoidable catastrophe? *Br J Anaesth* 80:131–132, 1998.

ANAESTHESIA FOR EAR, NOSE AND THROAT SURGERY

General anaesthetic problems

- Competition with the surgeon for airway, loss of access to the airway and airway compromise with packs, blood, pus or tissue.
- Spontaneous ventilation has the advantage that the reservoir bag provides a good monitor of respiration and any disconnection hidden by the drapes is immediately obvious.
- Extubate in a head-down, left lateral position to prevent aspiration of blood and debris and to protect the airway in the immediate postoperative period.

Ear surgery

Myringotomy

This is a short, relatively painless operation. Premedication is not usually necessary.

Chronic otitis media is often associated with upper respiratory tract infection. Morbidity not increased with uncomplicated URTI if mask rather than intubation used. Need postoperative O_2 if oxygen saturation <93% on room air.

Middle ear surgery

Careful positioning is required to avoid obstruction of venous drainage of the head. Tympanoplasty and mastoidectomy usually require identification of facial nerve. Therefore, avoid long-acting neuromuscular blocking drugs.

Use hypotensive anaesthesia to minimize bleeding. Maximum recommended safe dose of adrenaline = 0.1 mg/10 min.

Avoid N_2O which diffuses into the middle ear to cause expansion, or on cessation diffuses out of the middle ear to cause negative pressure and disruption of ossicles.

Consider prophylactic antiemetics.

Nasal surgery

Anaesthesia of the nasal cavities

Moffatt's solution

- 2 mL 8% cocaine
- 2 mL 1% bicarbonate
- 1 mL 1:1000 adrenaline.

Give with head extended over trolley, with half into each nostril.

Sluder's technique. Four applicators are dipped into adrenaline and cocaine solution, and placed on middle turbinates under anterior and posterior ends.

Packing of nasal cavities. Spray nasal cavities with 4–10% cocaine and then pack with gauze soaked in 4–5% cocaine solution.

Gauze must contact area behind middle meatus (greater and lesser palatine nerves) and ethmoidal plate (anterior ethmoidal nerve).

Throat surgery

Tonsillectomy

Avoid premedication if tonsils are large or there is a history of sleep apnoea. Use gas or i.v. induction. Either deep gaseous intubation (patient more drowsy postoperatively) or suxamethonium. Use throat pack and endotracheal tube. Spontaneous respiration tends to hypoventilation with risk of arrhythmias, especially with halothane.

Extubate awake (protective reflexes), with head-down in left lateral position.

Postoperative haemorrhage. Affects 0.5%; 75% of postoperative haemorrhages occur within 6 h of surgery. Main problems are:

- hypovolaemia
- full stomach
- residual effects of earlier GA
- upper airway oedema from previous surgery and intubation
- anxious child and parents.

Assessing the patient can be difficult. Tachycardia due to hypovolaemia may also be due to anxiety or pain. Blood loss is usually underestimated, as most is swallowed. Establish i.v. access, check BP sitting and lying (postural hypotension with hypovolaemia), check haematocrit and cross-match blood.

There are two approaches to induction:

- *Gas induction.* Head-down, left lateral position, head-down tilt. If cords are visualized once lightly anaesthetized, give suxamethonium and intubate. Deep gaseous intubation worsens hypotension if hypovolaemic.
- *Rapid sequence induction.* Head-down, left lateral position for intubation if practiced in this technique.

Both approaches need a selection of laryngoscope blades, stylettes, range of ETTs, two suction units (one may become blocked with clot), emergency tracheostomy kit and tipping trolley.

Pass NG tube and aspirate stomach prior to extubation.

Adenoidectomy

Usually performed in conjunction with tonsillectomy. Not as painful. May cause nasopharyngeal obstruction and obligate mouth breathing.

Obstructive sleep apnoea

Grossly hypertrophied tonsils can cause partial upper airway obstruction when awake and complete obstruction during sleep. Associated with obesity, micrognathia (e.g. Pierre–Robin syndrome) and neuromuscular disorders (e.g. cerebral palsy). May present as failure to thrive, snoring, daytime somnolence, developmental delay, recurrent chest infections and, if severe, cor pulmonale. Airway obstruction may persist post-tonsillectomy.

Peritonsillar abscess (quinsy)

The infected tonsil forms an abscess in the lateral pharyngeal wall with associated trismus and difficulty in swallowing. The abscess does not usually interfere with the airway, but there is a risk of rupture and aspiration of contents. Drainage under LA, otherwise treat as for epiglottitis. Consider tracheostomy under LA if abscess is likely to rupture on intubation.

NATIONAL PATIENT SAFETY AGENCY
Reducing the Risk of Retained Throat Packs after Surgery, April 2009

This Safer Practice Notice applies to all members of theatre teams and aims to reduce the risk of **throat packs** being **retained** after surgery is completed. Throat packs are often inserted by anaesthetists or surgeons to:

- absorb material created by surgery in the mouth
- prevent fluids or material from entering the oesophagus or lungs
- prevent escape of gases from around tracheal tubes
- stabilize artificial airways.

However, if a throat pack is retained after surgery is completed, it can lead to obstruction of the patient's airways. Data received by the Reporting and Learning System between 1 January 2006 and 31 December 2007 were analysed. A total of 38 incidents were identified, of which 24 were unintended retention of throat packs; one resulting in moderate harm.

Clinical risk managers responsible for anaesthesia and surgery should ensure that local policies and procedures are adapted to state that:

1. The decision to use a throat pack should be justified by the anaesthetist or surgeon for each patient. This person should assume responsibility for ensuring the chosen safety procedures are undertaken.
2. At least one visually-based and one documentary-based procedure is applied whenever a throat pack is deemed necessary.

Visual

- Label or mark patient: either the head, or exceptionally, on another visible part of the body, with an adherent sticker or marker.
- Label artificial airway (e.g. tracheal tube or supraglottic mask airway).
- Attach pack securely to the artificial airway.
- Leave part of pack protruding.

Documentary

- Formalized and recorded 'two-person' check of insertion and removal of pack.
- Record insertion and removal on swab board.
3. All staff are fully informed of the chosen procedures.

Bibliography

Chambers WA: ENT anaesthesia. In Nimmo WS, Rowbotham DJ, Smith G, editors: *Anaesthesia*, London, 1994, Blackwell Scientific Publications, pp 806–822.

National Patient Safety Agency: *Reducing the risk of retained throat packs after surgery*, 2009, 28 April. Ref: NPSA/2009/SPN001.

ANAESTHESIA AND LIVER DISEASE

Normal physiology

The liver receives 25% of cardiac output. Portal venous blood contributes 70% of total flow and 50–60% of oxygen. The portal venous system has little smooth muscle and is not as responsive to sympathetic tone as the hepatic artery. When portal flow decreases, hepatic artery flow increases. Autoregulation at a microvascular level is poorly developed in the liver but hepatocytes can extract more oxygen from the blood than can any other tissue.

Total hepatic blood flow is reduced by IPPV, PEEP, hypovolaemia, hypocarbia, general anaesthesia and epidurals.

Physiological changes in liver disease

CVS. Hyperdynamic circulation, ↓ systemic vascular resistance, portal hypertension, due to activation of renin–angiotensin system and intravascular and interstitial fluid accumulation. Alcoholic cardiomyopathy.

Respiratory. Restrictive lung disease, pleural effusions. Impaired hypoxic pulmonary vasoconstriction causing ↑ V/Q scatter and ↑ shunting, together with impaired respiration from ascites, causing hypoxia.

Haematology. Anaemia, thrombocytopenia, coagulopathy.

Renal. Hepatorenal syndrome (especially with sepsis and ↑ bilirubin). Prerenal failure causes acute tubular necrosis.

GI. Oesophageal varices, delayed gastric emptying. Increased gastric volume and acidity.

CNS. Encephalopathy, cerebral oedema.

Metabolic. Metabolic and respiratory alkalosis, hyper- or hypoglycaemia. Hyponatraemia (usually dilutional).

Pharmacokinetic and pharmacodynamic changes

- Early alcoholic liver disease induces liver enzymes, causing drug resistance. In late stages, impaired function causes drug sensitivity. Phase I metabolism is reduced more than phase II metabolism.
- Sodium and water retention and ascites increase V_D of water-soluble drugs.
- Hypoalbuminaemia increases free drug concentrations, e.g. barbiturates, propanolol, benzodiazepines etc.
- Increased CNS sensitivity to depressants due to increased blood–brain barrier permeability and altered CNS receptor kinetics.
- Decreased first pass of drugs due to shunting of portal blood flow into the systemic circulation, bypassing liver parenchyma.

Assessment of surgical risk

Child's (1963) classification assessed risk using albumin and bilirubin. Modified by Pugh et al (1973) (see Table 4.1). Perioperative mortality A<5%, B≈25%, C>50%.

Specific drugs

Anticholinergics. Little change in pharmacokinetics. Use normal doses.

Barbiturates. Increased sensitivity and prolonged excretion of thiopentone. Use <3–4 mg/kg.

Benzodiazepines. Lorazepam and oxazepam are metabolized by glucuronidation, which is minimally affected: therefore they are safe. Increased sensitivity to diazepam and midazolam due to impaired phase I reactions.

Table 4.1 Child–Pugh classification of surgical risk in patients with liver disease. Child–Pugh total score A, 5–6 points; B, 7–9 points; C, 10–15 points

Points	1	2	3
Serum bilirubin (μm.L^{-1})	<34	34–50	>50
Serum albumin (g.L^{-1})	>35	28–35	<28
Ascites	None	Controlled	Tense
Encephalopathy	None	Mild	Significant
INR	<1.7	1.7–2.3	>2.3

Propofol. Increased sensitivity. Use 2 mg/kg for induction.

Opioids. Increased sensitivity and prolonged half-life of morphine, diamorphine and pethidine. No change in remifentanil pharmacokinetics.

Muscle relaxants. Suxamethonium has prolonged action due to reduced plasma cholinesterase. Resistance to pancuronium due to increased V_D of these drugs. Atracurium is probably the drug of choice due to spontaneous degradation and little change in pharmacokinetics. Action of vecuronium is prolonged even with mild liver disease.

Anticholinesterases. Normal doses of neostigmine may be used.

Local anaesthetics. Reduced metabolism of amides. Reduced plasma cholinesterase prolongs elimination of esters.

Inhalational agents. Halothane > enflurane decrease hepatic blood flow. Little effect with isoflurane/sevoflurane/desflurane. Avoid halothane because of risks of hepatitis. Sympathomimetic effects of N_2O may reduce hepatic blood flow.

Other. Adrenaline and ephedrine increase hepatic blood flow. Sodium nitroprusside and β-blockers decrease hepatic blood flow.

Anaesthetic management

Preoperative

Assess cardiovascular and renal status. Optimize respiratory function with antibiotics, bronchodilators, physiotherapy and consider drainage of ascites. Correct coagulation with FFP, cryoprecipitate, vitamin K and platelets.

Premedication

Avoid if possible.

Monitoring

Routine monitoring, arterial line, CVP, urinary catheter, nerve stimulator, ± PCWP.

Induction

Use small amounts of thiopentone or midazolam.

Maintenance

Use isoflurane/sevoflurane/desflurane in oxygen. High F_iO_2 needed because of pulmonary shunting. Avoid hyperventilation which increases mean intrathoracic pressure, thus reducing hepatic blood flow, accelerates formation of ammonia, causing hepatic encephalopathy, and increases urinary potassium loss through respiratory alkalosis. Hepatic blood flow is proportional to mean arterial pressure. Keep CVP <5 mmHg to reduce haemorrhage secondary to venous congestion.

Neuromuscular blockade with atracurium or pancuronium. Reversal with normal doses of anticholinesterases. Avoid rocuronium which has prolonged action.

Maintain high urine output to protect against renal failure. Avoid excess sodium load in i.v. fluids to prevent dilutional hyponatraemia.

Hepatic disease reduces synthesis of coagulation factors and inhibitors, and causes quantitative and qualitative platelet defects and hyperfibrinolysis. Massive haemorrhage a particular risk with cirrhosis, steatosis, and after chemotherapy. Exacerbated by acidosis, hypothermia and hypocalcaemia. Use of cell salvage in malignancy is controversial. Anti-fibrinolytics (e.g. tranexamic acid) reduces perioperative blood loss.

Postoperative

IPPV may be necessary until patient is rewarmed and stabilized. Remove lines as soon as possible to reduce risk of infection. Analgesia with small doses of opioids. Remifentanil avoids accumulation of active opioid metabolites. Regional block may reduce requirements, provided clotting is normal.

Watch for hypoglycaemia as a result of impaired hepatic mobilization of glucose. Secondary hyperaldosteronism is common (sodium and water retention and oedema), which is minimized by restriction of sodium intake and treated with diuretics.

Bibliography

Fabbroni D, Bellamy M: Anaesthesia for hepatic transplantation, *Contin Edu Anaesth, Crit Care Pain* 6:171–175, 2006.

Hartog A, Mills G: Anaesthesia for hepatic resection surgery, *Contin Edu Anaesth, Crit Care Pain* 9:1–5, 2009.

Lai WK, Murphy N: Management of acute liver failure, *Contin Edu Anaesth, Crit Care Pain* 4:40–43, 2004.

ANAESTHESIA FOR OPHTHALMIC SURGERY

Physiology

Aqueous humour

Made by ciliary plexus and secreted into anterior chamber. Absorbed through the trabecular meshwork into the canal of Schlem.

Intraocular pressure (IOP)

Normal value 15–25 mmHg. Once the eye is opened, IOP is equal to atmospheric pressure. Hypoxia, hypercapnia, coughing and vomiting all increase IOP.

Oculocardiac reflex

Reflex pathway runs from the long and short ciliary nerves via the ciliary ganglion to the ophthalmic division of the trigeminal nerve (V) and then to the Gasserian ganglion. From here, the pathway runs to the trigeminal sensory nucleus in the brainstem, to the motor nucleus of the vagus (X) in the medulla, through the reticular formation and finally to the heart via the vagus nerve.

Causes bradycardia, asystole, PVCs, A–V block, VT and VF. It is more marked and frequent in children, particularly during squint surgery.

Reflex fatigues quickly with cessation of stimulus.

Prophylaxis with glycopyrrolate is as effective as atropine.

Effects of anaesthetic drugs on intraocular pressure

All volatile agents cause a dose-related decrease in IOP due to decreased extraocular muscle tone and increased aqueous humour outflow.

Etomidate and propofol lower IOP, as do (to a lesser degree) thiopentone, benzodiazepines, morphine and fentanyl. Ketamine increases IOP and causes blepharospasm and nystagmus.

Suxamethonium increases IOP, possibly by orbital smooth muscle contraction. Peak increase is 10 mmHg at 4 min, returning to baseline value by 6 min. Precurarization has a minimal effect on IOP. Rocuronium, pancuronium, vecuronium and atracurium all lower IOP.

Eye surgery

Requirements

- No coughing, straining or vomiting
- Soft, akinetic eye in central position.

Advantages of regional block over GA

- More suitable for day surgery
- Reduced anaesthetic morbidity (less nausea and sore throat)
- Safer for sick patients
- Better postoperative analgesia
- Faster patient turnover.

GA

More suitable for painful procedures, anxious patients, chronic cough, penetrating eye injuries, deaf and mentally handicapped patients, children and long operations. Assess other pathology associated with the eye disease, e.g. trauma, diabetes, myotonic dystrophy. Patient is often elderly with associated pathology, e.g. hypertension (47%), ischaemic heart disease (38%), hypothyroidism (18%), diabetes (16%), new malignancy (3%).

Premedication

- Opiates: respiratory depression increases IOP and causes nausea and vomiting
- Benzodiazepines: good
- Anticholinergics: do not $\uparrow$ IOP at premedication doses and are safe with narrow angle glaucoma.

Monitoring

Often in a dark room (to prevent glare interfering with surgical microscope) with minimal access to patient. Expose limb and illuminate a limb to allow access to a pulse and observe for cyanosis.

Induction

Propofol decreases IOP more than thiopentone and causes less nausea and vomiting. Laryngeal mask airway (LMA) results in less rise in IOP compared with ETT and less postoperative coughing and sore throat. If patient is ventilated, ETT avoids risks of regurgitation, but spray cord with local anaesthetic to reduce coughing. Tape ETT in place because a tie causes venous obstruction to drainage of head, raising IOP.

Smooth extubation to avoid coughing by extubating deep, deflating cuff before reversal and using lidocaine 1.5 mg/kg pre-extubation.

Ecothiopate (organophosphate – no longer available) inhibited plasma cholinesterase and prolonged action of suxamethonium. Avoid suxamethonium with myotonic dystrophy.

Keep IOP low by:

- 10° head-up tilt
- adequate neuromuscular blockade, which ensures low peak airway pressure

- keeping end-tidal CO_2 at the lower limit of normal (if IPPV)
- avoiding mechanical pressure on eyeball, e.g. lid retractors
- i.v. mannitol
- choroidal autoregulation – lost with systolic <90 mmHg.

Nitrous oxide. Intraocular bubbles of sulphur hexafluoride (SF_6) or perfluoropropane (C_3F_8) are used in surgery for detached retina to push the retina against the choroid. Nitrous oxide will cause rapid expansion of the bubble if used within 10 days.

Regional anaesthesia

The first local anaesthetic (LA) eye surgery using topical cocaine was performed by Koller in 1880. It is becoming more popular: 80% of all cataracts are now operated on under LA.

Absolute contraindications

- Changes in eye shape
- Orbital pathology
- Penetrating eye injury
- Previous retinal detachment surgery in that eye
- Uncooperative patient.

Relative contraindications

- Large eye (>26 mm)
- Warfarin (check INR <2.5).

Local anaesthetic solution

Use:

- equal volumes of lidocaine 2% and bupivacaine 0.75%
- hyaluronidase 5 units/mL
- ± adrenaline 1:200 000 (5 µg/mL) to prolong block.

Less painful injection if solution warmed to 35°C.

Retrobulbar and peribulbar blocks are equated with spinal and epidural blocks, respectively.

Retrobulbar block. First described by Atkinson in 1955. Patient looks straight ahead. Use a 25G 40 mm blunt needle.

1. Inject through inferior conjunctiva in a vertical line through edge of lateral border of iris. Advance needle in posterior direction to 1 cm then superomedially 2–3 cm to enter muscle cone (max. depth 25 mm) when the eye will bob downwards. Inject 4 mL LA solution.
2. Superior rectus block through upper lid in midline to depth of 15 mm.
3. Facial nerve block – there are several techniques:

- Van Lint: along lateral upper and lower orbital rims
- Atkinson: over zygomatic arch
- O'Brien: over temporomandibular joint.

The popularity of retrobulbar block has declined due to a greater risk of neurovascular damage compared with peribulbar block.

Peribulbar block. First described by Davis and Mandel in 1986. Aim to keep the needle always at a tangent to the globe, advancing the tip no further than the equator of the globe, outside the muscle cone. Uses larger dose of LA and has a longer onset time. Use a 25G 25 mm blunt needle.

1. Insert needle at fornix of conjunctiva at junction of lateral third and medial two-thirds, directed towards the floor of the orbit, and inject 4–10 mL LA.
2. Insert medial to the medial caruncle to a depth of 20 mm: inject 2–5 mL LA.

Compress eyeball for 10 min after injection to aid spread of LA using small pneumatic/lead balloon strapped over eye.
Block of facial nerve is not usually required.

Sub-Tenon's (episcleral) block Least painful of all blocks (99.1% patients report a painless injection). Topical LA to conjunctiva. Ask patient to look up and out. Using forceps, take a deep bite of conjunctiva and Tenon's capsule in the inferonasal quadrant, 5–7 mm from the limbus. Make a 2 mm opening halfway between the forceps and the globe, with scissors. A blunt, curved 19G, 25 mm sub-Tenon's cannula is passed into the tunnel and advanced slowly keeping the tip hugging the sclera until the syringe is vertical to a depth of 15–20 mm in the inferonasal quadrant. This delivers anaesthetic posterior to the equator of the globe. Globe akinesia not always obtained because of smaller volumes of LA. Chemosis and subconjunctival haemorrhage more common.

Complications of regional blocks

Of 60000 annual LA operations, life-threatening complications occur in 1:750. There are fewer complications with peribulbar block, but less akinesia.

- *Injection into optic nerve sheath* – solution may spread via optic chiasm to CNS, causing drowsiness, convulsions, cardiorespiratory arrest and loss of consciousness. Les risk with needles <25 mm length.
- *Muscle damage* – avoid inferior and lateral rectus muscles
- *Oculocardiac reflex*
- *Retrobulbar haemorrhage (arterial)* – avoid superior–medial quadrant. Avoid damaging arterial branches of ophthalmic artery on upper border of medial rectus muscle by directing needle 5° caudally
- *Venous haemorrhage* – reassure patient; generally not a problem
- *Chemosis* – worse with excessive LA volume. Massage orbit to reduce. May interfere with trabeculectomy surgery
- *Postoperative diplopia* – until LA worn off. Reassure patient
- *Respiratory deterioration* – patients with respiratory disease are prone to hypoxia and hypercarbia

- *Penetration of the eye*, causing:
  - intraocular haemorrhage
  - immediate/delayed retinal detachment
  - intraocular toxicity of local anaesthetic drugs and the following symptoms:
    - ▷ movement of the eye with the needle
    - ▷ acute pain
    - ▷ sudden loss of vision
    - ▷ loss of ocular tone.

Open eye injury and full stomach

There is a conflict between protection of the airway and prevention of increased IOP. Discuss with surgeons. Can surgery be delayed until stomach is empty?

A study of rapid sequence induction using suxamethonium in 228 patients failed to show any loss of vitreous through the penetrating wound (Libonati et al 1985).

Three approaches to rapid sequence induction:

1. Suxamethonium preceded by lidocaine 1.5 mg.kg^{-1} and a small dose of non-depolarizing drug
2. High-dose non-depolarizing muscle relaxant, e.g. vecuronium 0.2 mg.kg^{-1} or rocuronium 0.9 mg.kg^{-1}. Give anti-aspiration medication preoperatively (H$_2$ antagonist and metoclopramide) together with cricoid pressure
3. Awake intubation using topical anaesthesia.

LOCAL ANAESTHESIA FOR INTRAOCULAR SURGERY
Royal College of Anaesthetists and Royal College of Ophthalmologists 2001

General comments

- Day-care ophthalmic surgery under local anaesthesia (LA) is now preferred by patients and staff and is associated with the least disruption to the patient's normal activity.
- Multiprofessional teamwork is fundamental to day-care surgery. Appropriately trained nurses are increasingly performing tasks that were previously undertaken by medical staff, especially in relation to preoperative assessment and preparation.
- These guidelines may require to be fine-tuned to meet local requirements, but the following general aspects remain pertinent:
  - Record-keeping must be comprehensive, clear and unambiguous to comply with clinical audit and governance

- The results of preoperative assessment should be recorded on a checklist which is completed before the patient enters the operating theatre area
- Every Trust undertaking ophthalmic surgery should identify one anaesthetist with overall responsibility for the anaesthetic services to the eye department
- Good communication between members of the anaesthetic-surgical team is essential
- All intraocular surgery performed should be carried out in a facility which is appropriately equipped and staffed.

Preoperative assessment

- The preoperative assessment should be conducted according to locally designed protocols, which should include routes of communication about abnormalities or concerns.
- Preoperative assessment should normally be undertaken by specialist nurses with medical input as required.
- For the patient with no history of significant systemic disease and no abnormal findings on examination at the nurse-led assessment, no special investigations are indicated. Any patient requiring special tests may also need an opinion from a doctor.
- The patient should be provided with appropriate information, thereby reducing anxiety to a minimum.
- The preoperative assessment visit should take place within 3 months of the surgery.

Day of surgery

- Final simple preoperative checks must be made on the day of surgery. Recent changes in the patient's condition or therapy that might affect the surgical event must be identified.
- The LA must be administered by an appropriately trained anaesthetist, ophthalmologist or nurse.
- Nurses may administer topical or subconjunctival anaesthesia. In a few centres, nurses have been trained to administer sub-Tenon's blocks, but the administration by these professionals of peribulbar or retrobulbar injections is not recommended.
- Intravenous sedation should only be administered under the supervision of an anaesthetist, whose sole responsibility is to that list.
- Local staffing availability will dictate whether an anaesthetist can be provided for all ophthalmic lists. An anaesthetist is not essential when topical, subconjunctival or sub-Tenon's techniques without sedation are used.
- When peribulbar or retrobulbar techniques are used, an anaesthetist should be available in the hospital.
- No LA technique is totally free from the risk of serious systemic adverse events, although they may not be always a consequence of the technique itself, but of other patient factors.

- From prior to the administration of the LA to the end of the operation, continuous monitoring of ventilation and circulation by clinical observation and pulse oximetry is essential.
- A suitably trained individual must have responsibility for monitoring the patient throughout anaesthesia and surgery.
- All theatre personnel should participate in regular Basic Life Support (BLS) training, and there should always be at least one person present who has Advanced Life Support (ALS) training or equivalent.

Discharge and aftercare

- All patients, and especially those who are frail and elderly, are advised to have a friend or relative to accompany them to surgery and at discharge.
- Discharge criteria must be established for each unit.
- Written instructions should be given to the patient about what to do and who to contact in the event of problems or concern.

Training

High quality care requires that all personnel dealing with ophthalmic surgery under LA have specific training.

Bibliography

Canavan KS, Dark A, Garrioch MA: Sub-Tenon's administration of local anaesthetic: a review of the technique, *Br J Anaesth* 90:787–793, 2003.

Hamilton RC: Techniques of orbital regional anaesthesia, *Br J Anaesth* 75:88–92, 1995.

Johnson RW: Anatomy for ophthalmic anaesthesia, *Br J Anaesth* 75:80–87, 1995.

Libonati MM, Leahy JJ, Ellison N: The use of succinylcholine in open eye surgery, *Anesthesiology* 62:637–640, 1985.

Murgatroyd IH, Bembridge J: Intraocular pressure, *Contin Edu Anaesth, Crit Care Pain* 8:100–103, 2008.

Parness G, Underhill S: Regional anaesthesia for intraocular surgery, *Contin Edu Anaesth, Crit Care Pain* 5:93–97, 2005.

Raw D, Mostafa SM: Drugs and the eye, *BJA CEPD Rev* 1:161–165, 2001.

Royal College of Anaesthetists and Royal College of Ophthalmologists: *Local anaesthesia for intraocular surgery*, London, 2001, Royal College of Anaesthetists and Royal College of Ophthalmologists.

Thind GS, Rubin AP: Local anaesthesia for eye surgery, *Br J Anaesth* 86:473–476, 2001.

Vachon CA, Warner DO, Bacon DR: Succinylcholine and the open globe, *Anesthesiology* 99:220–223, 2003.

Vann MA, Ogunnaike BO, Joshi GP: Sedation and anesthesia care for ophthalmologic surgery during local/regional anesthesia, *Anesthesiology* 107:502–508, 2007.

ANAESTHESIA FOR ORTHOPAEDIC SURGERY

Epidemiology

Two main age groups:

1. Young males, due to trauma.
2. Elderly females, due to osteoporosis and osteoarthritis. Increasing numbers as the elderly population increases. Currently, 50 000 hip fractures in England p.a. Mean age 80 years, mean hospital stay 21 days, 5–24% mortality.

Anaesthetic management

Preoperative

Most elderly patients have co-existing diseases. Carry out cardiovascular and respiratory assessment. Treat other pathology as necessary, e.g. dehydration, diabetes, renal failure, infection. Osteoarthritis and joint immobility are common. Outcome is improved if surgery takes place between 24 and 36 h after admission. Excessive delays risk pressure sores, DVT and pulmonary embolus (PE), pneumonia and an overall increase in mortality. Therefore, do not prolong patient optimization longer than necessary.

Anaesthetic technique

Over the past decade, several studies have shown that regional anaesthesia is associated with reduced morbidity and mortality. Mechanisms may include:

- Better, earlier postoperative gas exchange (no difference by 24 h)
- Reduced blood transfusion requirements
- Reduced bleeding from bone, which may be of importance in preventing excess blood compromising bone cement fixation
- Improved cardiovascular stability
- Improved postoperative mental function
- Good postoperative analgesia
- Reduced incidence of DVT.

Preoperative autologous blood donation, cell salvaging and mild deliberate hypotension reduce transfusion requirements. Mild hypothermia (35.0 versus 36.6°C) has been shown to increase blood loss during hip arthroplasty.

Bone cement

Hypotension and cardiac arrest were initially attributed to free methylmethacrylate monomer forced into circulation during insertion of cement. However, they are now thought to be due to fat, air, platelet and marrow embolization with V/Q mismatching and release of vasoactive substances from the lungs. Severe pain during intramedullary nailing may also contribute.

Hypotension during cement insertion is more common with increasing age, uraemia and pre-existing hypertension. Incidence is reduced if normovolaemia is maintained during cement insertion.

Fat embolism syndrome (FES)

Fat is released into the circulation in most patients from long bones at the time of fracture or during intramedullary nailing to cause asymptomatic embolization. However, in 2% of patients following femoral fractures, 0.1% after hip/knee replacements, and as many as 90% of multiple trauma patients, the degree of embolization may be sufficient to cause a triad of symptoms (which are not always present):

1. Respiratory insufficiency
2. Cerebral decompensation
3. Skin petechiae.

Severe FES may cause cardiovascular collapse, multiorgan failure and death. Pathophysiological changes occur in three steps (Fig. 4.1). FES also reported with burns, acute pancreatitis, hepatic failure, bone marrow harvest and extracorporeal circulation.

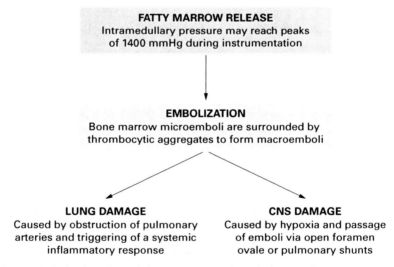

Figure 4.1 Pathophysiological changes in severe fat embolism syndrome.

Prophylaxis. Surgical measures to minimize intramedullary pressure. Ensure adequate hydration. Consider delaying medullary reaming in major trauma patients.

Treatment is non-specific and supportive. Early recognition is vital (desaturation, petechiae, confusion, hypotension). Consider bronchoalveolar lavage for diagnostic cytology. Oxygen, fluid management, anticoagulation. Steroids are unproven. Aspirin may improve blood gases, coagulation protein levels, and platelet count. Heparin is known to clear lipaemic serum by stimulating lipase activity and has been advocated for the treatment of FES, although may risk bleeding in trauma patients.

Postoperative hyponatraemia

Iatrogenic hyponatraemia is particularly common following orthopaedic surgery due to fluid overload from 5% dextrose, which after metabolism of dextrose leaves free water. Compounded by:

* thiazide diuretics – commonly used in the elderly to control hypertension, causing mild preoperative hyponatraemia
* surgical stress – causing a syndrome of inappropriate ADH secretion resulting in fluid retention and mild hyponatraemia for several days postoperatively
* impaired fluid homeostasis in elderly.

Some 20% of patients with symptomatic hyponatraemia die or suffer serious brain damage. Brain damage has been reported with sodium as high as 128 mmol/L. Postmenopausal women are usually not symptomatic until sodium <120 mmol/L.

Early symptoms. Weakness, nausea, vomiting and headache.

Late symptoms. Encephalopathy, convulsions, respiratory arrest, brain damage. Aim to raise serum sodium 1–2 mmol/L per hour until symptoms resolve. Risk of treatment is far less than risk of osmotic demyelination from treatment. Consider fluid restriction or hypertonic saline. Loop diuretics (e.g. furosemide) enhance free water excretion.

DVT prophylaxis

Without DVT prophylaxis, 50–80% of elderly patients will develop a DVT, and 1–5% die from pulmonary embolism. Compression stocking, aspirin and early mobilization all reduce DVT risk further.

NICE CLINICAL GUIDELINE 92
Venous Thromboembolism: Reducing the Risk of Venous Thromboembolism (Deep Vein Thrombosis and Pulmonary Embolism) in Patients Admitted to Hospital, January 2010

Assessing the risks of VTE and bleeding

1. Assess all patients to identify those who are at increased risk of venous thromboembolism (VTE)

Patients who are at risk of VTE

Medical patients

- If mobility significantly reduced for ≥3 days **or**
- If expected to have ongoing reduced mobility relative to normal state plus any VTE risk factor.

Surgical patients and patients with trauma

- If total anaesthetic + surgical time >90 min **or**
- If surgery involves pelvis or lower limb and total anaesthetic + surgical time >60 min **or**
- If acute surgical admission with inflammatory or intra-abdominal condition **or**
- If expected to have significant reduction in mobility **or**
- If any VTE risk factor present.

VTE risk factors (for women who are pregnant or have given birth within the previous 6 weeks, see full guidance for more detail)

- Active cancer or cancer treatment
- Age >60 years
- Critical care admission
- Dehydration
- Known thrombophilias
- Obesity (BMI >30 kg/m^2)
- One or more significant medical comorbidities (for example: heart disease; metabolic, endocrine or respiratory pathologies; acute infectious diseases; inflammatory conditions)
- Personal history or first-degree relative with a history of VTE
- Use of HRT
- Use of oestrogen-containing contraceptive therapy
- Varicose veins with phlebitis

2. Assess all patients for risk of bleeding before offering pharmacological VTE prophylaxis

Patients who are at risk of bleeding

All patients who have any of the following

- Active bleeding
- Acquired bleeding disorders (such as acute liver failure)
- Concurrent use of anticoagulants known to increase the risk of bleeding (such as warfarin with INR >2)
- Lumbar puncture/epidural/spinal anaesthesia within the previous 4 h or expected within the next 12 h
- Acute stroke
- Thrombocytopenia (platelets <75 × 10^9/L)
- Uncontrolled systolic hypertension (≥230/120 mmHg)
- Untreated inherited bleeding disorders (such as haemophilia or von Willebrand's disease)

3. Assess all patients for risk of bleeding before offering pharmacological VTE prophylaxis. Do not offer pharmacological VTE prophylaxis to patients with any of the risk factors for bleeding

4. Reassess risks of VTE and bleeding whenever the clinical situation changes.

Reducing the risk of VTE

- Encourage patients to mobilise as soon as possible.
- Offer one of the following to those at increased risk of VTE:
  - Fondaparinux sodium
  - Low molecular weight heparin
  - Unfractionated heparin for patients with renal failure.

Patient information and planning for discharge

- On admission, offer patients verbal and written information on VTE.
- As part of the discharge plan offer patient information on the symptoms and signs of VTE and the need for appropriate post-dicharge therapy.

Mechanical prophylaxis

- On admission to hospital, offer surgical inpatients mechanical VTE prophylaxis (see full guidance for more detail).
  - *Anti-embolism stockings*. Use thigh-length graduated compression/anti-embolism stockings, unless contraindicated (e.g. diabetic neuropathy, peripheral vascular disease, peripheral vascular disease).
  - *Foot impulse and intermittent pneumatic devices*. Intermittent pneumatic compression devices may be used as an alternative. These devices should be used for as much time as is possible.

Pharmacological prophylaxis

- Consider offering additional mechanical or pharmacological VTE prophylaxis if patient is at risk of VTE (Figs 4.2, 4.3).

Other anaesthetic-related issues

- Advise patients to consider stopping combined oral contraceptives 4 weeks before elective surgery.
- Carefully plan the timing of pharmacological prophylaxis if using regional anaesthesia to minimize the risk of haematoma.

Other strategies

- Do not allow patients to become dehydrated during their stay in hospital.
- Consider using regional anaesthesia if appropriate as it reduces the risk of VTE compared with GA.

Non-orthopaedic surgery

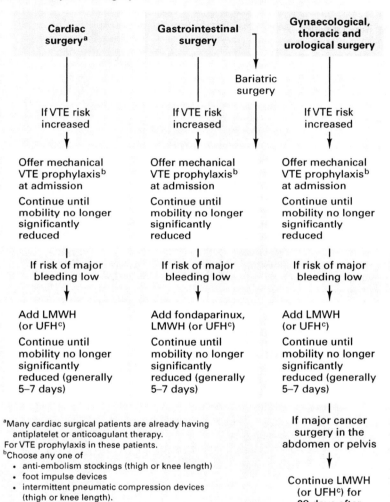

Figure 4.2 Non-orthopaedic surgery.

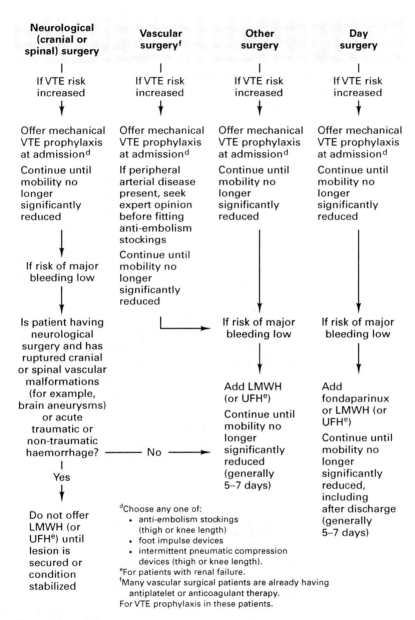

Neurological (cranial or spinal) surgery	Vascular surgery[f]	Other surgery	Day surgery
If VTE risk increased	If VTE risk increased	If VTE risk increased	If VTE risk increased
Offer mechanical VTE prophylaxis at admission[d]	Offer mechanical VTE prophylaxis at admission[d]	Offer mechanical VTE prophylaxis at admission[d]	Offer mechanical VTE prophylaxis at admission[d]
Continue until mobility no longer significantly reduced	If peripheral arterial disease present, seek expert opinion before fitting anti-embolism stockings	Continue until mobility no longer significantly reduced	Continue until mobility no longer significantly reduced
If risk of major bleeding low	Continue until mobility no longer significantly reduced	If risk of major bleeding low	If risk of major bleeding low
Is patient having neurological surgery and has ruptured cranial or spinal vascular malformations (for example, brain aneurysms) or acute traumatic or non-traumatic haemorrhage? — No →		Add LMWH (or UFH[e]) Continue until mobility no longer significantly reduced (generally 5–7 days)	Add fondaparinux or LMWH (or UFH[e]) Continue until mobility no longer significantly reduced, including after discharge (generally 5–7 days)
Yes			
Do not offer LMWH (or UFH[e]) until lesion is secured or condition stabilized			

[d]Choose any one of:
• anti-embolism stockings (thigh or knee length)
• foot impulse devices
• intermittent pneumatic compression devices (thigh or knee length).

[e]For patients with renal failure.

[f]Many vascular surgical patients are already having antiplatelet or anticoagulant therapy. For VTE prophylaxis in these patients.

Figure 4.2, cont'd

Orthopaedic surgery

Elective hip replacement	**Elective knee replacement**

At admission

Offer mechanical VTE prophylaxis with any one of:

- anti-embolism stockings (thigh or knee length), used with caution
- foot impulse devices
- intermittent pneumatic compression devices (thigh or knee length)

Continue until patient's mobility no longer significantly reduced

At admission

Offer mechanical VTE prophylaxis with any one of:

- anti-embolism stockings (thigh or knee length), used with caution
- foot impulse devices
- intermittent pneumatic compression devices (thigh or knee length)

Continue until patient's mobility no longer significantly reduced

1–12 hours after surgery

Provided there are no contraindications, offer pharmacological VTE prophylaxis

Continue pharmacological VTE prophylaxis for 28–35 days[a]

1–12 hours after surgery

Provided there are no contraindications, offer pharmacological VTE prophylaxis

Continue pharmacological VTE prophylaxis for 10–14 days[a]

Choose one of:

- dabigatran[b], started 1–4 hours after surgery
- fondaparinux, started 6 hours after surgical closure, provided haemostasis has been established
- LMWH (or UFH[c]), started 6–12 hours after surgery
- rivaroxaban[d], started 6–10 hours after surgery

[a]According to the summary of product characteristics for the individual agent being used.
[b]In line with 'Dabigatran etexilate for the prevention of venous thromboembolism after hip or knee replacement surgery in adults' (NICE technology appraisal guidance 157), dabigatran etexilate, within its marketing authorisation, is recommended as an option for the primary prevention of venous thromboembolic events in adults who have undergone elective total hip replacement surgery or elective total knee replacement surgery.
[c]For patients with renal failure.
[d]In line with 'Rivaroxaban for the prevention of venous thromboembolism after total hip or total knee replacement in adults' (NICE technology appraisal guidance 170), rivaroxaban, within its marketing authorisation, is recommended as an option for the prevention of venous thromboembolism in adults having elective total hip replacement surgery or elective total knee replacement surgery.

Figure 4.3 Orthopaedic surgery.

Bibliography

Connolly D: Orthopaedic anaesthesia, *Anaesthesia* 58:1189–1193, 2003.

Donaldson AJ, Thomson HE, Harper NJ, et al: Bone cement implantation syndrome, *Br J Anaesth* 102:12–22, 2009.

Gardner AC, Dunsmuir RA: What's new in spinal surgery? *Contin Edu Anaesth, Crit Care Pain* 8:186–188, 2008.

Gupta A, Reilly CS: Fat embolism, *Contin Edu Anaesth, Crit Care Pain* 7:148–151, 2007.

Jandziol AK, Griffiths R: The anaesthetic management of patients with hip fractures, *BJA CEPD Rev* 1:52–55, 2001.

Lane N, Allen K: Hyponatraemia after orthopaedic surgery, *BMJ* 318:1363–1364, 1999.

Mellor A, Soni N: Fat embolism, *Anaesthesia* 56:145–154, 2001.

NICE: Venous thromboembolism: reducing the risk of venous thromboembolism (deep vein thrombosis and pulmonary embolism) in patients admitted to hospital, 2010. January 2010 http://guidance.nice.org.uk/CG92.

ANAESTHESIA AND RENAL FAILURE

Acute renal failure

Table 4.2 Diagnosis of acute renal failure

	Prerenal	Renal
Urine: plasma (U:P) osmolality	>2:1	<1:2
U:P urea	>20	<10
U:P creatinine	>40	<10
Urine Na+ (mEq/L)	<20	>60

There is no agreed definition of acute renal failure, but it can be described as the sudden deterioration in renal function with concomitant electrolyte, acid–base and fluid balance disturbance.

Chronic renal failure

Chronic renal failure is defined as a glomerular filtration rate (GFR) <60 mL. $min^{-1}.1.73\,m^{-2}$, for ≥3 months.

Causes of chronic renal failure:

- Diabetes mellitus
- Glomerulonephritis
- Pyelonephritis
- Renovascular disease
- Polycystic kidneys
- Hypertension

The 2006 UK Renal Registry Report documented the UK annual incidence of new patients accepted for renal replacement therapy as approx 100 patients/million p.a.

Pharmacokinetic and pharmacodynamic changes

- Decreased active tubular excretion and decreased GFR
- Decreased protein binding secondary to hypoalbuminaemia
- Phase I hepatic metabolism (reduction, hydrolysis, etc.) reduced by uraemia. Phase II metabolism (conjugation) reduced by accumulating drug metabolites
- Competition for protein binding by accumulation of endogenous substances and drug metabolites
- Impaired salt and water excretion.

These changes result in hypertension, water retention, peripheral oedema and hyperdynamic circulation; also accumulation of ionized, water-soluble compounds, e.g. non-depolarizing neuromuscular blockers, digoxin, atropine, neostigmine, water-soluble β-blockers, e.g. atenolol.

Common conditions associated with chronic renal failure

CVS. Hypertension, LVF exacerbated by A–V fistula, accelerated atherosclerosis causing ischaemic heart disease and peripheral vascular disease. Pericardial effusion and cardiomyopathy secondary to uraemia and dialysis.

Respiratory. Peritoneal dialysis causes diaphragmatic splinting, atelectasis and shunting. Respiratory infection is common. Fluid overload between periods of dialysis, causing pulmonary congestion.

GI. Delayed gastric emptying and increased gastric acid secretion. High risk of aspiration. GI bleeding. Deranged liver function secondary to transfusion-related hepatitis.

Neurological. Peripheral and autonomic neuropathy. Mild uraemic encephalopathy.

Haematology. Normochromic normocytic anaemia due to decreased erythropoietin, bone marrow depression from anaemia, iron, folate and B_{12} deficiency and increased red cell fragility. Decreased O_2 delivery compensated for by ↑ CO, metabolic acidosis and ↑ 2,3-DPG, shifting O_2 dissociation curve to the right. Defective platelet function, increased factor VIII and fibrinogen, and decreased antithrombin III result in hypercoagulable state despite increased bleeding time.

Post-dialysis. Residual heparinization for 10h post-dialysis. Large fluid shifts may cause hypotension, nausea and vomiting.

Other. Metabolic acidosis, hyperkalaemia, hypomagnesaemia, hypocalcaemia, hyperphosphataemia, bone decalcification and carbohydrate intolerance.

Specific drugs

1. *Anticholinergics*. Atropine and glycopyrrolate are both water-soluble and therefore accumulate. Hyoscine has minimal renal excretion.

2. **Barbiturates**. Decreased dose requirements of thiopentone due to decreased protein binding and increased blood–brain barrier permeability.
3. **Ketamine**. Increases renal blood flow through altered autoregulation but reduces urine output. May worsen hypertension.
4. **Benzodiazepines**. Slight decrease in dose requirement due to reduced protein binding; more marked with those that are more highly protein-bound, e.g. diazepam.
5. **Etomidate**. Decreased dose requirement due to reduced protein binding.
6. **Propofol**. Little change in pharmacokinetics.
7. **Opioids**. *Morphine* effect is prolonged due to accumulation of renally excreted metabolite morphine-6-glucuronide. *Pethidine* causes excitation due to accumulation of renally excreted metabolite norpethidine.
   Fentanyl, alfentanil and *remifentanil* have unaltered pharmacokinetics.
8. **Muscle relaxants**
   - *Suxamethonium*. Prolonged action due to plasma cholinesterase depletion with dialysis. Also increases K^+ by 0.5 mmol/L (same degree as healthy adults), which may be dangerous in the presence of hyperkalaemia.
   - Clearance of non-depolarizing drugs depends upon degree of renal excretion:
     - >70% – gallamine, pancuronium, pipecuronium
     - <25% – vecuronium, atracurium, mivacurium.
   - *Atracurium*. Little change in pharmacokinetics. Considered by many to be the muscle relaxant of choice. Accumulation of laudanosine to levels >17 μg/mL causes fits in dogs but the highest level recorded in a patient is 8.65 μg/mL.
   - *Vecuronium*. Accumulates with repeated doses.
   - *Mivacurium, doxacurium, pipecuronium*. All are renally excreted and therefore action is prolonged.
   - *Rocuronium* is a medium-duration steroid mostly excreted by the liver. Does not appear to have prolonged action in renal failure. May be a useful alternative to atracurium.
9. **Anticholinesterases**. Impaired renal excretion results in significant prolongation of action of anticholinesterases, outlasting non-depolarizing neuromuscular blockers. Neuromuscular blockers may also be prolonged with acidosis and hypokalaemia.
10. **Local anaesthetics**. Reduced protein binding increases risk of toxicity.
11. **Inhalational agents**
    - *Indirect effects*. Decreased myocardial function, reducing GFR.
    - *Direct effects*. Renal toxicity of fluoride ion (methoxyflurane, enflurane) causes high-output renal failure. Minimum toxic level is 50 μmol/L. Enflurane in renal failure may reach 40 μmol/L.

Anaesthetic management for chronic renal failure patients

Preoperative

Measure baseline creatinine clearance. Preoperative haemodialysis to correct fluid and electrolytes, avoid cannulae in limbs (in case they are needed for fistula formation), correct hypertension and dehydration, control diabetes, administer anti-aspiration premedication.

Monitoring

ECG, invasive BP, pulse oximetry, CVP, urinary catheter, ± PCWP. Regular blood glucose.

Induction

Thiopentone, etomidate or propofol is suitable. Suxamethonium may increase K^+ 0.5 mmol.L^{-1}. Intravenous opioids (fentanyl/alfentanil/remifentanil) useful to blunt stress response to intubation in hypertensive patients.

Maintenance

Patients with CRF are acidotic, so avoid spontaneous respiration. F^- produced by metabolism of methoxyflurane was nephrotoxic. F^- levels with enflurane reached 75% of nephrotoxic threshold. Much less F^- produced by sevoflurane >isoflurane, with levels below nephrotoxic threshold. Desflurane does not increase F^- levels. N_2O is safe. Effective antihypertensive drugs are GTN or trimetaphan. Sodium nitroprusside in end-stage renal failure (ESRF) may cause cyanide toxicity.

Use neuromuscular blockers whose excretion is independent of renal function (e.g. atracurium, vecuronium, rocuronium). Pancuronium and morphine prolonged as mostly renal excretion.

Keep well hydrated. Replace fluid loss with salt-containing solutions (avoid Hartmann's as this contains K^+). Low threshold for blood transfusion since patient is already anaemic.

Regional anaesthesia

Spinal and epidural anaesthesia can maintain renal blood flow if hypotension is avoided. Bladder innervation via SNS from T_{12}–L_3 and PNS from S_2–S_4. Therefore, aim for regional anaesthesia extending T_{10}–S_4.

Other

Aminoglycoside antibiotics increase furosemide nephrotoxicity and potentiate non-depolarizing neuromuscular blockers.

NSAIDs impair production of prostaglandins (PGE_1) and prostacyclins (PGI_2), which modulate the vasoconstrictor effects of angiotensin II, noradrenaline and vasopressin. In the presence of renal disease or hypovolaemia, NSAIDs reduce renal blood flow and thus glomerular filtration rate. May worsen renal function or cause acute renal failure. May also cause oedema, heart failure and hypertension secondary to sodium retention.

Postoperative

Patient is usually extubated immediately postoperatively. Monitor CVP and renal function closely.

Renal transplantation
Common indications for renal transplantation

- Diabetes
- Hypertensive nephropathy
- Polycystic disease
- Chronic glomerulonephritis
- Interstitial nephritis.

Anaesthesia for renal transplantation

Renal transplantation was first performed in 1906, but introduction of immunosuppressive drugs in the 1960s established this procedure as treatment of choice for end-stage renal failure. There are approximately 1800 renal transplants p.a. in the UK. Organ survival at 2 years is now 80% (cadaveric) – 90% (living donor); patient survival is 95%.

Dialyze pre-transplant to correct acid–base status and hyperkalaemia. Preoperative erythropoietin aims to maintain Hb $9.5\,g.dL^{-1}$, but may cause hypertension. Immunosuppressive drugs (cyclosporine, azathioprine, steroids, muromonab) may themselves cause morbidity. GA is usually the anaesthetic of choice as regional techniques risk bleeding and complicate assessment of intravascular volume. The kidney is usually transplanted into the right iliac fossa. Vascular anastomosis is performed prior to ureteric anastomosis. Avoid hypotension. If BP is low despite adequate filling (CVP $\geq 10–12\,mmHg$), consider low dose dopamine ($<5\,\mu g.kg^{-1}.min^{-1}$). Vasoconstriction ($\alpha$-effects) at higher rates may reduce renal blood flow, so change to dobutamine or dopexamine. Give diuretics to promote immediate renal function; mannitol may cause $\uparrow K^+$ and $\downarrow\downarrow Na^+$ in renal failure. Avoid NSAIDs for postoperative analgesia.

Bibliography

Craig RG, Hunter JM: Recent developments in the perioperative management of adult patients with chronic kidney disease, *Br J Anaesth* 101:296–310, 2008.

Rabey PG: Anaesthesia for renal transplantation, *BJA CEPD Rev* 1:24–27, 2001.

Short A, Cumming A: ABC of intensive care. Renal support, *BMJ* 319:41–44, 1999.

ANAESTHESIA FOR UROLOGICAL SURGERY

Transurethral resection of the prostate

Specific problems

- Increased age-related pathology
- Pharmacokinetic and pharmacodynamic changes related to age
- Risks from diathermy to pacemakers
- Lithotomy position
- Risk of hypothermia
- Fluid overload and hyperglycinaemia following bladder irrigation
- Haemorrhage from surgery and release of urokinase
- Bacteraemia.

Anaesthetic techniques

Both GA and spinal anaesthesia cause decreased BP and cardiac output after induction, with changes more marked with GA. Spinal anaesthesia is regarded as the technique of choice for TURP, although there are no proven difference in outcomes between GA and regional techniques.

General anaesthesia. Fit elderly patients can be managed with a laryngeal mask and spontaneous ventilation, but those with significant respiratory or cardiovascular disease are best managed by intubation and IPPV or regional technique.

Regional anaesthesia

- Need sensory block from T_{10} to S_4
- Not suitable if patient is unable to lie still or has a cough
- Allows early warning of TURP syndrome because patient is awake
- Increased intravascular space may reduce risk of TURP syndrome
- Reduced blood loss. Reduced incidence of DVT
- Good postoperative analgesia
- Incidence of postdural puncture headache (PDPH) is low in the elderly
- Crystalloid preloading has no effect on the incidence of hypotension. More effective to use vasopressors to maintain blood pressure.

Lithotomy position

Lithotomy position may result in hypoventilation and hypoxaemia due to a fall in FRC with age and supine position, and compression of lungs by abdominal contents. Thus, awake surgery may not be tolerated by all patients.

Lithotomy position increases the risk of gastric aspiration, particularly in obese patients and those with hiatus hernia. There is a further risk in the elderly due to impaired protective upper airway reflexes.

Increased CVP in the lithotomy position may cause angina or precipitate heart failure.

Bladder irrigation

Glycine 1.5% is slightly hypotonic (osmolality = $220\,mOsm.L^{-1}$). It is used because it is non-conductive, thus preventing dispersion of the diathermy current. Fluid absorbed through open venous sinuses in the prostate causes the TURP syndrome, characterized by:

- *Fluid overload*. Proportional to height of irrigation fluid. Absorption may be as rapid as $30\,mL/min$. Limit height of irrigation fluid to $60\,cm$ with irrigation time no more than 1 h. Spiking irrigation fluid with ethanol and measuring expired ethanol concentration has been used to measure the degree of fluid absorption. The amount of fluid absorbed correlates well with hyponatraemia.

  Spinal anaesthesia can increase speed and volume of irrigation fluid absorbed compared with general anaesthesia. Probably due to lowered hydrostatic pressure in the prostatic veins.

  Symptoms due to fluid overload and dilutional hyponatraemia include bradycardia, hypertension progressing to hypotension, heart failure, headache, mental confusion and convulsions.

  Treat with fluid restriction and hypertonic saline. Rapid correction of Na^+ may cause central pontine myelinosis. Correction of no more than $12\,mmol/$day is suggested as safe.

- *Hyperglycinaemia*. Glycine is an inhibitory neurotransmitter in the brain and spinal cord. Temporary blindness may be due to inhibition of retinal transmission. Metabolism of glycine to ammonia may contribute to neurological symptoms. Glycine is also cardiotoxic. Addition of ethanol to irrigation fluid and measurement of expired ethanol have also been used to assess degree of glycine absorption.

- *Haemolysis*. Now distilled water has been replaced by glycine, this is no longer a problem.

Haemorrhage

Assess blood loss by measuring Hb in irrigation fluid collected from washout. Average blood loss is $500\,mL$.

Release of prostatic urokinase triggers conversion of plasminogen to plasmin with resulting fibrinolysis. This phenomenon may account for persistent bleeding in some patients. Plasminogen activators may be of benefit in extreme cases.

Bacteraemia

Urinary outflow obstruction predisposes to urinary tract infection. Prophylactic antibiotics are necessary if infection is present or if there is a risk of endocarditis.

Bibliography

O'Donnell A, Foo ITH: Anaesthesia for transurethral resection of the prostate, *Contin Edu Anaesth, Crit Care Pain* 9:92–96, 2009.

5 Metabolism

ENDOCRINOLOGY

Diabetes

Prevalence is increasing throughout the world, partly related to increasing obesity. Better glycaemic control has been shown to improve morbidity and mortality. The World Health Organization defines diabetes as a random plasma glucose >11.1 mmol.L^{-1} or fasting glucose >7.0 mmol.L^{-1}.

- Type 1: β-pancreatic cell destruction
- Type 2: defective insulin secretion and insulin resistance.

Pathophysiology

CVS. Results in micro- and macrovascular disease, accelerated atherosclerosis and cardiomyopathy. Autonomic neuropathy causes increased HR and BP during induction of anaesthesia. Increased need for inotropic support following CABG. Increased platelet aggregation.

Respiratory. Reduced FEV1 and FVC. Reduced sensitivity to hypoxia and hypercapnia. Increased risk of chest infections, decreased pulmonary diffusing capacity, central and peripheral obstructive sleep apnoea, aspiration pneumonia.

CNS. Neuropathy impairs neuromuscular transmission. Decreased response to tetanic stimulation.

Renal. Chronic failure is common, heralded by the onset of microalbuminuria. Progress of chronic renal failure can be limited with good diabetic control.

GI. Delayed gastric emptying and gastroparesis are secondary to autonomic neuropathy.

Other. Poor wound healing, increased risk of infection. Juvenile-onset diabetics may have reduced atlanto-occipital movement, making intubation difficult. Autonomic neuropathy impairs thermoregulation.

Drugs

Sulfonylureas, e.g. glibenclamide and tolbutamide, stimulate release of insulin by increasing β-cell sensitivity to glucose.

Biguanides, e.g. metformin, reduce basal glucose production.

Thiazolidinediones, e.g. pioglitazone, rosiglitazone, reduce peripheral insulin resistance, leading to a reduction of blood-glucose concentration and inhibit hepatic gluconeogenesis. Contraindicated in patients with ischaemic heart disease. NICE (May 2008) has recommended that, when glycaemic control is inadequate with existing treatment, a thiazolidinedione can be added to a sulphonylurea, and/or metformin.

Modifiers of glucose absorption, e.g. acarbose suppresses breakdown of complex carbohydrates in the gut.

Perioperative management

If possible, avoid drugs that may interfere with glycaemic control. Ketamine causes hyperglycaemia, β-blockers result in a slower recovery from hyperglycaemia and ganglion-blocking drugs reduce sympathetic-mediated gluconeogenesis. Sympathomimetics and diuretics antagonize insulin. β-blockers, clonidine, monoamine oxidase inhibitors (MAOIs) and salicylates potentiate insulin. Epidurals/spinals have minimal effect on glucose.

Check anion gap (= $[Na^+ + K^+] - [HCO_3^- + CL^-]$) in ketoacidotic patients. Above $16\,mEq/L$ is due to ketone bodies in ketoacidosis, lactic acid in lactic acidosis, increased organic acids from renal failure or a combination of these.

Avoid lactate-containing solutions, e.g. Hartmann's.

Assess degree of stability by:

- frequency of hypoglycaemic attacks
- variations in insulin dosage
- glycosylated Hb <10%.

Control regimens

There are several different regimens. Omission of insulin avoids hypoglycaemia but risks severe hyperglycaemia and catabolism. Insulin infusion produces more stable blood glucose levels than bolus administration and is more physiological. Tight control of perioperative blood glucose may improve wound healing and reduce the risk of infection.

Alberti regimen (Alberti and Thomas 1979). Safe because glucose and insulin are provided together.

- 500 mL 10% glucose
- 10 mmol KCl
- 10 U soluble insulin (e.g. Actrapid)
- Give over 4 h with 2-hourly BM stix.

If glucose is:

- <5 mmol, use 5 U/bag
- 5–10 mmol, as above
- >10 mmol, use 15 U/bag
- >20 mmol, use 20 U/bag.

Infusion regimen. Provides the tightest control of all regimens and is now becoming the method of choice for insulin-dependent diabetic patients. Separate infusions of glucose and insulin risk hypo/hyperglycaemia if one stopped without the other.

GUIDELINES FOR THE MANAGEMENT OF DIABETIC PATIENTS UNDERGOING SURGERY
British National Formulary 59

Perioperative control of blood-glucose concentrations in patients with type 1 diabetes is achieved via an adjustable, continuous, intravenous infusion of insulin. Detailed local protocols should be available to all healthcare professionals involved in the treatment of these patients; in general, the following steps should be followed:

- Give an injection of the patient's usual insulin on the night before the operation;
- Early on the day of the operation, start an intravenous infusion of glucose containing potassium chloride (provided that the patient is not hyperkalaemic) and infuse at a constant rate appropriate to the patient's fluid requirements (usually 125 mL per hour); make up a solution of soluble insulin in sodium chloride 0.9% and infuse intravenously using a syringe pump piggy-backed to the intravenous infusion. Glucose and potassium infusions, and insulin infusions should be made up according to locally agreed protocols;
- The rate of the insulin infusion should be adjusted according to blood-glucose concentration (frequent monitoring necessary) in line with locally agreed protocols. Other factors affecting the rate of infusion include the patient's volume depletion, cardiac function, and age.

Protocols should include specific instructions on how to manage resistant cases (such as patients who are in shock or severely ill or those receiving corticosteroids or sympathomimetics) and those with hypoglycaemia.

If a syringe pump is not available, soluble insulin should be added to the intravenous infusion of glucose and potassium chloride (provided the patient is not hyperkalaemic), and the infusion run at the rate appropriate to the patient's fluid requirements (usually 125 mL per hour) with the insulin dose adjusted according to blood-glucose concentration in line with locally agreed protocols.

Insulinoma

Small β-islet cell tumours of the pancreas producing marked hypoglycaemia from insulin release. May be precipitated by food or starvation.

Diagnose by Whipple's triad:

1. Plasma glucose <2.5 mmol.L^{-1}
2. Symptoms and signs of hypoglycaemia with fasting or exercise
3. Symptoms relieved by glucose.

Diazoxide may suppress insulin release. Discontinue preoperatively and initiate glucose infusion with BM stix every 15 min and every 5 min during tumour manipulation. Hyperglycaemic rebound may occur after tumour removal.

Suppressed islet cells take several days to recover, so monitor glucose for this period.

Cushing's syndrome

Caused by excess cortisol from steroid therapy, adrenal hyperplasia, adrenal carcinoma or ectopic ACTH. Cushing's disease is due to an ACTH-secreting pituitary tumour.

Symptoms and signs. Moon face, 'buffalo hump', thin skin, hirsutism, easy bruising, hypertension (85%), myocardial hypertrophy causing impaired LV function, diabetes (60%), osteoporosis (50%), pancreatitis (2%), muscle weakness, poor wound healing.

Perioperative problems. Careful positioning due to osteoporosis and fragile skin. Congestive cardiac failure, hyperglycaemia, hypertension.

Postoperative problems. Sleep apnoea (20%), steroids risk wound breakdown and infection.

Addison's disease

Adrenocortical insufficiency due to autoimmune disease, TB, adrenal infiltration with amyloid, tumour, leukaemia, pituitary failure or surgical adrenalectomy.

Symptoms and signs. Tiredness, lethargy, weight loss, nausea, hyperpigmentation, muscle weakness, hypotension, hyponatraemia, hyperkalaemia and hypoglycaemia.

Perioperative problems. Hypotension, low intravascular volume and small heart causing heart failure with minor fluid overload. Hyperkalaemia (care with suxamethonium) and hypoglycaemia. Remember steroid replacement.

Acromegaly

This is characterized by excess growth hormone secretion resulting in soft tissue overgrowth.

Anatomical. Visual field defects, epiglottis and tongue overgrowth, recurrent laryngeal nerve palsy, headaches, rhinorrhoea, myocardial hypertrophy causing impaired LV function.

Endocrine. Causes diabetes and hypertension, osteoarthritis and osteoporosis, muscle weakness, peripheral neuropathy.

Surgery. Via transfrontal craniotomy or transethmoidal approach.

Perioperative: 25% have enlarged thyroid which may compress the trachea.

Postoperative. Addison's disease, hypothalamic damage, CSF leak, diabetes insipidus, sleep apnoea.

Thyroid disease

Hyperthyroidism

Symptoms. Excitability, tremor, sweating, weight loss, palpitations, exophthalmos.

Signs. Tachycardia, atrial fibrillation (AF), heart failure, sweating, neuropathy, proximal myopathy and autoimmune diseases.

Diagnosis. Thyroid-stimulating hormone (TSH), free T_3/T_4, resin uptake, thoracic inlet X-ray/CT.

Hypothyroidism

Symptoms. Tiredness, lethargy, cold sensitivity, obesity, dry skin, constipation.

Signs. Anaemia, hypoglycaemia, bradycardia, pericardial effusion, hypothermia, polyneuropathy, hyponatraemia, impaired hepatic drug metabolism.

Diagnosis. TSH, free T_3/T_4, autoantibodies.

Anaesthetic management of thyroid disease

Aim for euthyroid patient, but risk of thyroid storm still remains in treated hyperthyroid patients. Antithyroid drugs (carbimazole, propylthiouracil) block T_3/T_4 synthesis but take 6 weeks to be effective. β-blockers are effective to control T_3/T_4-induced sympathetic stimulation, particularly thyroid storm. Check cord movement preoperatively. Assess tracheal compression and deviation by X-ray of thoracic inlet and CT scan. Thyroid hypertrophy may cause superior vena cava (SVC) obstruction and, if malignant, may invade surrounding structures. Exclude other autoimmune diseases.

Check that the patient can be manually ventilated before administration of a neuromuscular blocker. Enlarged tongue may make intubation difficult. Consider awake fibreoptic intubation. Use armoured tube. Avoid atropine if hyperthyroid. Isoflurane/sevoflurane cause least increase in T_4 of any volatile agent. CVS and respiratory depressant effects of drugs are magnified in hypothyroidism. Remifentanil provides good analgesia intraoperatively, contributes to the hypotensive anaesthetic required to provide a bloodless surgical field, and obtunds laryngeal reflexes to reduce the need for further doses of muscle relaxant.

Thyroid replacement therapy may precipitate myocardial ischaemia. Take care with fluid overload. There is a tendency to hypothermia with hypothyroidism. Provide eye care.

Extubate light, following direct inspection of the vocal cords. Damage to both nerves results in cords fixed in adduction. Postoperative airway obstruction may occur due to peritracheal haematoma or tracheal oedema. Thyroid resection risks postoperative hypoparathyroidism (causing hypocalcaemia) and hypothyroidism.

Hypoparathyroidism

Usually occurs following thyroidectomy. Symptoms include paraesthesia, muscle cramps, tetany, laryngeal stridor, CNS irritability and convulsions. Similar symptoms arise with metabolic/respiratory alkalosis.

Severe hypocalcaemia indicated by:

Trousseau's sign. Tourniquet inflated above arterial pressure causes carpopedal spasm.

Chvostek's sign. Percussion of the facial nerve produces facial muscle contraction.

Treat with 10–20 mL 10% calcium chloride.

Hyperparathyroidism

Symptoms and signs are due to hypercalcaemia: renal stones (50%), polyuria, bone pain (10%), osteoporosis and fractures; abdominal pain (5%), vomiting, pancreatitis and ulcers; psychoses. Hypercalcaemia worsens digitalis toxicity.

INTRAOPERATIVE NERVE MONITORING DURING THYROID SURGERY
National Institute for Health and Clinical Excellence, March 2008

Guidance

The evidence on intraoperative nerve monitoring during thyroid surgery raises no major safety concerns. In terms of efficacy, some surgeons find intraoperative nerve monitoring helpful in performing more complex operations such as reoperative surgery and operations on large thyroid glands. Therefore, it may be used with normal arrangements for consent, audit and clinical governance.

Phaeochromocytoma

Pathology

Arises from chromaffin cells which secrete noradrenaline >> adrenaline. May be part of multiple endocrine neoplasia (MEN) syndrome. 10% are extra-adrenal.

Symptoms

Continuous or paroxysmal hypertension, headache, sweating, palpitations. Dilated and hypertrophic cardiomyopathies.

Noradrenaline causes systolic and diastolic hypertension with reflex bradycardia; adrenaline causes systolic hypertension, diastolic hypotension and tachycardia. Intraoperative cardiovascular instability is related to preoperative catecholamine levels.

Diagnosis

Liquid chromatography allowing direct measurement of urine adrenaline, noradrenaline and dopamine levels has generally replaced older methods, e.g. urine vanillyl mandelic acid (VMA).

Preoperative

Aim to:

- lower BP and prevent paroxysmal hypertensive crises
- increase intravascular volume
- decrease myocardial dysfunction.

Block catecholamine synthesis with α-methyltyrosine. Preoperative α- and then β-blockade, e.g. phenoxybenzamine ($\alpha_1 > \alpha_2$ blockade) followed by β-blocker if tachycardia persists. Consider ACE inhibitors and calcium-channel blockers.

Monitoring

Arterial line, CVP ± PCWP, glucose and temperature.

Induction and maintenance

Combined regional and GA advocated. Minimize sympathetic response to intubation. Suxamethonium causes abdominal muscle contraction, compressing tumour and releasing catecholamines. Induction with fentanyl, propofol and neuromuscular blockade. Maintenance with isoflurane in O_2/air/N_2O and fentanyl/alfentanil. Remifentanil also used successfully.

Avoid atropine, and histamine-releasing drugs. Droperidol causes hypertension. Draw up antihypertensive drugs for immediate administration, e.g. nitroprusside, phentolamine, labetalol.

Manipulation of the tumour causes catecholamine release with hypertension, tachycardia and pulmonary oedema. Ligation of the tumour reduces catecholamine release to cause severe hypotension, corrected with fluid loading ± noradrenaline infusion. Decrease in catecholamines also causes hypoglycaemia, so check plasma glucose frequently.

Postoperative

Of the patients, 50% remain hypertensive for several days postoperatively, as catecholamine levels do not return to normal for 7–10 days.

Carcinoid tumour

Pathology

Vasoactive amines are released from enterochromaffin cells of neural crest. Asymptomatic if the tumour lies proximal to liver portal flow where amines are deactivated. Secondaries in liver secrete amines (5HT, bradykinin, prostaglandins, histamine, substance P, neurotensin, neuropeptide K, pancreatic polypeptide), which escape into venous blood to cause hypertension (5HT), hypotension (bradykinin), flushing, wheezing, pulmonary stenosis, tricuspid regurgitation and diarrhoea.

Diagnosis

Measure urinary 5-hydroxyindoleacetic acid (5-HIAA). Chromogranin A is an important general tumour marker for all types of carcinoid tumors. Somatostatin receptor scintigraphy and positron emission tomography are used for staging and localization of the tumour.

Preoperative

Block amine production preoperatively with α-methyldopa. Preoperative octreotide also reduces amine secretion. Correct fluid and electrolyte balance. Give antibiotic prophylaxis for endocarditis if there is heart valve involvement.

Monitoring

Potential for wide swings in BP. Therefore, carry out invasive BP and CVP monitoring. Consider pulmonary artery pressure measurement if there are cardiac complications.

General anaesthesia

Avoid histamine-releasing drugs, which may cause cardiovascular instability and worsen wheeze. Benzodiazepine premedication and benzodiazepine + fentanyl induction provide good cardiovascular stability. Etomidate and propofol are also suitable.

Suxamethonium causes 5HT and histamine release. Vecuronium or if liver failure, atracurium, are the most suitable neuromuscular blocking drugs. Isoflurane produces good cardiovascular control and is rapidly eliminated postoperatively.

If regional techniques are used, avoid hypotension, which causes histamine release.

Use amine antagonists to control BP perioperatively:

- ketanserin or methysergide antagonize 5HT
- aprotinin antagonizes bradykinin production (but not now available – more effective to use preoperative octreotide and steroids)
- chlorphenamine antagonizes histamine
- give boluses of octreotide if patient is hypotensive during surgery.

Perioperative hyperglycaemia may occur. Use of catecholamines to treat perioperative cardiovascular collapse may precipitate peptide release and impair resuscitation efforts.

Postoperative

Hypotension may occur up to 3 days postoperatively and usually responds to octreotide. Good analgesia with continuous epidural infusion or fentanyl patient-controlled analgesia (PCA).

Perioperative Steroid Supplementation

Normal steroid response to surgery is dependent upon the magnitude and duration of the operation. Plasma cortisol increases rapidly, reaching a peak at 4–6 h and declining over a 48–72 h period. Major surgery is associated with as much as 100 mg endogenous cortisol release.

Therapy with glucocorticoids results in suppression of the hypothalamic–pituitary–adrenal (HPA) axis. Failure of cortisol secretion is due primarily to inhibition of synthesis of corticotrophin (ACTH). The HPA axis can be assessed preoperatively by the following:

1. *Random cortisol*
2. *Short synacthen test* – plasma cortisol is measured 0, 30 and 60 min after an injection of synthetic ACTH. Normal function results in cortisol levels >500 nmol/L
3. *Insulin tolerance test* – 0.1 U/kg insulin injected into fasting patient. Resulting hypoglycaemia (<2.2 mmol/L) causes release of ACTH from the pituitary. Normal function results in cortisol levels >500 nmol/L.

Anaesthetic implications

There is no evidence that aiming for cortisol levels higher than normal baseline values is of any benefit in patients with suppressed HPA function (i.e. those on steroid therapy). The current recommendations are summarized in Table 5.1.

Table 5.1 Recommendations for perioperative steroid supplementation

Preoperative		Additional steroid cover
Patients currently taking steroids		
<10 mg/day	Assume normal HPA function	Additional steroid cover not required
>10 mg/day	Minor surgery	25 mg hydrocortisone on induction
	Moderate surgery	Usual preoperative steroids + 25 mg hydrocortisone on induction + 100 mg/day for 24 h
	Major surgery	Usual preoperative steroids + 25 mg hydrocortisone on induction + 100 mg/day for 48–72 h
Patients stopped taking steroids		
<3 months		Treat as if on steroids
>3 months		No perioperative steroids necessary

Equivalent steroid doses

- Hydrocortisone 20 mg
- Prednisolone 5 mg
- Methylprednisolone 4 mg
- Betamethasone 0.75 mg
- Dexamethasone 0.75 mg.

Bibliography

Alberti KG, Thomas DJ: The management of diabetes during surgery, *Br J Anaesth* 51:693–703, 1979.

Annane D, Bellissant E, Bollaert PE, et al: Corticosteroids in the treatment of severe sepsis and septic shock in adults: a systematic review, *JAMA* 301:2362–2375, 2009.

Bacuzzi A, Dionigi G, Del Bosco A, et al: Anaesthesia for thyroid surgery: perioperative management, *Int J Surg* 6:S8, 2008.

British National Formulary 59, http://bnf.org.bnf/extra/current/450062.htm. The reader is reminded that the BNF is constantly revised; for the latest guidelines please consult the current edition at www.bnf.org.

Holdcroft A: Hormones and the gut, *Br J Anaesth* 85:58–68, 2000.

Lipshutz AKM, Gropper MA: Perioperative glycemic control – an evidence-based review, *Anesthesiology* 110:408–421, 2009.

Malhotra S, Sodhi V: Anaesthesia for thyroid and parathyroid surgery, *Contin Edu Anaesth, Crit Care Pain* 7:55–58, 2007.

Mihai R, Farndon JR: Parathyroid disease and calcium metabolism, *Br J Anaesth* 85:29–43, 2000.

NICE: *Intraoperative nerve monitoring during thyroid surgery*, 2008, March, National Institute for Health and Clinical Excellence. www.nice.org.uk/IPG255distributionlist.©c

Nicholson G, Burrin JM, Hall GM: Peri-operative steroid supplementation, *Anaesthesia* 53:1091–1104, 1998.

Pace N, Buttigieg M: Phaeochromocytoma, *BJA CEPD Rev* 3:20–23, 2003.

Robertshaw HJ, Hall GM: Diabetes mellitus: anaesthetic management, *Anaesthesia* 61:1187–1190, 2006.

Smith M, Hirsh NP: Pituitary disease and anaesthesia, *Br J Anaesth* 85:3–14, 2000.

Vaughan DJ, Brunner MD: Anesthesia for patients with carcinoid syndrome, *Int Anesthesiol Clin* 35:129–142, 1997.

Webster NR, Galley HF: Does strict glucose control improve outcome? *Br J Anaesth* 103:331–334, 2009.

MALIGNANT HYPERTHERMIA

Malignant hyperthermia (MH) is defined as a fulminant hypermetabolic state of skeletal muscle. The UK incidence is 1:200 000 in adults and 1:15 000 in children. Inheritance is autosomal dominant. There is a mortality of about 10% (improved from 24% in the 1970s).

The first description was published in the *Lancet* by Denbrough (Australia) in 1960. Animal model in Landrace pigs.

Signs

Early. Tachypnoea, rise in end-tidal CO_2, tachycardia, hypoxaemia, fever ($>2°C.h^{-1}$), masseter spasm.

Late. Generalized muscle rigidity ($>75\%$ cases), metabolic and respiratory acidosis, hyperkalaemia, increased muscle enzymes (CPK, LDH, SGOT) and myoglobinaemia.

Disease associations

ENT and trauma surgery (?because triggering agents used more often). Possibly myopathies and periodic paralysis. Kyphoscoliosis, pes cavus, squint and inguinal hernia are not now thought to be associated.

Triggering factors

- *Definite* – suxamethonium (may accelerate the onset of MH when using volatiles), all volatile agents (including isoflurane, desflurane and sevoflurane).
- *Possible* – atropine (may make attack more fulminant); phenothiazines (?neuroleptic malignant syndrome mistaken for MH).
- *Unsure* – stress, exercise.

Safe drugs

Opioids, all local anaesthetics, nitrous oxide, non-depolarizing neuromuscular blockers, benzodiazepines, propofol, thiopentone (delays onset of MH in animals), etomidate, ketamine, droperidol and metoclopramide.

Pathophysiology

Muscle contraction results from flooding of the cytoplasm by Ca^{2+} entering across the plasma membrane through voltage-gated Ca^{2+} channels and released from the sarcoplasmic reticulum (SR) through ryanodine-sensitive Ca^{2+} channels (Fig. 5.1). These channels occur in pairs where folds in the SR meet the sarcolemma of the t-tubule. The ryanodine (Ry_1) receptor is a large protein molecule comprising four identical monomers that sits between the two Ca^{2+} channels. Depolarization results in charge movement in the voltage-operated Ca^{2+} channels which activates the Ry_1 receptor to open and Ca^{2+} is released into the myoplasm. Volatile anaesthetic agents may increase the leak of Ca^{2+} through the Ry_1 protein, which does not cause clinical symptoms. In myopathic muscle, this leak may be sufficient to trigger a final common pathway with activation of contractile elements, ATP hydrolysis, O_2 consumption, CO_2 production, lactate and heat generation, uncoupling of oxidative phosphorylation, and cell breakdown with loss of myoglobin, CPK and K^+ to cause the clinical picture of MH.

All Landrace pigs have a defective ryanodine receptor, resulting from an arginine to cysteine mutation. Similar mutations have been found in about 5% of human MH cases, and glycine to arginine mutations have also been documented. The defective gene for mutations of the ryanodine receptor is located

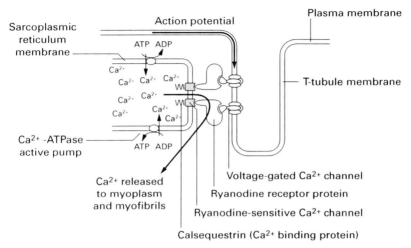

Figure 5.1 Mechanism of excitation–contraction coupling and calcium release in skeletal muscle.

on or near the long arm of chromosome 19 (19q13.1 region). However, a number of MH families are not linked to this chromosome. There is evidence that mutations in other cytoplasmic proteins that contribute to the functioning of the Ry protein may also cause defective Ca^{2+} homeostasis (e.g. calsequestrin). Mutation of the $\alpha_2\delta$ subunit of voltage-gated Ca^{2+} channels has also been documented in some patients with MH. In many cases, no genetic defects have been identified.

Dantrolene may bind to multiple sites other than the Ry protein. There is evidence that it may actually increase Ca^{2+} release, explaining why patients with MH treated with dantrolene may undergo a recrudescence of hypermetabolism.

GUIDELINES FOR THE MANAGEMENT OF A MALIGNANT HYPERTHERMIA CRISIS
Association of Anaesthetists of Great Britain and Ireland 2007

Diagnosis
Consider MH if the following are together:
1. Unexplained, unexpected increase in end-tidal CO_2
2. Unexplained, unexpected tachycardia
3. Unexplained, unexpected increase in oxygen consumption.

Take measures to halt the MH process
1. Remove trigger drugs, turn off vaporizers, use high fresh gas flows (oxygen), use a new, clean non-rebreathing circuit, hyperventilate.

Maintain anaesthesia with intravenous agents such as propofol until surgery completed.

2. Dantrolene: give 2–3 mg.kg^{-1} i.v. initially and then 1 mg.kg^{-1} PRN.
3. Use active body cooling but avoid vasoconstriction. Convert active warming devices to active cooling, give cold intravenous infusions, cold peritoneal lavage, extracorporeal heat exchange.

Monitor

ECG, SpO2, end tidal CO_2, invasive arterial BP, CVP, core and peripheral temperature, urine output and pH, arterial blood gases, potassium, haematocrit, platelets, clotting indices, creatine kinase (peaks at 12–24 h).

Treat the effects of MH

1. Hypoxaemia and acidosis: 100% O_2, hyperventilate, sodium bicarbonate.
2. Hyperkalaemia: sodium bicarbonate, glucose and insulin, i.v. calcium chloride (if *in extremis*).
3. Myoglobinaemia: forced alkaline diuresis (aim for urine output >3 mL. kg^{-1}.h^{-1}, urine pH >7.0).
4. Disseminated intravascular coagulation: fresh frozen plasma, cryoprecipitate, platelets.
5. Cardiac arrhythmias: procainamide, magnesium, amiodarone (avoid calcium channel blockers which interact with dantrolene).

ICU management

1. Continue monitoring and symptomatic treatment.
2. Assess for renal failure and compartment syndrome.
3. Give further dantrolene as necessary (recrudescence can occur for up to 24 h).
4. Consider other diagnoses, e.g. sepsis, phaeochromocytoma, myopathy.
5. Continue monitoring and symptomatic treatment.

Late management

1. Counsel patient and/or family regarding implications of MH.
2. Refer patient to MH unit.

Treatment

Admit patient to ITU. Do not stop treatment until symptoms have completely resolved, otherwise MH may recur (morbidity $\propto$ duration of symptoms). Continue dantrolene 1 mg/kg i.v. q.d.s. for up to 48 h (same dose can be given p.o. after 24 h).

Dantrolene. Each vial contains 20 mg orange dantrolene crystals and 3 g mannitol to aid solubility. Made up with 60 mL water to pH 9.5. Side-effects include phlebitis, nausea and vomiting, muscle weakness, uterine atony, placental transfer with fetal weakness, potentiation of non-depolarizing neuromuscular blockers, hyperkalaemia and CVS collapse.

Differential diagnosis

Overheating (blankets, heating mattress etc.), infection, thyrotoxicosis, phaeochromocytoma, transfusion reaction, CNS trauma, neuroleptic malignant syndrome, MAOIs, cocaine, tricyclics, atropine, glycopyrrolate, droperidol, ketamine, alcohol withdrawal and ecstasy.

Perioperative management of patients with known MH

Elective surgery. Run O_2 at 8L/min through machine for at least 12h preoperatively. Fit with new breathing circuit. Avoid triggering agents. Regional/local blocks are safe. Only use dantrolene prophylaxis (2.5 mg/kg i.v. preoperatively) if there is a risk of stress-induced MH or hypermetabolic state (e.g. thyrotoxicosis) because of dantrolene side-effects.

Dental patient. Any major surgery must be performed in hospital.

Obstetric patient. Stress of labour and delivery may increase susceptibility but dantrolene prophylaxis causes both increased blood loss due to uterine atony and fetal weakness. Best managed with early epidural. Rapid sequence induction must avoid suxamethonium (e.g. vecuronium 0.25 mg/kg). Obstetric drugs (terbutaline, oxytocin etc.) not shown to trigger MH.

Masseter muscle rigidity

There are three groups of patients:
1. *Normal jaw stiffness*
2. *Jaw tightness interfering with intubation* – change to safe drugs, carefully monitor and continue
3. *True masseter muscle rigidity* – jaw not able to be opened; 50% of children and 25% of adults are subsequently found to be MH-susceptible. Therefore, stop anaesthetic immediately and monitor closely for 24h. Postoperative CPK >20000 is highly suggestive of MH.

Screening

MH is autosomal dominant, so all parents, siblings and children should be screened. Muscle biopsy taken for *in vitro* halothane and caffeine contracture tests. The latter has been shown to have 97% sensitivity (3% false negatives) and 78% specificity (22% false positives). Genetic testing is now available to identify the 15 associated mutations identified on the myoplasmic RYR1 (ryanodine receptor) domain of the RYR gene.

Bibliography

Adnet P, Lestavel P, Krivosic-Horber R: Neuroleptic malignant syndrome, *Br J Anaesth* 85:129–135, 2000.

Association of Anaesthetists of Great Britain and Ireland 2007, Guidelines for the management of a malignant hyperthermia crisis, Reproduced with the kind permission of the Association of anaesthetists of Great Britain and Ireland.

Hopkins PM: Malignant hyperthermia. Advances in clinical management and diagnosis, *Br J Anaesth* 85:118–128, 2000.

Robinson RL, Hopkins PM: A breakthrough in the genetic diagnosis of malignant hyperthermia, *Br J Anaesth* 86:166–168, 2001.

ANAESTHESIA FOR THE MORBIDLY OBESE PATIENT

Prevalence of obesity continues to rise in both developed and developing countries (UK 700 000 people; USA 100 million). It is associated with a wide spectrum of medical and surgical pathologies.

Definition

Body mass index (BMI) = weight (kg)/height (m)^2. Normal = 22–28 kg/m^2.

- *Obesity* = BMI >30. Affects ≈25% of the population.
- *Morbid obesity* (MO) = BMI >35, or weight >ideal body weight (IBW) + 45 kg. Affects 1% of the population.

Pathophysiology

CVS. Increased blood volume, increased cardiac output by increased stroke volume, left ventricular hypertrophy; hypertension; increased O2 consumption; cardiac autonomic dysfunction increasing risk of sudden death; fatty infiltration causing conduction blocks and arrhythmias. Hypertension. Increased risk of ischaemic heart disease and stroke.

Airway. Large tongue, high and anterior larynx, multiple chin skin folds and large breasts limit neck and head flexion/extension; fatty pharyngeal tissue narrows the airway.

Respiratory. Increased work of breathing, decreased compliance, decreased FRC <CC causes V/Q mismatch and hypoxia, obstructive sleep apnoea progressing to Pickwickian syndrome (cor pulmonale, hypoxia, hypercapnia, polycythaemia). Increased O_2 consumption and low FRC cause faster desaturation.

GI. Increased gastric acidity and volume (90% of MO patients have gastric pH <2.5 and volume >25 mL). Incompetent lower oesophageal sphincter and hiatus hernia are common. Impaired liver function is common.

Renal. Increased GFR, increased renal clearance of drugs, microalbuminuria.

Other. Glucose intolerance, hyperlipidaemia and malignancies, osteoarthritis of weight-bearing joints.

Pharmacokinetic and pharmacodynamic changes

- Water-soluble drugs have similar V_D, clearance and half-life.
- Fat-soluble drugs, e.g. thiopentone, benzodiazepines and lignocaine, have ↑ V_D, ↑ half-life but normal clearance. Prolonged recovery does not occur with fat-soluble anaesthetic agents.
- Plasma protein levels and plasma protein binding are not changed significantly by obesity.

- Impaired hepatic and renal function may alter drug metabolism and elimination. Increased GFR increases clearance of drugs not biotransformed before renal excretion.

Drug doses

Some drug dosages may need to be altered for morbidly obese patients (see Table 5.2).

- High plasma cholinesterase levels, so use suxamethonium 1.5 mg/kg lean weight.
- Vecuronium dose should be based on lean body weight for normal recovery times.
- Atracurium dose should be based on absolute weight for normal recovery times.

Table 5.2 Changes in drug doses for morbidly obese patients

Unchanged dose per total weight	Unchanged dose per lean weight	Larger absolute dose but smaller dose per total weight
Midazolam	Vecuronium	Thiopentone
Diazepam	Propofol	
Suxamethonium	Remifentanil	
Pancuronium		
Atracurium		
Fentanyl		
Alfentanil		
Lignocaine		

Perioperative management

OR preparation

Equipment must be able to cope with weight. Positioning and padding of the patient should be done with care. Excessive extension of head and limbs as they hang off the obese trunk may cause nerve injury. Lumbar support reduces backache. Powerful ventilator may be needed.

Premedication

Avoid intramuscular route. Sedative premed may cause respiratory depression in morbidly obese. Give antacid, H_2 antagonists and metoclopramide. Give anticholinergic if awake intubation is planned.

Monitoring

Use arterial line in all but the shortest cases (blood pressure cuffs overestimate BP if undersized). Capnograph, pulse oximeter, temperature, peripheral nerve stimulator (may need percutaneous electrodes). Consider arterial line and pulmonary artery catheter if there is cardiorespiratory disease.

Airway management

Endotracheal intubation is necessary because maintaining an airway with a face mask is difficult. There is a need for IPPV due to hypoventilation and risk of aspiration; 13% of MO patients are difficult intubations because of the presence of a fat pad at the back of the neck, and/or because of deposition of fat into the soft tissues of the neck. Such patients may also be at greater risk of acid reflux, and appropriate antacid prophylaxis should be instituted. Consider topically anaesthetizing upper airway and larynx in an attempt to visualize cords prior to induction. Awake intubation is recommended if >1.75 of IBW.

General anaesthesia

Rapid sequence induction with cricoid pressure. Dose on ideal body mass. Keep well relaxed. Balanced anaesthesia is recommended, using volatiles (sevoflurane gives quicker recovery than desflurane), opioids (remifentanil), non-depolarizing neuromuscular blockers ± extradural anaesthesia. N_2O has low fat solubility and minimal metabolism, but its use limits F_iO_2.

Lithotomy, head-down and subdiaphragmatic packs may further impair respiration. IPPV is usually necessary. Use large tidal volumes based on IBW at 8–10 breaths/min. P_aCO_2 <4 kPa increases shunt fraction. PEEP may improve oxygenation but lowers cardiac output and may reduce O_2 delivery.

Reversal

Neuromuscular block must be fully reversed and patient awake with protective upper airway reflexes before extubation.

Postoperative

Consider elective admission to ITU because of high risk of cardiorespiratory complications. Postoperative hypoxaemia may last for 6 days after intra-abdominal surgery so consider supplemental O_2 therapy on ward. Nurse at 30° head-up to reduce pressure of gut on diaphragm. High incidence of DVT, so use thromboprophylactic measures. Increased dose of anaesthetic drugs increases risk of renal and hepatic side-effects. Consider thromboprophylaxis.

Postoperative analgesia. There is perhaps a lesser need for opioid analgesics. Intramuscular injections are likely to be intrafat. Most reliable route is i.v., e.g. PCA. Epidural local anaesthetic or epidural opioid is associated with fewer postoperative respiratory complications and faster discharge home compared with i.v. opioids. Obstructive sleep apnoea syndrome is worse with opioids.

Regional/local anaesthesia

Local blocks may be difficult because of hidden anatomical landmarks. Use nerve stimulator. Epidural and subarachnoid blocks may not be as difficult as anticipated because there is less fat in the midline over the spine. Doses reduced by 20–25%, except normal doses for obstetric epidurals. Blocks above T_5 may cause respiratory compromise. Give supplemental O_2.

Never perform regional/local block unless able and ready to convert to a GA.

PERIOPERATIVE MANAGEMENT OF THE MORBIDLY OBESE PATIENT
Association of Anaesthetists of Great Britain and Ireland 2007

Key recommendations

All trained anaesthetists should be competent in the management of morbidly obese patients and familiar with the equipment and protocols in the hospitals in which they work.

All patients should have their height and weight recorded. Where possible this should be measured rather than relying on the patient's estimate. The body mass index (BMI) should be calculated and recorded.

Although BMI is not an ideal measure of risk, it is the most useful of the currently available markers and is a simple measure to apply.

Every hospital should have a named consultant anaesthetist and a named theatre team member who will ensure that appropriate equipment and processes are in place for the perioperative management of morbidly obese patients.

Protocols including details of the availability of equipment should be readily to hand in all locations where morbidly obese patients may be treated.

Mandatory manual handling courses should include the management of the morbidly obese.

Preoperative assessment is a key component in the assessment and management of risk.

Early communication between those who will be caring for the patient is essential and scheduling of surgery should include provision for sufficient additional time, resources and personnel.

The absolute level of the BMI should not be used as the sole indicator of suitability for surgery or its location.

OBESITY: GUIDANCE ON THE PREVENTION, IDENTIFICATION, ASSESSMENT AND MANAGEMENT OF OVERWEIGHT AND OBESITY IN ADULTS AND CHILDREN

National Institute for Health and Clinical Excellence, December 2006 (http://www.nice.org.uk/CG043)

NICE indications for surgery:

- BMI >40 kg.m^{-2}
- The patient is receiving or has received specialist obesity management.

When:

- All appropriate non-surgical measures have failed.
- The patient has received specialist obesity management.
- The patient is fit for anaesthesia and surgery.
- The patient agrees to long-term follow-up.

Bariatric surgery also recommended as a first-line option if BMI >50 kg.m^{-2} if surgical treatment appropriate. Consider orlistat or sibutramine before surgery if the waiting time is long.

Bibliography

Association of Anaesthetists of Great Britain and Ireland: Peri-Operative Management of the Morbidly Obese Patient. Reproduced with the kind permission of the Association of Anaesthetists of Great Britain and Ireland, 2007.

Cheah MH, Kam PCA: Obesity: basic science and medical aspects relevant to anaesthetists, *Anaesthesia* 60:1009–1021, 2005.

Lotia S, Bellamy MC: Anaesthesia and morbid obesity, *Contin Edu Anaesth, Crit Care Pain* 8:151–156, 2008.

NICE: *Obesity* – guidance on the prevention, identification, assessment and management of overweight and obesity in adults and children, 2006, December, National Institute for Health and Clinical Excellence. www.nice.org.uk/CG043.

Ogunnaike BO, Jones SB, Jones DB: Anesthetic considerations for bariatric surgery, *Anesth Analg* 95:1793–1805, 2002.

Pieracci FM, Barie PS, Pomp A: Critical care of the bariatric patient, *Crit Care Med* 34:1796–1804, 2006.

Saravanakumar K, Rao SG, Cooper GM: Obesity and obstetric anaesthesia, *Anaesthesia* 61:36–48, 2006.

METABOLIC RESPONSE TO STRESS

The stress response is an evolutionary response that has evolved to protect the body from injury and enhance chances of survival. Comprises a cardio-vascular, thermoregulatory and metabolic response. It was first described by Cuthbertson in 1929.

The **metabolic response** is initiated by:

- *Afferent neuronal input* (somatic and autonomic) from operative site triggering neuroendocrine response
- *Release of interleukins* and histamine from damaged tissue, triggering synthesis of acute-phase proteins (cytokines [IL-1β, IL-2, IL-6], tumour necrosis factor, C-reactive protein, fibrinogen, complement and interferons) involved in haemostasis, tissue repair and regeneration.

This **neurohumoral response** (Fig. 5.2) converges on the hypothalamus to trigger:

- *sympathetic response* (rapid) – release of adrenaline and noradrenaline
- *hormonal response* (slow)
  - increased catabolic hormones: ACTH, prolactin, glucagon, catecholamines, GH
  - decreased anabolic hormones: insulin, testosterone, T_3
- *metabolic response* – increased breakdown of carbohydrate, lipid and protein and reduced peripheral glucose utilization. Results in thermogenesis, hyperglycaemia, acute-phase protein synthesis, leucocytosis, salt and water retention, and mineral and electrolyte imbalance. Decreased skeletal muscle protein, plasma divalent cations and zinc.

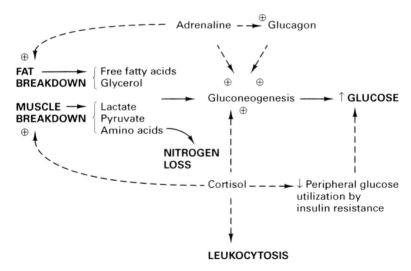

Figure 5.2 Metabolic changes triggered by the stress response.

Effects of surgery

Rapid increase in cytokines (particularly interleukin IL-6), proportional to degree of tissue damage. Laparoscopy is associated with reduced IL-6 levels compared with open laparotomy, but adrenaline and noradrenaline release is the same in both groups, i.e. visceral afferent stimulus is the main factor triggering the neuroendocrine response and is only ablated by complete block of sensory fibres.

Effects of anaesthesia on the stress response

Opioids

Low dose fentanyl ($<15\,\mu g.kg^{-1}$) does not modify cytokine response to surgery. High-dose fentanyl ($>50\,\mu g.kg^{-1}$) inhibits cortisol and GH responses to pelvic surgery but $>100\,\mu g.kg^{-1}$ is required for upper abdominal surgery. High-dose opioids suppress most hormonal responses to surgery but not those triggered by cardiopulmonary bypass.

Induction agents

Etomidate inhibits 11β-, 17α- and 18β-hydroxylase and increases mortality in critically ill patients sedated with the drug. A single induction dose is not associated with adverse effects. Midazolam reduces adrenocortical response to major upper abdominal surgery.

Volatiles

Less effective than narcotics in suppressing the stress response. May contribute to hyperglycaemia by inhibiting insulin release.

Regional anaesthesia

Only affects those aspects of the stress response that are mediated by afferent neuronal stimulation. There is no evidence that neuronal blockade can decrease the inflammatory response to surgery. Complete afferent blockade (somatic and autonomic) is required to prevent the neuroendocrine response. Complete neuronal block can only be achieved for limbs, pelvic organs and the eye. Extradural block for pelvic surgery does not affect IL-6 levels but prevents anterior pituitary hormone changes and blocks catecholamine-mediated metabolic changes. Less effective for upper abdominal and thoracic procedures, probably because of incomplete blockade of afferent fibres.

Benefits of modifying the stress response

It is generally agreed that it is beneficial to decrease stress response in patients with cardiovascular disease. Neonates undergoing cardiac surgery show a decreased stress response when anaesthesia is supplemented with sufentanil and may suffer fewer postoperative complications.

There is no evidence that limiting the endocrine and metabolic responses to surgery is of benefit in all patients. However, regional anaesthesia may reduce complications in elderly high-risk patients (decreased CVS and respiratory complications, reduced hospital stay) but further studies are needed.

Patients on steroid therapy require supplementary doses perioperatively. However, excess may cause side-effects, particularly:

- impaired wound healing
- increased risk of infection
- hyperglycaemia
- stress ulcers
- fluid retention causing hypertension
- psychiatric disturbance.

Bibliography

Burton D, Nicholson G, Hall G: Endocrine and metabolic response to surgery, *Contin Edu Anaesth, Crit Care Pain* 4:144–147, 2004.
Desborough JP: The stress response to trauma and surgery, *Br J Anaesth* 85:109–117, 2000.

THERMOREGULATION

Physiology
Normal thermoregulation

- Closely controlled at $37 \pm 0.2°C$
- Small deviation causes large physiological impact.

Afferent input

Warm receptors

- Quiescent at normothermia and increase rate of firing as temperature increases
- Unmyelinated C fibres.

Cold receptors

- Fire continuously and increase rate of firing as temperature decreases
- $A\delta$ nerve fibres.

Five main areas each supply approximately 20% of sensory thermal input (Fig. 5.3). Core structures comprise 80% of this input, whereas the periphery is only 20% of the total input.

Central control

- Integration of afferent input begins in the spinal cord
- Further integration in the pre-optic nuclei of the anterior hypothalamus
- Reflex spinal cord pathways may control some responses
- Impaired control in elderly, obese, malnourished and severely ill.

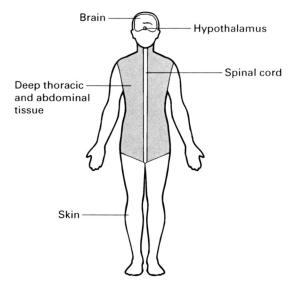

Figure 5.3 Sensory thermal input to the hypothalamus.

Efferent mechanisms

Hypothermia

- *Cutaneous vasoconstriction*
  - reduces heat loss from radiation and convection
  - regulated by α-adrenergic action on arteriovenous shunts.
- *Non-shivering thermogenesis*
  - doubles heat production in infants
  - probably of little significance in adults.
- *Shivering*
  - doubles heat production in adults.

Hyperthermia

- *Sweating*
  - mediated by postganglionic, cholinergic nerves
  - blocked by atropine or nerve blocks
  - non-athletes can sweat up to 1 L/h.
- *Active vasodilation*
  - mediated by an unknown protein released from sweat glands
  - cutaneous blood flow can reach 7.5 L/min
  - less effective than sweating at heat loss.

Measurement

Nasopharyngeal and tympanic membrane temperature are good indicators of brain temperature. Axillary temperature is a less accurate measure of core temperature. Changes in rectal temperature lag behind changes at other core sites. Also blood temperature (via pulmonary artery catheter), bladder temperature and oesophageal temperature. Skin temperature is dependent upon skin blood flow.

Perioperative hypothermia

Perioperative hypothermia develops in three phases (see Figs 5.4 and 5.5):

1. *Change in temperature distribution.* GA causes peripheral vasodilation with ↑ peripheral temperature and ↓ core temperature, redistributing heat from core to periphery. Temperature (heat) content remains constant.
2. *Linear phase.* Slow decrease for 2–3 h as heat loss exceeds production. Heat is lost by radiation (40%), convection (30%), evaporation (20%) and conduction (10%) (Fig. 5.6). Heat loss is accelerated by naked patient in cold environment, cold skin preparation, cold i.v. fluids and cold gases from ventilator. GA decreases basal metabolic rate (BMR) with 15% less heat production and impairment of compensatory mechanisms. The greatest influence on heat loss is the operating room temperature.
3. *Plateau phase.* Temperature becomes constant as thermoregulatory vasoconstriction limits heat loss to a rate equal to heat production.

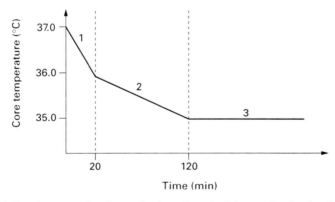

Figure 5.4 Development of perioperative hypothermia. 1, heat redistribution; 2, linear phase; 3, plateau phase.

Effects of general anaesthesia

GA inhibits behavioural responses to hypothermia, decreases metabolic rate, inhibits hypothalamic function and attenuates homeostatic reflexes. The threshold at which compensatory mechanisms to hypothermia are activated

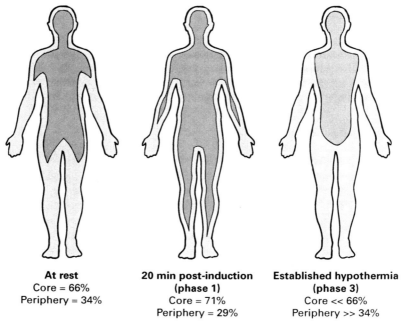

At rest
Core = 66%
Periphery = 34%

20 min post-induction (phase 1)
Core = 71%
Periphery = 29%

Established hypothermia (phase 3)
Core << 66%
Periphery >> 34%

Figure 5.5 Perioperative changes in core and peripheral compartment size.

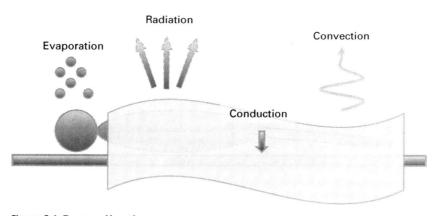

Radiation

Evaporation

Convection

Conduction

Figure 5.6 Routes of heat loss.

is lowered by about 2.5°C and the threshold for mechanisms protecting from hyperthermia is increased by about 1.0°C, i.e. widening of thresholds with ↑ MAC (Fig. 5.7).

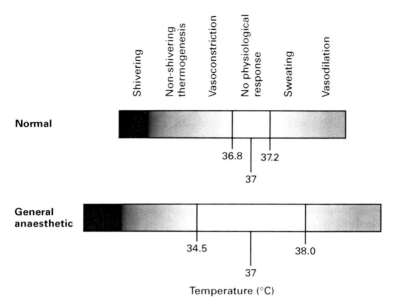

Figure 5.7 Changes in thermoregulatory thresholds.

Thermoregulatory thresholds vary depending upon the anaesthetic agents used:

Vasoconstriction threshold
- all volatiles decrease threshold to 34.5°C
- propofol, fentanyl and nitrous oxide appear to have similar effects
- gain and maximum intensity are generally preserved.

Shivering threshold
- rarely seen during general anaesthesia because shivering threshold is decreased to below that of core temperature.

Effects of regional anaesthesia

Less pronounced lowering of thermoregulatory threshold and similar three-phase pattern of hypothermia to that seen with GA. However, sympathetic inhibition below the level of the block prevents thermoregulatory vasoconstriction in the lower half of the body so the core temperature plateau (phase 3) may not be established because heat loss continues to exceed heat production.

Despite a marked core hypothermia, shivering is rarely seen, even in awake patients. This may be because the continuously firing cold receptors are blocked, fooling the hypothalamus into overestimating the peripheral temperature.

Effects of hypothermia

CVS

- Decreased CO below 32°C, bradycardia and reduced MAP
- Vasoconstriction occurs below 32°C, increasing afterload and thus increasing myocardial work
- Increased PR interval, widening of QRS complex, prolonged QT interval. Risk of VF below 28°C. J waves on ECG
- Increased cardiac ischaemia and perioperative mortality.

Respiratory

- Decreased CO_2 production
- Increased anatomical and physiological dead space
- Diaphragm fatigue
- Metabolic acidosis, causing pulmonary hypertension.

GI

- Decreased hepatic and renal blood flow, prolonging action of anaesthetic drugs
- Decreased liver metabolism, prolonging action of anaesthetic drugs.

Metabolism

- Decreased metabolic rate 8% per °C
- Shivering increases O_2 consumption by up to 800%. Resultant increased muscle blood flow may accelerate heat loss
- Hypothermia shifts O_2 dissociation curve to the left, reducing O_2 delivery
- Increased stress response and increased nitrogen loss postoperatively
- Hyperglycaemia secondary to increased glycogenolysis and reduced insulin production
- Reduced drug metabolism. Hypothermia increases neuromuscular resistance to non-depolarizing muscle relaxants, but increased sensitivity occurs as hypothermia progresses.

CNS

- Decreased MAC
- CNS protection below 24°C
- Pupils become fixed and dilated <30°C
- Risk of intraventricular haemorrhage in neonates.

Other

- Poor wound healing and increased risk of infection due to immunosuppression secondary to decreased white cell function and count.
- Increased postoperative bleeding due to increased prothrombin time (PT), partial thromboplastin time (PTT), and decreased platelet count and function.
- Increased risk of DVT and PE.

Shivering following general anaesthesia

Shivering during recovery from anaesthesia may be due to not only true core hypothermia, but also differential recovery of the brain and spinal cord from anaesthesia; quicker cord recovery resulting in an uninhibited spinal clonic tremor. Risk factors for postoperative shivering include male gender, anticholinergic premed, and type of induction agents (propofol << thiopentone). Associated with difficulty in monitoring the patient, tachycardia and hypertension (sympathetic stimulation), raised intraocular pressure and exacerbation of pain.

Shivering is reduced with radiant heat, pethidine, tramadol, alfentanil, fentanyl, clonidine and doxapram.

Techniques to avoid heat loss

- Maintain ambient temperature >24°C and ambient humidity >50%
- Prevent draughts
- Prevent skin contact with cold surfaces
- Prevent exposure of patients by use of drapes, blankets and head covering
- Silver blankets reflect heat and may reduce heat loss
- Cover exposed bowel
- Use warm fluids for washout of body cavities
- Warm i.v. fluids
- Use low fresh gas flow (FGF) in circle system
- Use heat and moisture exchanger or warmed and humidified inspiratory gases
- Use warming mattress/blankets, forced-air convective warming (Bair Hugger)
- Use radiant heat.

INADVERTENT PERIOPERATIVE HYPOTHERMIA
NICE Clinical Guideline 65, April 2008

Introduction

Hypothermia is defined as a patient core temperature of <36.0°C. The perioperative pathway is divided into three phases:

1. Preoperative phase: the 1 h before induction of anaesthesia.
2. Intraoperative phase: total anaesthesia time.
3. Postoperative phase: the 24 h after entry into the recovery area in the theatre suite.

There was sufficient evidence of clinical effectiveness and cost-effectiveness for recommendations to be made on the use of forced air warming to prevent and treat perioperative hypothermia.

Perioperative care

- Patients should be informed that:
  - staying warm before surgery will lower the risk of postoperative complications
  - the hospital environment may be colder than their own home
  - they should bring additional clothing to help them keep comfortably warm
  - they should tell staff if they feel cold at any time during their hospital stay.

Preoperative phase

- Each patient should be assessed for their risk of inadvertent perioperative hypothermia and potential adverse consequences before transfer to the theatre suite. Patients should be managed as higher risk if any two of the following apply:
  - ASA grade II–V. The higher the grade, the greater the risk
  - Preoperative temperature <36.0°C and pre-operative warming is not possible because of clinical urgency.
  - Undergoing combined general and regional anaesthesia
  - Undergoing major or intermediate surgery
  - At risk of cardiovascular complications.
- If the patient's temperature is <36.0°C:
  - Forced air warming should be started preoperatively on the ward or in the emergency department (unless there is a need to expedite surgery because of clinical urgency, for example bleeding or critical limb ischaemia)
  - Forced air warming should be maintained throughout the intraoperative phase.

Intraoperative phase

- The patient's temperature should be measured and documented before induction of anaesthesia and then every 30 min until the end of surgery.

- Induction of anaesthesia should not begin unless the patient's temperature is ≥36.0°C (unless there is a need to expedite surgery because of clinical urgency, for example bleeding or critical limb ischaemia).
- Intravenous fluids (500 mL or more) and blood products should be warmed to 37°C using a fluid warming device.
- Patients who are at higher risk of inadvertent perioperative hypothermia and who are having anaesthesia for <30 min should be warmed intraoperatively from induction of anaesthesia using a forced air warming device.
- All patients who are having anaesthesia for >30 min should be warmed intraoperatively from induction of anaesthesia using a forced air warming device.

Postoperative phase

- The patient's temperature should be measured and documented on admission to the recovery room and then every 15 min.
  - Ward transfer should not be arranged unless the patient's temperature is ≥36.0°C.
  - If the patient's temperature is <36.0°C, they should be actively warmed using forced air warming until they are comfortably warm.

Bibliography

Buggy DJ, Crossley AW: Thermoregulation, mild perioperative hypothermia and post-anaesthetic shivering, Br J Anaesth 84:615–628, 2000.

NICE: Inadvertent perioperative hypothermia, NICE clinical guideline 65, 2008. www.nice.org.uk/CG065.

Sessler DI: Temperature monitoring and perioperative thermoregulation, Anesthesiology 109:318–338, 2008.

6 General

ANAESTHESIA FOR THE ELDERLY

People over 65 years of age have conventionally been regarded as elderly and this is still used as a social definition. For GA purposes, elderly is defined as over 80 years, based on physiological parameters. In the UK, there are currently 2.4 million people over 80 years of age. By 2040, this number is expected to increase to 4.4 million. Operations in this age group are more common as the numbers of elderly increase.

Physiology
CVS

- Reduced cardiac output and cardiac reserve, ↑ SVR, ↑ circulation time
- Reduced sympathetic and parasympathetic responses
- Loss of vascular compliance causes systolic > diastolic hypertension.

Respiratory

- ↓ lung total surface area, ↓ compliance
- ↑ closing capacity, ↑ FRC, ↑↑ RV, ↓ expiratory reserve volume (ERV), ↓ VC
- ↓ response to CO_2.

Renal

- ↓ renal blood flow, GFR and concentrating ability
- ↓ active tubular excretion.

GI

- GI tract – prolonged gastric emptying, ↑ acid reflux, ↓ gastric acidity, ↓ blood flow, ↓ mucosal surface area. However, little overall effect on oral drug absorption
- ↓ hepatic blood flow, ↓ hepatic metabolism (↓ liver mass, not ↓ microsomal enzyme activity). ↓ plasma albumin, thus decreased plasma binding, e.g. benzodiazepines, barbiturates.

CNS

- ↓ cerebral blood flow
- ↓ cognitive, motor and sensory function (20% of those >80 years age suffer from dementia).

Other

- Decreased bone mass and strength, periodontal disease, and reduced subcutaneous fat, increasing the chance of peripheral nerve injury. Chronic and iron deficiency anaemia. Impaired temperature homeostasis. Decrease in basal metabolic rate decreases drug metabolism.
- Among the elderly, 47% are hypertensive, 31% have renal disease, and 22% have heart failure/cardiomegaly.

Pharmacokinetic and pharmacodynamic changes

- ↓ lean body mass
- ↓ total body water
- ↑ total body fat
- ↓ blood volume.

Therefore, ↓ V_D for water-soluble drugs, ↑ V_D for fat-soluble drugs.

- ↓ protein binding but effect minimal (except pethidine)
- ↓ hepatic and renal clearance so reduced clearance of drugs excreted by these routes
- ↓ MAC
- ↓ blood:gas solubility (?changes in cholesterol, triglycerides and albumin)
- Faster inhalational induction with ↓ cardiac output and ↓ blood:gas solubility countered by ↑ intrapulmonary shunting and ↓ cerebral blood flow
- Prolonged recovery due to decreased tissue perfusion and higher proportion of body fat acting as drug reservoir
- Drug interactions more likely due to polypharmacy. One-third of patients >75 years are taking ≥3 drugs/day.

Specific drugs

Anticholinergics. Increased V_D atropine with ↑ half-life. Causes central anticholinergic syndrome unlike glycopyrrolate because of passage across blood–brain barrier.

Barbiturates. Larger V_D with prolonged clearance; 30–40% ↓ dose requirement.

Benzodiazepines (Table 6.1). Increased CNS sensitivity. High protein binding of diazepam results in greater free drug in elderly in contrast to lesser change in dose requirements of midazolam. The latter may cause severe hypotension in the elderly (Committee on Safety of Medicines warning).

Table 6.1   Half-life of benzodiazepines

	$t_{1/2}$ (h)	
	Young adult	Elderly
Diazepam	24	72
Midazolam	2.8	4.3

Propofol. 50% reduced dose requirement. More enhanced CVS depression and greater hypotensive effect (diastolic > systolic). Reduce hypotension on induction by slower rate of injection. Propofol reduces postoperative mental confusion compared with other induction agents.

Volatiles. MAC decreases linearly with age. Volatiles with rapid elimination, e.g. desflurane, may reduce postoperative mental confusion. Isoflurane, desflurane and sevoflurane have fewer cardiovascular side-effects than other volatiles.

Opioids (Table 6.2). Smaller V_D with higher initial plasma concentrations. Increased elimination half-life ($\downarrow$ clearance greater than $\downarrow$ V_D). Decreased protein binding of pethidine with increasing age.

Muscle relaxants. Reduced plasma cholinesterase but minimal effect on hydrolysis. There are conflicting results for atracurium and vecuronium. Probably little change in initial dose requirements but prolonged elimination. No change in dose requirements or elimination of cisatracurium, but 30% increase in time to effective block. Pancuronium and gallamine cause tachycardia, worsening any myocardial ischaemia.

Anticholinergics. No change in dose but slower onset of action and prolonged muscarinic side-effects.

Local anaesthetics. Decreased elimination of lidocaine and bupivacaine with increased risk of toxicity.

Table 6.2   Half-life of opioids

	$t_{1/2}$ β (min)	
	Young adult	Elderly
Alfentanil	90	130
Fentanyl	250	925

Regional anaesthesia

In the elderly, regional anaesthesia decreases postoperative mental confusion and allows immediate recognition of angina, TIAs and mental confusion during TURP. Although some studies show benefits from regional anaesthesia, e.g. reduced incidence of MI, DVT, confusion, postoperative hypoxia, and decreased blood loss, others have reported increased risk of CVA and intraoperative hypotension. Meta-analysis shows trend towards reduced early mortality using regional anaesthesia.

Central anticholinergic syndrome

- Occurs with atropine, hyoscine and promethazine
- Causes confusion, amnesia, agitation, ataxia, hallucinations and coma
- Reverse with physostigmine 1 mg/kg i.v.

General principles of anaesthetic management

- Avoid premedication. Use temazepam if necessary
- Take care with placement of i.v. cannulae
- Reduce all drug doses and allow time for induction agents to circulate
- Decrease % MAC of volatiles and increase F_iO_2
- Avoid fluid overload which increases morbidity (NCEPOD)
- Take care with immobile joints (especially the neck) and bony prominences
- Elderly patients particularly susceptible to perioperative hypothermia
- Pressure sores prolong hospital stay, and may cause sepsis, which can be fatal.
- Preventative measures are especially important during prolonged operations and may be compounded by periods of hypotension with poor skin perfusion.

ANAESTHESIA AND PERIOPERATIVE CARE OF THE ELDERLY
Association of Anaesthetists of Great Britain and Ireland 2001

Summary

1. Elderly surgical patients of ≥80 years of age present a specific challenge to anaesthetists, who need to acquire and maintain skill and expertise in the management of such patients. Departments should have a lead clinician with an interest in the care of the elderly.
2. The number of elderly patients is increasing and age should not be a bar to surgery. Recognition of this must be incorporated into service provision. Twenty-four hour recovery facilities, high dependency unit (HDU) and intensive therapy unit (ITU) beds should be available at all hospitals for these patients.
3. Preoperative assessment will benefit from cross-specialty advice involving anaesthetists, surgeons and physicians. The development of this team approach requires time and resources that must be recognized and provided by management.

4. The provision of certain intraoperative equipment, such as active warming devices and anti-pressure sore apparatus, is mandatory for the elderly and budgets must permit the purchase and replacement of such equipment for both theatres and wards.
5. Age does not obtund the perception of pain. Acute and chronic pain management teams should be aware of the particular problems in the treatment of the elderly.
6. The increase in time and resources that the elderly require, particularly with respect to higher nursing ratios in ward and recovery areas, must be recognized.
7. Thromboembolic disease is common in this age group and requires extra resources.

Bibliography

Association of Anaesthetists of Great Britain and Ireland: *Anaesthesia and perioperative care of the elderly*, 2001. Reproduced with the kind permission of the Association of anaesthetists of Great Britain and Ireland.

Dodds C, Murray D: Pre-operative assessment of the elderly, *BJA CEPD Rev* 1:181–184, 2001.

Rivera R, Antognini JF: Perioperative drug therapy in elderly patients, *Anesthesiology* 110:1176–1181, 2009.

ANAPHYLACTIC REACTIONS

History

- 2640BC – Egyptian hieroglyphics describe the sudden death of a Pharaoh following a wasp sting
- 1902 – Richet and Porter describe the death of dogs following a second injection of sea anemone toxin.

Epidemiology

The average number of reported suspected anaphylactic reactions related to anaesthesia is 55 p.a. compared with an average of 319 for all drugs. A total of 10% of anaesthetic reports were of fatalities, compared with 3.7% for all drugs reported. It is estimated, however, that there may be as many as 175–1000 severe reactions in the UK each year (1:5000–25000 anaesthetics), with an overall mortality of 3.4%.

Some 90% occur within 10 min of drug administration. It is more common in females (5:1 neuromuscular blocking drugs; 3:1 thiopentone).

Types of allergic reaction

Anaphylactic reaction

This is an exaggerated response to a foreign protein, associated with the release of vasoactive substances, e.g. type I hypersensitivity reaction, histamine, serotonin or complement activation (classical pathway). Tends to be self-perpetuating and therefore more severe.

Anaphylactoid reaction

Clinically identical to an anaphylactic reaction but is not mediated by sensitizing IgE antibody, e.g. direct stimulation of histamine release or complement activation (alternate pathway). May be equally as severe but tends to be short-lived.

Hypersensitivity reactions

- *Type I* – anaphylactic; previous sensitization. Mediated via mast cells and IgE
- *Type II* – cytotoxic; antibodies directed against the cell membrane
- *Type III* – immune complex
- *Type IV* – delayed-type hypersensitivity; T-cell mediated.

Mast cells

Found in perivascular tissue, gut mucosa, lung and skin. Up to 10% of their total weight is histamine. Stimulation causes release of histamine, eosinophil and neutrophil chemotactic factors, leukotrienes, prostaglandins, platelet-activating factor and kinins.

Hypersensitivity to drugs (Fig. 6.1)

In a French study (Laxenaire 2001), overall incidence of reactions was 1 in 13 000 anaesthetics, while the incidence of anaphylaxis to neuromuscular blocking agents was 1 in 6500 anaesthetics. Causes included neuromuscular blocking drugs (62%), latex (17%), antibiotics (8%), hypnotics (5%), colloids (3%) and opioids (3%).

Cross-reactivity may occur between drugs with similar structures, causing a type I hypersensitivity reaction to a drug to which the patient has not previously been exposed. In 70% of patients found to be allergic to a neuromuscular blocking drug, cross-reactivity was found to others; 17% of those allergic to a neuromuscular blocking drug had not had anaesthesia before.

Opioids

Usually cause anaphylactoid reactions. Mostly morphine. Reactions to synthetic opioids are rare.

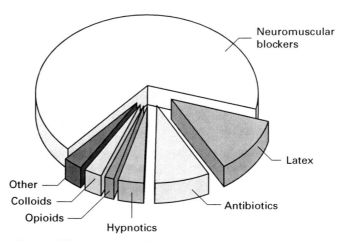

Figure 6.1 Causes of life-threatening allergic reactions during anaesthesia. (Data from Laxenaire 2001.)

Antibiotics

Cause 15% of anaesthesia-related reactions. Mostly cephalosporins and penicillins, which share a ß–lactam ring. Patients who are allergic to penicillin or amoxicillin have a higher incidence of allergic reaction to first generation cephalosporins (cephalexin, cefadroxil, cephradine) but not later generations (cefuroxime, cefotaxime, ceftazidime, ceftriaxone).

Induction agents

Of reactions to thiopentone, 20% are anaphylactic; the remainder are anaphylactoid (90% direct histamine release, 10% complement activation) – methohexitone > thiopentone > propofol > etomidate. Specific IgE interaction may occur against the isopropyl groups on propofol, although most adverse reactions to propofol are non-immunological.

Muscle relaxants

Muscle relaxants are the commonest cause of drug reactions. Steroid-based compounds (rocuronium, vecuronium, pancuronium) cause anaphylactic reactions, whereas benzylisoquiniliniums (doxacurium, mivacurium, atracurium) tend to cause anaphylactoid reactions. The neuromuscular blocking drugs implicated were (in decreasing order of frequency) vecuronium, atracurium, succinylcholine (suxamethonium), pancuronium, rocuronium, mivacurium and gallamine.

Colloids

Reactions to colloids (dextrans, hydroxyethyl starch (HES), gelatins) make up 4% of all perioperative anaphylactic reactions. Anaphylaxis from colloids may take place immediately or it may be delayed.

Latex

Latex originates from the sap of the rubber tree *Hevea braziliensis*, but is chemically modified to enhance stretch and durability. Allergy to latex proteins emerged as an occupational disease in the 1980s. Overall prevalence = 1%. High-risk groups include patients exposed to repeated bladder catheterizations, repeated laparotomies, and patients with an occupational exposure to latex (e.g. healthcare workers 2–17%). Latex allergy accounted for 10% of anaphylactic reactions during surgery in 1996, increasing to 16% by 2000. Risk factors include male gender, non-Caucasian race, young age, atopy (asthma, allergic rhinitis, eczema and hay fever), spinal cord abnormality and food allergies (particularly banana or kiwi fruit; also chestnuts, potato, tomato and avocado). Latex exposure is associated with three clinical syndromes:

- Irritant dermatitis
- Delayed (type IV) hypersensitivity reaction
- Acute (type I) allergic reaction (often delayed 30–60 min after latex exposure).

Under the Control of Substances Hazardous to Health Regulations 2002 (COSHH), employers are responsible for risk assessment and minimization of exposure. NHS guidelines published in 2008, 'Latex allergy – Occupational aspects of management', recommend minimizing use of latex products in hospitals.

Other drugs

Chlorhexidine is a commonly applied topical antiseptic. Severe life-threatening reactions have been reported following mucosal and parenteral exposure. Reactions to cutaneous applications perioperatively are often missed and underestimated.

Clinical symptoms (Fig. 6.2)

Awake patients may experience a metallic taste and a sense of impending doom. Commonest symptoms are hypotension (80%), rash/erythema (50%) and bronchospasm (36%). Tachycardia due to chronotropic effects of histamine and secondary release of adrenaline and noradrenaline. SVR is decreased by as much as 80% due to direct effect of histamine. Other symptoms include:

CVS. Arrhythmias, pulmonary hypertension

Respiratory. Pharyngeal and laryngeal oedema (24%), rhinitis, pulmonary oedema

GI. Nausea and vomiting, diarrhoea, abdominal colic

Other. Generalized oedema (7%).

Factors which increase severity included asthma, β-blockade and neuraxial anaesthesia. All of these states are associated with reduced endogenous catecholamine response.

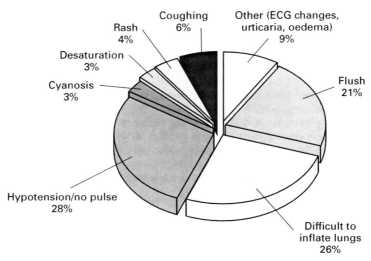

Figure 6.2 The first clinical feature of an anaphylactic reaction. (Data from Whittington and Fisher 1998.)

Treatment

SUSPECTED ANAPHYLACTIC REACTIONS ASSOCIATED WITH ANAESTHESIA
Association of Anaesthetists of Great Britain and Ireland and the British Society of Allergy and Clinical Immunology. Revised guidelines 2009 (4E)

Treatment
Immediate management
- Use the ABC approach (airway, breathing, circulation).
- Remove all potential causative agents and maintain anaesthesia, if necessary, with an inhalational agent.
- Call for help and note the time.
- Maintain the airway, give 100% oxygen. Intubate the trachea if necessary and ventilate the lungs with oxygen.
- Elevate the patient's legs if there is hypotension.
- If appropriate, start CPR immediately, according to ALS guidelines.
- Give adrenaline i.v.:
  – Adult dose: 50 µg (0.5 mL of a 1:10 000 solution)
  – Child dose: 1.0 µg.kg⁻¹ (0.1 mL.kg⁻¹ of a 1:100 000 solution).

- Give saline 0.9% or lactated Ringer's solution at a high rate via an i.v. cannula or an appropriate gauge (large volumes may be required):
  - Adult: 500–1000 mL
  - Child: 20 mL.kg⁻¹.
- Plan transfer of the patient to an appropriate Critical Care area.

Secondary management

- Give chlorphenamine i.v.
  - Adult: 10 mg
  - Child 6–12 years: 5 mg
  - Child 6 months – 6 years: 2.5 mg
  - Child <6 months: 250 μg.kg⁻¹.
- Give hydrocortisone i.v.
  - Adult: 200 mg
  - Child 6–12 years: 100 mg
  - Child 6 months – 6 years: 250 mg
  - Child <6 months: 25 mg.
- If the blood pressure does not recover despite an adrenaline infusion, consider the administration of an alternative i.v. vasopressor according to the training and experience of the anaesthetist, e.g. metaraminol.
- Treat persistent bronchospasm with an i.v. infusion of salbutamol. If a suitable breathing system connector is available, a metered-dose inhaler may be appropriate. Consider giving i.v. aminophylline or magnesium sulphate.

Investigations

- Take blood samples (5–10 mL clotted blood) for mast cell tryptase:
  - Initial sample as soon as feasible after resuscitation has started – do not delay resuscitation to take the sample
  - Second sample at 1–2 h after start of the symptoms
  - Third sample either at 24 h or in convalescence. This is a measure of baseline tryptase levels as some individuals have a higher baseline.
- Ensure that the samples are labelled with the time and date.
- Liaise with the hospital laboratory about analysis of samples.

Later investigations to identify the causative agent

The anaesthetist who gave the anaesthetic or supervising anaesthetic consultant is responsible for ensuring that the reaction is investigated. The patient should be referred to a specialist Allergy or Immunology Centre. The patient, surgeon and general practitioner should be informed. Reactions should be notified to the AAGBI National Anaesthetic Anaphylaxis Database. All suspected adverse reactions should be reported to the Medicines and Healthcare Products Regulatory Agency.

Other tests

Mast cell tryptase is the principal protein content of mast cell granules and is released, together with histamine and other amines, in anaphylactic and anaphylactoid reactions. Its concentration in the plasma or serum is raised between 1 and 6 h after reactions which involve mast cell degranulation. Thus post-mortem analysis of plasma tryptase may yield meaningful results. The normal value of basal plasma tryptase is <1 ng/mL. Plasma tryptase levels >20 ng/mL may be seen after anaphylactic reactions.

In reactions to anaesthetic drugs, the analysis of mast cell tryptase appears to be a specific and sensitive diagnostic test for anaphylactic and anaphylactoid reactions. It is the most useful acute test available at present but requires further validation in mild/moderate reactions.

Skin prick tests to general anaesthetic drugs (which show the presence of specific IgE antibodies to these drugs) should be carried out 4–6 weeks after the reaction. For a limited number of anaesthetic drugs, specific IgE antibodies in the serum can be measured. Currently, the only commercial assay available is for suxamethonium.

Methylhistamine is the principal metabolite of histamine and is excreted in the urine. Raised urinary concentrations occur after reactions which involve systemic histamine release.

Latex allergy can be assessed by history supported by skin testing or measuring specific IgE, e.g. by radioallergosorbent (RAST) or CAP (the CAP system is an alternative to RAST. It is a fluoroimmunoassay for the measurement of antigen-specific antibodies and is usually more sensitive than RAST).

Prophylaxis

Prophylaxis with antihistamines (H_1 and H_2) does not reduce the incidence of allergic reactions, but reduces mortality if they occur.

Screening

There is no method of predicting sensitivity to anaesthetic drugs. A history of previous exposure is not necessary for an anaphylactic reaction. The use of test doses of intravenous drugs is not an appropriate method of testing for anaphylaxis. Anaphylaxis has resulted from very small doses.

Anaesthesia for the atopic patient

There is some evidence that mast cells may degranulate more readily in atopic patients, but no evidence that atopic patients are any more susceptible to drug-mediated allergic reactions. Consider using drugs with low incidence of reaction, i.e. ketamine, etomidate and pancuronium.

Bibliography

Association of Anaesthetists of Great Britain and Ireland and the British Society of Allergy and Clinical Immunology: *Revised guidelines (4E), Suspected anaphylactic reactions associated with anaesthesia*, 2009. Reproduced with the kind permission of the Association of anaesthetists of Great Britain and Ireland.

Fischer SSF: Anaphylaxis in anaesthesia and critical care, *Curr Allergy Clin Immunol* 20:136–139, 2007.

Hepner DL, Castells MC: Latex allergy: an update, *Anesth Analg* 96:1219–1229, 2003.

Laxenaire MC, Mertes PM; Groupe d'Etudes des Réactions Anaphylactoïdes Peranesthésiques: Anaphylaxis during anaesthesia. Results of a two-year survey in France, *Br J Anaesth* 87:549–554, 2001.

Romano A, Pascal D: Recent advances in the diagnosis of drug allergy, *Curr Opin Int Med* 6:443–447, 2007.

Whittington T, Fisher MM: *Balliere's clinical anesthesiology*, vol 12, London, 1998, Elsevier, pp 301–321.

Wildsmith JAW, McKinnon RP: Histaminoid reactions in anaesthesia, *Br J Anaesth* 74:217–228, 1995.

BLOOD

Blood donors

Some 17 million units of blood are donated in Europe each year. Each unit is screened for antibodies to:

- syphilis
- hepatitis B and C
- HIV 1 & 2
- ± CMV.

Blood groups

The ABO blood groups are summarized in Table 6.3.

Table 6.3   Summary of ABO blood groups

Group	(%)	Erythrocyte antigens	Antibodies	
O	47	Nil	Anti-A, anti-B	Universal donor
A	42	A	Anti-A	
B	8	B	Anti-A	
AB	3	AB	Nil	Universal recipient

Coagulation cascade

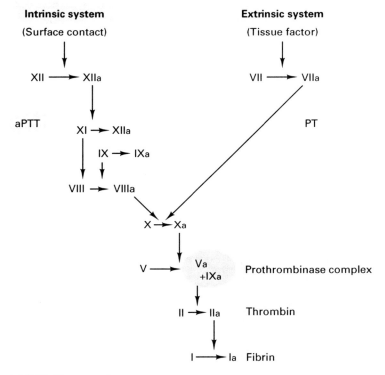

Figure 6.3 Clotting cascade.

Products
Whole blood

- 500 mL per bag with a haematocrit of 0.40
- No functioning platelets after 2–3 days; ↓ 2,3-DPG by 2 weeks
- Normal concentrations of albumin and clotting factors, except factors V and VIII, which are reduced to 10–20% of normal
- Not sterilized, so there is a risk of transmitted pathogens.

Red cell concentrate (packed cells): 2.2×10^6 units used p.a. in the UK

- 250 mL per bag with haematocrit of 0.60
- No functioning platelets; 2,3-DPG levels maintained for 14 days
- Storage is 35 days with SAGM (saline, adenine, glucose, mannitol); 42 days with A-CPD (adenine, citrate, phosphate, dextrose).

Platelet concentrates: 260 000 units used p.a. in the UK

- Usually as a pool of 5–6 single unit donations; 4 units of platelets contain 1 unit FFP
- High incidence of transfusion-related acute lung injury (TRALI) associated with platelet transfusions. Usually due to an interaction between leucocyte antibodies in donor plasma and the corresponding antigen in the patient
- Infection risk. Increased by multiple donors and platelets >3 days old
- Use ABO-compatible platelets. Maximum storage is 5 days at 4°C.

Fresh frozen plasma (FFP): 300 000 units used p.a. in the UK

- Prepared from plasma from single donation; 150 mL per bag
- Contains all clotting factors, albumin and gammaglobulin
- Use within 24 h of thawing if kept at 4°C
- Must be ABO-compatible and Rh(D)-negative if recipient is a Rh(D) fertile female
- Risk of anaphylactic reactions.

Cryoprecipitate: 100 000 units used p.a. in the UK

- Precipitates from FFP when slowly thawed; supplied as 6–8 units
- High in factor VIII, fibrinogen and von Willebrand factor
- Indicated for DIC and von Willebrand's disease.

Human albumin solution

Prepared by fractionation of multiple units of plasma giving 96% albumin and 4% globulin. Available as 4.5 or 20% (hyperoncotic) solution. Each 20 g of albumin requires 20 000 blood donations. Pasteurized at 60°C for 10 h to kill all microorganisms including viruses.

Factor VIII concentrate

- Freeze-dried protein as 250 units
- Sterilized to inactivate viruses.

Factor IX concentrate

- Freeze-dried protein as 250 units
- Sterilized to inactivate viruses
- Also contains factors II and X.

Immunoglobulin products

- Fractionation of plasma to produce pool with >90% IgG
- No risk of viral transmission
- Used for immune thrombocytopenia and immunodeficiency states.

Recombinant blood products
Recombinant FVIIa

rFVIIa initially developed to treat bleeding in haemophiliacs. FVIIa binds to tissue factor on damaged vascular beds to activate FIX and FX. The subsequent conversion of prothrombin to thrombin, activates platelets FVIII, FV and FXI and results in a large thrombin burst to transform fibrinogen to fibrin (Fig. 6.3). A recent meta-analysis of seven randomized clinical trials showed a reduction in blood transfusion requirements with no major safety concern (Ranucci 2008). Concerns remain regarding possible risks of thrombotic events.

Transfusion reactions
Acute

- *Haemolysis* – due to antibodies directed against red cells
- *Fever* – donor leucocytes attack host red cells
- *Anaphylaxis* – due to antibodies directed against recipient IgA
- *Transfusion-related acute lung injury* – due to donor antibodies directed against leucocytes. Clinically identical to ARDS
- *Hyperkalaemia* – 5–10 mmol K$^+$ in a unit of blood stored for 4–5 weeks. Effects of additional K$^+$ are exacerbated by acidosis and hypothermia. Hyperkalaemia is usually transient
- *Citrate toxicity* – citrate is added as a preservative to bind excess calcium and prevent clotting. Metabolized to bicarbonate. Excess causes metabolic alkalosis
- *Acid–base disturbance* – citrate from preservative and lactate from red cells
- *Hypocalcaemia* – citrate anticoagulant binds ionized calcium; ↓ BP, ↓ pulse pressure. Give CaCl$_2$ only if there are symptoms/signs (not Ca^{2+} gluconate, which must be metabolized to release free Ca^{2+})
- *Febrile reaction* – due to bacterial contamination
- *Microemboli* – aggregates of all cellular components, increase with age of blood. Cause complement activation, haemolysis and thrombocytopenia. Removed by 170 μm filter; +/– 40 μm screen and depth filters
- *Hypothermia* – left shift of O$_2$ dissociation curve, platelet and clotting dysfunction
- *Air embolus*
- *Fluid overload.*

Delayed

- *Haemolytic transfusion reaction* – from red cell antibodies
- *Graft-versus-host disease*
- *Alloimmunization* (reaction to minor foreign antigens) – 10% of all transfusion reactions:
    - red cell antibodies including anti-Rh(D)

- leucocyte antibodies
- platelet antibodies

- *Viral infection* – hepatitis B (<1:20 000 units) and C (<1:1 000 000 units), HIV (<1:4 000 000 units), cytomegalovirus, parvovirus (causes aplastic anaemia in sickle cell patients)
- *Other infections* – syphilis, malaria, trypanosomiasis
- *Prions* – risk of acquiring variant Creutzfeldt–Jakob disease (vCJD) is unknown. To minimize risk, UK National Blood Service leuco depletes blood, obtains plasma for fractionation from countries other than the UK and excludes donors who themselves received transfusions before 1980. At present, no test for vCJD exists.
- *Tumour recurrence* – increased risk
- *Sensitization* – resulting in antibody formation and subsequent difficulties with cross-matching
- *Iron overload* – occurs with repeated transfusions.

Massive blood transfusion

Defined as the acute administration of more than 1.5 times the patient's blood volume, or replacement of the patient's total blood volume within 24 h.
   Blood groups for urgent transfusion are:

- Rh(D)-negative if patient not cross-matched
- Uncross-matched blood (type-specific) if patient's blood group is known

Blood transfusions can be avoided by:

- reducing blood loss – hypotensive anaesthesia, antifibrinolytic agents
- tolerating a lower haematocrit

GUIDELINES FOR AUTOLOGOUS BLOOD TRANSFUSION
British Committee for Standards in Haematology Blood Transfusion Task Force 1997

Summary

The purpose of all forms of autologous transfusion (acute preoperative haemodilution and preoperative donation or intraoperative cell salvage) is to avoid the transfusion of allogeneic blood and the associated risks. Autologous transfusion procedures are not usually acceptable to Jehovah's Witnesses, although some accept intraoperative cell salvage.

Intraoperative cell salvage

Indications. Elective and emergency surgery with expected blood loss >20% total body volume.
   Contraindications. Bacterial contamination of wound, malignant disease and sickle cell disease.

Acute preoperative haemodilution and preoperative donation

Indications. Elective surgery with expected blood loss >20% total body volume.

Contraindications. Aortic stenosis, unstable angina, and moderate to severe left ventricular impairment (Napier et al, 1997).

BLOOD TRANSFUSION AND THE ANAESTHETIST – RED CELL TRANSFUSION

Association of Anaesthetists of Great Britain and Ireland, June 2008

Summary

1. The decision to transfuse should always be made on an individual patient basis.
2. Patients need not be transfused to achieve a 'normal' haemoglobin concentration.
3. Anaesthetists should play a lead role in good preoperative assessment and preparation.
4. Departmental guidelines should be drawn up on matters of blood transfusion and be readily available for reference.
5. A permanent record of the administration of each unit of red blood cells is required by European law.
6. Record the reason for preoperative and postoperative transfusions in the clinical notes.
7. Local surgical blood ordering schedules, once developed, need to be reviewed at regular intervals by auditing red cell use.
8. Every Hospital Transfusion Committee is advised to include a representative from the Department of Anaesthesia.

BLOOD TRANSFUSION AND THE ANAESTHETIST – BLOOD COMPONENT THERAPY

Association of Anaesthetists of Great Britain and Ireland, December 2005

Recommendations

- Assessment of haemostasis in the preoperative period can reduce perioperative blood loss.
- Red cell concentrates do not contain coagulation factors or platelets, so the use of blood components (fresh frozen plasma (FFP) and platelets) needs to be considered early in managing a patient with massive haemorrhage.

- Emergency use of blood components requires assessment of haemostasis in advance of administration even if empirical use is necessary.
- The use of near-patient testing devices can improve decision making on the use of blood components.
- Thawed FFP can be stored at 4°C and can be used safely within 24 h.
- Thawed FFP kept at room temperature must be infused within 4 h.
- Vitamin K ± prothrombin complex concentrate (PCC) is recommended to reverse warfarin. FFP is indicated when there is severe bleeding or when PCC is unavailable.
- Platelet transfusion in the bleeding patient, or a patient requiring urgent surgery, is indicated at a platelet count $<50 \times 10^9.L^{-1}$ but in stable non-bleeding patients in intensive care, a trigger of $10 \times 10^9.L^{-1}$ is acceptable.
- Component therapy should not be used to make regional anaesthesia possible if there are alternative anaesthetic methods available.

BLOOD TRANSFUSION AND THE ANAESTHETIST – INTRAOPERATIVE CELL SALVAGE
Association of Anaesthetists of Great Britain and Ireland, September 2009

Recommendations
- The use of intraoperative cell salvage (ICS) reduces the demand on allogeneic (donor) red cells and is a cost-effective measure.
- Trusts should provide the resources required to set up and maintain an ICS service in a safe and appropriate manner.
- Each Trust needs to ensure there is a clinical lead for ICS.
- A member of the theatre management team is responsible for ensuring overall management and facilitation of the ICS service.
- All personnel using ICS must be adequately trained and competent in its use.
- Preoperative assessment clinics should provide information on ICS to patients.
- All ICS cases undertaken require documentation and audit of use to enable future service planning and quality assurance.

Operative indications
- Anticipated blood loss >1000 mL or >20% estimated blood volume.
- Patients with a low HB or increased risk factors for bleeding.
- Patients with multiple antibodies or rare blood types.
- Patients with objections to receiving allogeneic (donor) blood.

Substances that should not be aspirated in the ICS system
- Antibiotics not licensed for i.v. use
- Iodine
- Topical clotting agents
- Orthopaedic cement.

Special circumstances

Malignancy – Concerns regarding reinfusion of malignant cells. Recent studies of the use if ICS during surgery for hepatocellular and bladder/ prostate cancer have shown no difference in recurrence rates or long-term survival in patients receiving ICS; conversely, there is good evidence that allogeneic blood transfusion is an independent factor for postoperative infection and disease recurrence. The use of ICS in urological malignancies was approved by NICE in 2008.

Obstetrics – No proven cases of amniotic fluid embolus caused by reinfusion of salvaged blood. The use of ICS in obstetrics was approved by NICE in 2005.

Bowel contamination – Concern regarding infection risk if contaminated blood (with microorganisms) is reinfused. A RCT of ICS in abdominal trauma showed no increased infection risk when using ICS. Some case reports have suggested that reinfused blood in these patients may cause hypotension.

- transfusing autologous blood – prior donation, use of cell saver
- artificial blood
- erythropoietin.

Antifibrinolytic agents

Antifibrinolytic agents, e.g. tranexamic acid (aprotinin was withdrawn because of concerns about excess mortality and renal failure), bind to plasminogen and plasmin to interfere with their ability to split fibrinogen. Prostatic plasminogen activator is released during prostate surgery to cause bleeding, inactivated by antifibrinolytic agents. Antifibrinolytic agents may reduce bleeding in cardiac surgery following cardiopulmonary bypass.

Artificial blood (Fig. 6.4)

Perfluorocarbons. Inert carbon chains with oxygen solubility 20 times that of plasma. One study showing that perfluorocarbon emulsion may limit transfusion requirements, but trend towards greater morbidity and mortality (Spahn et al 2005).

Recombinant Hb (rHb1.1). Modified human haemoglobin tetramer cross-linked with a glycine bridge between the alpha subunits. Produced from *E. coli* or yeast. Cross-linking prevents renal excretion. Cleared by the reticuloendothelial system within 24 h.

Purified Hb. From expired red cells, e.g. diaspirin cross-linked haemoglobin. Now abandoned because of higher mortality in some trauma studies.

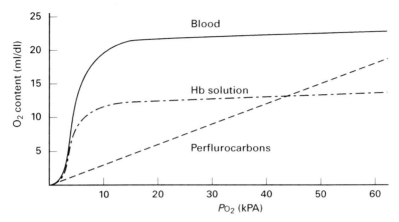

Figure 6.4 Oxygen dissociation curve for oxygen-carrying molecules.

Jehovah's Witnesses

For the life of the flesh is in the blood: and I have given it to you upon the altar to make atonement for your souls: for it is the blood that maketh an atonement for the soul. Therefore I said unto the children of Israel, No soul of you shall eat blood, neither shall any stranger that sojourneth among you eat blood.

(Leviticus 17: 10–12; see also Genesis 9: 3–4 and Acts 15: 28–29).

There are an estimated 145 000 Jehovah's Witnesses in the UK. They refuse administration of all blood and usually all blood products. They will allow blood to be retransfused if it has not lost contact with the circulation, e.g. cardiopulmonary bypass. The Children and Young Persons Act 1933 states that parents have a duty of care to their children which is not fulfilled if permission for a life-saving blood transfusion is withheld. Doctors can apply to the courts for permission to give blood against the parents' wishes, but in an emergency, blood can be given to children without consulting the courts. Children under the age of 16 can consent to a blood transfusion if they understand the issues involved, but may not refuse blood.

Clinical issues

Anaesthetists have the right to refuse to anaesthetize an elective case (when referral can be made to other colleagues) but must anaesthetize an emergency case if failure to do so would harm the patient. Ideally, consultant staff should be involved with patient care.

Preoperative assessment should take place as early as possible. Anaemia should be treated. Use of iron supplements and erythropoietin should be considered. Patients must be seen alone to avoid undue influence from other family/church members. The patient must be made fully aware of the risks of refusal of blood products. It must be clarified which blood products and techniques (e.g. cell saver) are acceptable.

Intraoperative management

Blood loss >500 mL in adults is associated with increased mortality. Techniques to minimize blood loss include positioning to avoid venous congestion, hypotensive anaesthesia, use of tourniquets, meticulous haemostasis, use of vasoconstrictors, acute hypervolaemic haemodilution and use of a cell saver. Antifibrinolytics (e.g. tranexamic acid) may also reduce blood loss. Recombinant factor VIIa has been used successfully in these patients.

Postoperative care

- Early detection and correction of postoperative oozing
- Consider elective ventilation to increase oxygen delivery
- Active cooling reduces oxygen demand and increases dissolved oxygen carriage
- Hyperbaric oxygen therapy may also be of benefit.

MANAGEMENT OF ANAESTHESIA FOR JEHOVAH'S WITNESSES

Association of Anaesthetists of Great Britain and Ireland 2005 (2E)

Recommendations

1. Wherever possible, consultant staff (anaesthetists and surgeons) should be directly involved throughout the care of Jehovah's Witness patients.
2. Departments of anaesthesia should review their procedure for being alerted at an early stage of the scheduling of Jehovah's Witness patients for elective surgery.
3. Departments should keep a regularly updated list of those senior members prepared to care for followers of the Jehovah's Witness faith.
4. In an emergency, an anaesthetist is obliged to care for a patient in accordance with the patient's wishes.
5. Properly executed Advance Directives must be respected and special Jehovah's Witness consent forms should be widely available for use as required.
6. All Jehovah's Witnesses must be consulted individually, whenever possible, to ascertain what treatments they will accept.
7. Discussions with individual Jehovah's Witness patients should be fully documented and their acceptance or rejection of treatments recorded and witnessed.
8. In the case of children, local procedures for application to the High Court for a 'Specific Issue Order' should be reviewed and available for reference.
9. A 'Specific Issue Order' or equivalent should only be applied for when it is felt to be entirely necessary to save the child in an elective or semi-elective situation.
10. In a life-threatening emergency in a child unable to give competent consent, all life-saving treatment should be given, irrespective of the parents' wishes.

Consumptive coagulopathies

Disseminated intravascular coagulation (DIC)

Consumptive coagulopathy associated with activation of both coagulation and fibrinolytic pathways. Commonest causes are sepsis, obstetric-related conditions or shock. Treatment should be guided by clinical signs and coagulation results, to include platelet concentrate, fresh frozen plasma, cryoprecipitate (a source of fibrinogen) and red cells. Antifibrinolytic agents may risk permanent clot formation. Use of heparin is controversial, but may be of benefit in amniotic fluid embolism.

Thromboelastography

Thromboelastography (TEG) was first described in 1948, but the risks of blood product transfusion and financial costs have led to a renewed interest in improving coagulation management.

Principles of TEG

TEG uses the viscoelastic changes of blood that are associated with fibrin polymerization. Clot formation is induced by putting whole blood in a low shear environment (which mimics sluggish venous flow). The patterns of shear-elasticity alteration reveal the kinetics of clot formation and growth, and the strength and stability of the formed clot. The kinetics of clot formation reflects the adequacy of quantitative factors available, while the clot strength/stability reveals the ability of the clot to perform the work of haemostasis.

The thrombelastograph consists of a larger vertical cylinder within which sits a smaller cylinder. The outer cylinder (cuvette) of the thrombelastograph oscillates at a fixed frequency. The internal cylinder (pin) of the thrombelastograph is free to move. As the blood sample placed between the cylinders clots, it forms a mechanical bond between the inner and outer cylinders of the thrombelastograph such that the oscillatory motion of the outer cylinder is transmitted to the inner cylinder. The stronger the clot, the greater the adhesion between the two cylinders and the larger the transmitted oscillation of the inner cylinder. The oscillations of the smaller cylinder are amplified to create a TEG trace.

TEG endpoints (Fig. 6.5)

R time

The time from the start of measurement until the start of clot formation. Reflects the initiation of clotting, thrombin formation, and the start of fibrin polymerization. Prolonged R time is caused by:

- Factor deficiency
- Heparin
- Severe thrombocytopenia
- Severe hypofibrinogenaemia.

Short R time is caused by:

- Hypercoagulable states.

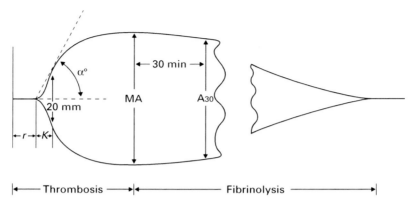

|←——— Thrombosis ———→|←——————— Fibrinolysis ———————→|

Figure 6.5 A thromboelastograph tracing, showing the endpoints used for TEG analysis.

K time

The time from starting clot formation until amplitude of 20 mm is reached. Represents fibrin polymerization, stabilization of the clot with platelets and FXIII. Prolonged by:

- Factor deficiency
- Thrombocytopaenia
- Thrombocytopathy
- Hypofibrinogenaemia.

Shortened by:

- Hypercoagulable state.

Angle (α)

Measures the rapidity of fibrin build-up and cross-linking (clot strengthening). Increased angle is caused by:

- Hypercoagulable state.

Decreased α is caused by:

- Hypofibrinogenaemia
- Thrombocytopaenia.

Maximum amplitude (MA)

A direct function of fibrin and platelet bonding via GPIIb/IIIa, reflecting ultimate clot strength. Correlates with platelet numbers and function, and fibrinogen levels.
Increased by:

- Hypercoagulable state.

Decreased by:

- Thrombocytopaenia

- Thrombocytopathy
- Hypofibrinogenaemia.

LY30 or LY60

Measures percentage decrease in amplitude at 30 or 60 min post-MA, indicating the degree of fibrinolysis. (Normal range <7.5%.)

This TEG trace is charted over time, producing a distinct shape according to the coagulation profile (Fig. 6.6).

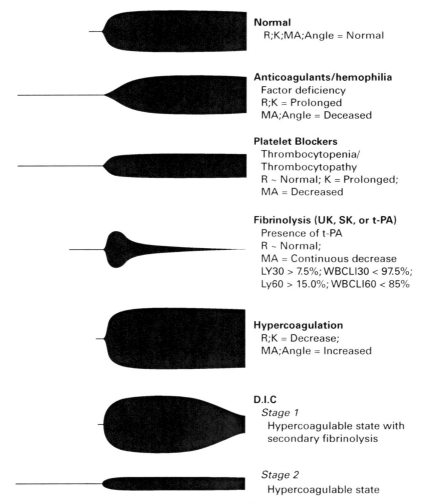

Normal
  R;K;MA;Angle = Normal

Anticoagulants/hemophilia
  Factor deficiency
  R;K = Prolonged
  MA;Angle = Deceased

Platelet Blockers
  Thrombocytopenia/
  Thrombocytopathy
  R ~ Normal; K = Prolonged;
  MA = Decreased

Fibrinolysis (UK, SK, or t-PA)
  Presence of t-PA
  R ~ Normal;
  MA = Continuous decrease
  LY30 > 7.5%; WBCLI30 < 97.5%;
  Ly60 > 15.0%; WBCLI60 < 85%

Hypercoagulation
  R;K = Decrease;
  MA;Angle = Increased

D.I.C
  Stage 1
    Hypercoagulable state with
    secondary fibrinolysis

  Stage 2
    Hypercoagulable state

Figure 6.6 Common patterns of abnormal TEG profiles.

Advantages of TEG

- Provides initial results within 10–20 min
- Good at differentiating between surgical and coagulopathic bleeding (negative predictive value >90%)
- Has been shown to reduce transfusion requirements.

Limitations of TEG

- Poor at detecting platelet dysfunction (TEG uses celite or kaolin activation of the clotting cascade. This results in supra-physiological thrombin generation, which is sufficient to activate even platelets inhibited by aspirin or clopidogrel)
- Whole blood TEGs are performed at 37°C, masking any anticoagulant effects of hypothermia.

Bibliography

Association of Anaesthetists of Great Britain and Ireland: *Management of anaesthesia for Jehovah's Witnesses*, 2nd ed, 2005. Reproduced with the kind permission of the Association of anaesthetists of Great Britain and Ireland.

Association of Anaesthetists of Great Britain and Ireland: *Blood Transfusion and the Anaesthetist – Red Cell Transfusion*, June 2008. Reproduced with the kind permission of the Association of anaesthetists of Great Britain and Ireland.

Association of Anaesthetists of Great Britain and Ireland:: *Blood Transfusion and the anaesthetist – blood component therapy*, Dec 2005, Reproduced with the kind permission of the Association of anaesthetists of Great Britain and Ireland.

Association of Anaesthetists of Great Britain and Ireland: *Blood Transfusion and the anaesthetist – introperative cell salvage*, Sept 2009, Reproduced with the kind permission of the Association of anaesthetists of Great Britain and Ireland.

Bux J: Transfusion-related acute lung injury (TRALI): a serious adverse event of blood transfusion, *Vox Sang* 89:1–10, 2005.

Contreras M, editor: *ABC of Transfusion*, ed 3, London, 1998, BMJ Publishing.

Mackman N: The role of tissue factor and factor VIIa in hemostasis, *Anesth Analg* 108:1447–1452, 2009.

Martlew VJ: Peri-operative management of patients with coagulation disorders, *Br J Anaesth* 85:446–455, 2000.

Maxwell MJ, Wilson MJA: Complications of blood transfusion, *Contin Edu Anaesth, Crit Care Pain* 6:225–229, 2006.

Milligan LJ, Bellamy MC: Anaesthesia and critical care of Jehovah's Witnesses, *Contin Edu Anaesth, Crit Care Pain* 4:35–39, 2004.

Napier JA, Bruce M, Chapman J, et al; British Committee for Standards in Haematology Blood Transfusion Task Force: Autologous Transfusion Working Party: Guidelines for autologous transfusion. II. Perioperative haemodilution and cell salvage, *Br J Anaesth* 78:768–771, 1997.

Ramanarayanan J, Krishnan GS, Hernandez-Ilizaliturri FJ: Factor VII, 2008, www.emedicine.com/med/topic3493.htm.

Ridley S, Taylor B, Gunning K: Medical management of bleeding in critically ill patients, 7:116–121, 2007.

Serious Hazards of Transfusion Annual Report: 2008, www.shot-uk.org.

Shore-Lesserson L: Evidence based coagulation monitors: heparin monitoring, thromboelastography, and platelet function (Review), *Semin Cardiothorac Vasc Anesth* 9:41–52, 2005.

Silverman TA, Weiskopf RB: Planning Committee and the Speakers: Hemoglobin-based oxygen carriers: current status and future directions, *Anaesthesiology* 111:946–963, 2009.

Spahn DR, Tucci MA, Makris M: Is recombinant FVIIa the magic bullet in the treatment of major bleeding? *Br J Anaesth* 94:553–555, 2005.

Spahn DR, Rossaint R: Coagulopathy and blood component transfusion in trauma, *Br J Anaesth* 95:130–139, 2005.

Tanaka KA, Key NS, Levy JH: Blood coagulation: hemostasis and thrombin regulation, *Anesth Analg* 108:1433–1446, 2009.

BURNS

Epidemiology

There are 10 000 burns admissions p.a. in the UK, of which 600 are fatal; 35% of burn injuries occur in children. Most burns are scalds (children), flame burns and flash burns (adults); also electrical and chemical burns. Cold injury (frostbite) is rare in the UK.

Systemic effects of burns

Tissue damage is due to both direct thermal injury and secondary damage from inflammatory mediators.

CVS. Initial reduction in cardiac output due to hypovolaemia and myocardial depressant factor. Substantial amounts of water, sodium and protein are lost within 48 h due to leakage from capillary beds. This increased capillary permeability may cause generalized oedema in large burns (>30%). Hypermetabolic state leads to an increased cardiac output within a few days. Hypertension is common secondary to catecholamines and renin activation. Responds to ACE inhibitors.

Respiratory. Reduced chest wall compliance, reduced FRC, reduced pulmonary compliance. Mucosal damage from upper airway burn.

Renal. Renal failure due to reduced GFR (inadequate resuscitation), myoglobinuria, haemoglobinuria and sepsis.

GI. Impaired liver function due to hypovolaemia, hepatotoxins and hypoxia. Curling's ulcers form in the stomach.

CNS. Encephalopathy, seizures.

Haematology. Bone marrow suppression, anaemia, thrombocytopenia and coagulopathy.

Skin. Increased heat, fluid and electrolyte loss. Loss of protective antimicrobial barrier.

Metabolism. Full-thickness burn causes water loss of 200 mL/m^2 per hour; 500 calories are used to evaporate 1000 mL water. Therefore there is an increased energy demand.

Inhaled carbon monoxide and cyanide reduce tissue oxygen delivery.

Stress response causes a hypermetabolic state with accelerated nitrogen turnover, negative nitrogen balance, hyperinsulinaemia and insulin resistance. Large nutritional requirements necessitate early high-calorie feeding.

Pharmacokinetic and pharmacodynamic changes

- Suxamethonium risks significant hyperkalaemia, probably due to extrajunctional migration of the ACh receptor, resulting in the entire myocyte cell membrane acting as a receptor. Earliest post-burn hyperkalaemic response described at 9 days, lasting for up to 10 weeks. Resistance to non-depolarizing neuromuscular blockers is due to increased V_D and upregulation of ACh receptors. These changes are proportional to the size of burn and may persist for at least 2 years after the burn has healed
- Renal and hepatic failure reduce drug clearance
- Increased tolerance to narcotics and sedatives despite decreased clearance
- Hypocalcaemia is common.

Patient assessment

Initial evaluation

Assess airway (A), breathing (B) and circulation (C). Establish venous access. Perform a secondary survey and exclude any other injuries. Assess neurological status (D) and expose the patient fully (E).

Wear protective clothing if there are chemical burns.

Treatment of burn injury

Airway

Direct thermal injury, toxic gases and smoke inhalation cause:

- upper airway oedema and obstruction
- lung parenchymal damage
- carbon monoxide poisoning
- cyanide poisoning (burning plastic).

Breathing

Monitor respiratory function, especially if there is inhalational injury. Indicators of an upper airway burn include voice changes, CXR changes, carboxyhaemoglobinaemia >15%, or compromised arterial blood gases.

Humidify inspired gases if there is upper airway burn. Intubate immediately if severe airway burn, since facial oedema will develop rapidly over the initial 24 h following a facial burn and may make intubation very difficult.

Carbon monoxide poisoning. 1000 deaths p.a. in the UK. The symptoms of CO poisoning are given in Table 6.4. HbCO results in over reading of the pulse oximeter. The half-life of carbon monoxide (250 times the affinity of O_2 for Hb) is:

- room air – 5 h
- 100% O_2 1 h.

Table 6.4 Symptoms of carbon monoxide poisoning

%HbCO	Symptoms
0–10	None
10–20	Headache, malaise
30–40	Nausea and vomiting, slowing of mental activity
>60–70	CVS collapse, death. Consider hyperbaric O_2 therapy

Hyperbaric oxygen treatment is recommended with COHb >20%, loss of consciousness at any stage, neurological signs/symptoms arrhythmias, or pregnancy. Reduces the risk of serious neurological deficit and shortens recovery.

Cyanide poisoning. Causes metabolic acidosis, raised lactate, arterial hypoxaemia and increased anion gap. Consider treatment with cyanide-chelating agents (dicobalt edetate) or agents accelerating cyanide metabolism (sodium thiosulphate).

Circulation

Risk of profound hypovolaemia with hypotension. Early fluid shifts result in loss of fluid from the plasma into the extracellular tissue around the burn. This fluid is similar in composition to plasma with equal electrolyte content but with slightly less protein. If crystalloid is used for resuscitation, larger volumes are necessary and may result in tissue oedema. Fluid loss is maximal in the first few hours and returns to basal levels by 36 h.

Blood loss during surgical debridement may be rapid and exceed 2 mL/kg per 1% of burn desloughed.

Extent and depth of burn

Burn size. This is estimated using the 'Rule of Nines' (Fig. 6.7).

Depth of burn

Superficial. Damage to epidermis. Erythema but no blistering. Painful. Heals in 2–3 days.

Partial thickness. Destruction of epidermis and dermis with formation of blisters. If deep, may also include islets of fat. Painful. Heals within 10 days as fresh epidermis grows out from hair follicles but deep partial thickness burns may be slow to heal.

Full thickness. Complete loss of epidermis and dermis down to subcutaneous fat. Loss of pain receptors renders burn painless. The burn is either white or charred with eschar. Heals by wound contraction and thus if circumferential may require escharotomies in the acute stage.

Fluid replacement. Formal fluid resuscitation is commenced in adults with >15% burns or in children with >10% burns. Ringer's lactate is the crystalloid of choice. Hypertonic saline may reduce fluid volumes and oedema, but some

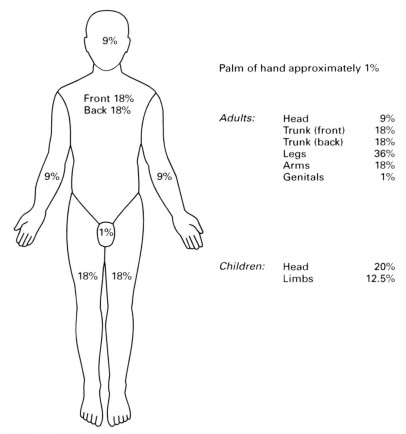

Palm of hand approximately 1%

Adults:		
	Head	9%
	Trunk (front)	18%
	Trunk (back)	18%
	Legs	36%
	Arms	18%
	Genitals	1%

Children:		
	Head	20%
	Limbs	12.5%

Figure 6.7 'Rule of Nines' for assessing burn area.

studies have shown that it causes hypernatraemia, renal failure and increased mortality.

These regimens are given in addition to the normal daily fluid requirements (usually given as 5% dextrose or dextrose saline). Volumes may need increasing if clinical indicators show inadequate resuscitation (mental status, vital signs, urine output, capillary refill, CVP, etc.).

Check electrolytes, haematocrit and plasma and urine osmolality every 4 h. Low volume urine with osmolality >450 suggests continuing hypovolaemia. Transfuse blood if haematocrit <0.3.

Common fluid replacement formulae:

- *Parkland (commonest in UK)*
    - 4 mL/kg crystalloid × % burn
    - (½ given over first 8 h, ¼ over next 8 h, ¼ over next 8 h).

- *Muir and Barclay (Mount Vernon formula)*
  - 0.5 mL/kg colloid (PPF/albumin) × % burn given over 4, 4, 4, 6 and 6 h.
- *Brook*
  - 0.5 mL/kg colloid and 1.5 mL/kg crystalloid × % burn
  - (½ given over first 8 h, ¼ over next 8 h, ¼ over next 8 h).

Infection

May worsen depth of burn, risks spreading to become a systemic infection and may destroy any skin grafts. Patients at high risk both from loss of protective skin barrier and from generalized immunosuppression.

Nurse in as clean an area as possible because of high risk of infection. Take measures to avoid cross-infection. Use topical antimicrobial prophylaxis with silver sulphadiazine cream (Flamazine).

Antibiotic cover is necessary to cover dressing changes. Systemic antibiotics should not be given routinely.

Hypothermia

Impaired homeostatic control and heat loss through burns result in rapid onset of hypothermia, accelerated by general anaesthesia and cold fluids. Keep room at 30°C to minimize energy requirements and ensure use of blood warmer and heated mattress.

Multiple anaesthetics

Are required for dressing changes and skin grafting. Monitoring (e.g. ECG dot placement) may be difficult with extensive burns. Venous access may have to be gained through burnt tissue or by a cutdown.

Nutrition and GI

Early feeding is vital because of high catabolic state. NG tube may be necessary for feeding and to prevent acute gastric dilatation. Gastric stasis is common, in which case a nasojejunal tube is necessary. Calculate amount of feed needed according to Sutherland or modified Curreri formula. Aim for a calorie:nitrogen ratio of 100:1. Give gastric stress ulcer prophylaxis. Monitor blood sugar closely.

Analgesia

Any burns less than full thickness require large doses of opioid analgesia.

Surgical management

Superficial burns usually heal spontaneously within 10 days and do not require surgery.

Partial-thickness burns require frequent debridement and may require grafting if unhealed by 3 weeks.

Full-thickness burns require early debridement and grafting. Although early debridement of a large area further traumatizes the patient and may result in loss of a large blood volume, a delay in debridement risks wound colonization and septic shock and prolongs the catabolic state following injury. If full-thickness burns are not grafted, they may never heal, or if they do they will result in contractures.

Bibliography

Black RG, Kinsella J: Anaesthetic management of burns patients, *BJA CEPD Rev* 1:177–180, 2001.

Brazeal BA, Traber DL: Pathophysiology of inhalation injury, *Curr Opin Anaesth* 10:65–67, 1997.

Hilton P, Hepp M: The immediate care of the burned patient, *BJA CEPD Rev* 1:113–116, 2001.

Latenser BA: Critical care of the burn patient: the first 48 hours, *Crit Care Med* 37:2819–2826, 2009.

MacLennan N, Heimbach DM, Cullen BF: Anesthesia for major thermal injury, *Anesthesiology* 89:749–770, 1998.

Pitkin A, Davied N: Hyperbaric oxygen therapy, *BJA CEPD Rev* 1:150–157, 2001.

DAY-CASE ANAESTHESIA

Advantages

- More convenient for patient
- Reduced morbidity (pneumonia, DVT, etc.)
- Reduced risk of hospital-acquired infections
- Cost savings
- Increased hospital efficiency.

Patient selection

Social – Responsible adult to care for the patient for 24 h postoperatively with easy access to a telephone. Suitable home situation.

Medical factors – All patients should be seen in advance of their surgery by someone trained in pre-assessment for day surgery. Consultant led, nurse run pre-assessment clinics provide a suitable method to attain this.

Patients should be fully fit or any illness should be well controlled. Generally limited to ASA I and II patients. Elderly and ASA III patients may be considered suitable if their systemic disease is well controlled preoperatively. Patients with morbid obesity are probably best treated as in-patients. Length of anaesthesia is directly related to postoperative morbidity. Healthy full-term infants <6 months are suitable for day-case surgery. Infants <50 weeks post-conceptual age are unsuitable because of risk of postoperative apnoea, poor gag reflex and poor temperature control.

Personnel factors – Good liaison between GP, hospital and community nurses.

General anaesthesia

Requirements of a general anaesthetic

- Safe and effective anaesthesia
- Minimal side-effects
- Rapid recovery
- Good postoperative analgesia.

Premedication

May impair coordination for 5–12h postoperatively, therefore avoid if possible. Insufficient evidence to recommend the use of routine prophylactic anti-emetics in day surgery practice, except in certain patient groups (strong history of PONV, laparoscopic sterilization, laparoscopic cholecystectomy and tonsillectomy).

Airway

Laryngeal mask airway (LMA) reduces the incidence of postoperative sore throat and avoids the need for intubation. Ventilation with LMA appears safe but does not protect against gastric aspiration. For patients at risk of aspiration, use cuffed endotracheal tube. Endotracheal intubation using propofol/alfentanil may avoid the need for neuromuscular blockers.

Induction agents

Thiopentone may impair motor skills for up to 8h. Children induced with thiopentone are more sleepy for the first 30 min postoperatively compared with gas induction with halothane.

Etomidate is rapidly metabolized but is associated with a higher incidence of nausea and vomiting.

Propofol recovery is faster than thiopentone, methohexitone, etomidate, isoflurane, enflurane or halothane and causes less nausea and vomiting. More CVS depression than barbiturates. High incidence of pain on injection reduced with lidocaine or opioid and injection into a large vein. At 24h, patients given propofol are more alert, less drowsy and less tired than those given thiopentone.

Midazolam is highly suitable for sedation during local procedures due to minimal cardiorespiratory depression and rapid clearance. However, CNS recovery is more rapid with propofol.

Opioids

Short-acting opioids may reduce volatile requirements and actually decrease postoperative recovery time. Decrease pain on injection and movement with etomidate and methohexitone. Emergence is more rapid with alfentanil than with fentanyl. Use with prophylactic antiemetics, although there is less nausea and vomiting if combined with propofol.

Inhalational agents

Desflurane has the lowest blood:gas solubility of the current volatile agents (0.42) and therefore undergoes the fastest elimination with rapid recovery. Too irritant for gas induction.

Sevoflurane (blood:gas solubility = 0.6) is less pungent and can be used for gas induction with rapid elimination. Because both undergo rapid equilibration, a more rapid adjustment of anaesthetic depth is possible. Both allow more rapid recovery than a propofol infusion and cause less residual impairment of cognitive function. Neither causes nausea or vomiting. Both are more expensive than *isoflurane* and have not been shown to enable earlier discharge home.

Muscle relaxants

Use of neuromuscular blockers may reduce recovery time by decreasing volatile requirements.

Suxamethonium can cause myalgia for up to 4 days.

Intubating dose of mivacurium (0.2 mg/kg) causes maximum blockade within 3 min and spontaneous recovery by 20–30 min. Mivacurium 0.08 mg/kg produces maximum blockade in 4 min and 95% recovery of twitch height within 25 min. It has the fastest recovery of any non-depolarizer, usually avoiding the use of reversal drugs.

Brief laparoscopic procedures may be possible with spontaneous ventilation and face mask.

Neostigmine and glycopyrrolate increase the incidence of postoperative nausea and vomiting.

Recovery

Postoperative waking is faster with sevoflurane and desflurane.

Postoperative nausea, vomiting and headaches are associated with N_2O, etomidate, fentanyl and volatiles. Droperidol causes increased postoperative drowsiness.

Evidence of benefit for the elderly population with studies showing a reduction in postoperative cognitive dysfunction.

Local/regional anaesthesia

Avoids complications of GA, reduces aspiration risk and provides good postoperative analgesia. Cognitive defects are present at 3 days postoperatively in GA patients but are not present following local infiltration.

Day-case techniques include topical anaesthesia (including EMLA), Bier's block, field infiltration, peripheral nerve blocks, regional blocks.

Spinal headaches are more common in the young, especially with early ambulation. Use fine Sprotte or Whitacre needles (<24G). Discharge times using spinal for inguinal hernia are significantly longer than with field block.

Fluid management

Allow clear fluids up to 2 h preoperatively. This minimizes preoperative thirst and discomfort, avoids hypoglycaemia (particularly in children) and reduces hypotension on induction. Consider i.v. fluids if surgery is scheduled to last >30 min; blood loss >300 mL or there is a risk of nausea and vomiting (e.g. squint surgery).

ENT surgery

Day-case adenotonsillectomy for children is safe and cost-effective. Children undergoing tonsillectomy for airway obstruction are at continuing risk of obstruction in the postoperative period, so admit overnight.

Discharge criteria
General anaesthetic

- Awake, orientated and tolerating oral fluids
- Urine passed
- Stable observations for 60 min
- Responsible adult to accompany patient home.

Regional anaesthetic

- As above, but also ensure regression of motor, sensory and sympathetic blockade
- Suitable criteria include normal perianal (S_{4-5}) sensation, plantar flexion of the foot and proprioception in the big toe.

Postoperative complications

Adequate analgesia to take home is particularly important. The 30-day postoperative mortality is 1:11 000. Incidence of stroke, MI and pulmonary embolus is extremely low, and less than would be expected in a similar population undergoing surgery involving a hospital stay.

Unanticipated postoperative admission rate is approximately 1%, mostly due to bleeding and inadequate pain relief; 3–12% patients discharged contact their GP/hospital due to bleeding, inadequate pain relief and headaches/dizziness.

DAY SURGERY
Association of Anaesthetists of Great Britain and Ireland.
Revised 2005

Summary

- Day surgery is a continually evolving specialty performed in a range of ways across different units. The NHS plan target of 75% of elective surgery being performed as day cases means that this will form a high proportion of the work of most Departments of Anaesthesia.
- Pre-assessment clinics should be consultant-led and nurse-run. The assessment criteria should be developed in conjunction with the local Department of Anaesthesia.
- Fitness for a procedure should relate to the patient's health as found at pre-assessment and not limited by arbitrary limits such as ASA status or age. Whatever surgery is to be undertaken as a day-case, the decision must be based on proven safety and quality.
- Good quality advice leaflets, assessment forms and protocols are in use in many centres and are available to other units.
- Each anaesthetist should develop techniques that permit the patient to undergo the surgical procedure with minimum stress, maximum comfort and optimize their chance of early discharge.
- Central neural blockade can be used for day-stay surgery.
- Effective audit is an essential component of good day stay anaesthesia.

Bibliography

Association of Anaesthetists of Great Britain and Ireland Revised Edition: *Day surgery*, 2005. Reproduced with the kind permission of the Association of anaesthetists of Great Britain and Ireland.

DoH: *Day surgery. Operational guide*, London, 2002, Department of Health.

Jackson IJB: The management of pain following day surgery, *BJA CEPD Rev* 1:48–51, 2001.

Marshall SI, Chung F: Discharge criteria and complications after ambulatory surgery, *Anesth Analges* 88:508–517, 1999.

NHS Modernisation Agency: *National good practice on pre-operative assessment for day surgery*, London, 2002, NHS.

Rawi N: Analgesia for day-case surgery, *Br J Anaesth* 87:73–87, 2001.

DEPTH OF ANAESTHESIA

Guedel classification

Described for spontaneous respiration with diethyl ether in 1937.

- **Stage 1: Analgesia** – beginning of induction to loss of consciousness
  - Regular, small-volume respiration
  - Pupils normal.
- **Stage 2: Excitement** – loss of consciousness to onset of automatic breathing
  - Irregular respiration
  - Divergent, dilated pupils
  - Active laryngeal/pharyngeal reflexes
  - Eyelash reflex abolished.
- **Stage 3: Surgical anaesthesia** – automatic respiration to respiratory paralysis:
  - *Plane 1*: Regular, large-volume respiration
    - ▷ Central, pinpoint pupils. Cessation of eye movements
    - ▷ Eyelid reflex abolished
  - *Plane 2*: Thoracic component of respiration decreased
    - ▷ Loss of corneal reflex
  - *Plane 3*: Respiration becoming diaphragmatic. Small volume
    - ▷ Laryngeal reflexes depressed
    - ▷ Pupils normal
  - *Plane 4*: Irregular diaphragmatic, small-volume respiration
    - ▷ Dilated pupils
    - ▷ Carinal reflex depressed.
- **Stage 3:** More recent classification, replacing that of Guedel:
  - *Light anaesthesia*: until cessation of eyeball movement
  - *Medium anaesthesia*: increasing intercostal muscle paralysis
  - *Deep anaesthesia*: diaphragmatic respiration.
- **Stage 4: Coma**
  - Apnoea, hypotension.

Monitoring depth of anaesthesia

Autonomic responses. BP, pulse and variability, sweating, dilated pupils.

Isolated forearm technique of Tunstall (1977). Tighten tourniquet on upper arm above systolic pressure before injection of neuromuscular blocker.

Spontaneous skeletal muscle activity. Abolished with neuromuscular blockers.

EEG. Difficult to use and interpret because of specific effects of different anaesthetic agents. A drug-independent EEG parameter has not yet been identified. Fourier analysis (decomposes EEG into its component sine waves) correlates well with sedation but not depth of anaesthesia. Bispectral index monitoring (BIS) is based on bispectral processing that determines the harmonic and phase relations among the various EEG frequencies. Values may vary depending on anaesthetic drugs used. May be a useful adjunct for reducing the risk of awareness.

Evoked potentials. Auditory, visual and electrical. Measure change in latency and amplitude of EEG responses.

Oesophageal smooth muscle provoked contraction. Provoked with balloon dilation in lower third of oesophagus. Unaltered with neuromuscular blockers. Different volatiles affect the response in different ways.

Awareness during anaesthesia

Occurs in 0.1–1% of paralysed patients, and 0.3% of patients undergoing fast-track cardiac anaesthesia. Single case report of a patient aware during spontaneous respiration. Commonest during obstetric GA, often at intubation.

Causes

- Use of minimal dose of induction agents and no opioids for lower segment caesarean section (LSCS) to avoid fetal depression
- Use of minimal drugs if patient seriously ill
- Prolonged attempts at intubation during which induction agent wears off and patient remains paralysed
- VOC with percentage of volatile within the circle lower than that set on the vaporizer
- Vaporizer exhausted of volatile
- Vaporizer not seated correctly on back bar, causing loss of volatile
- Leak within the breathing circuit
- Disconnection
- Total intravenous anaesthesia:
  - infusion not commenced immediately after induction agent given
  - incorrect infusion rates, too low to be used without the addition of N_2O and opioids
  - pump failure or occlusion of line
- Hypermetabolic states with increased volatile requirement, e.g. thyrotoxicosis.

Bibliography

Drummond JC: Monitoring depth of anaesthesia, *Anesthesiology* 93:876–882, 2000.

Kissin I: Depth of anesthesia and bispectral index monitoring, *Anesth Analg* 90:1114–1117, 2000.

Tempe D: In search of a reliable awareness monitor, *Anesth Analg* 92:801–804, 2001.

GENERAL TOPICS

ASA grading (1963)

I – Healthy. No systemic disease
II – Mild/moderate systemic disease not limiting patient's activities
III – Severe systemic disease causing functional limitation
IV – Severe systemic disease which is a constant threat to life
V – Moribund patient unlikely to survive >24 h with/without surgery
E – Additional coding for Emergency surgery.

CEPOD classification of diseases

- *Immediate* – resuscitation simultaneous with surgical treatment, e.g. ruptured aortic aneurysm
- *Urgent* – operation performed as soon as possible after resuscitation, e.g. congenital diaphragmatic hernia
- *Scheduled* – early operation but not immediately life-saving, e.g. cancer surgery
- *Elective* – operation at a time convenient to surgeon, anaesthetist and patient, e.g. plastic surgery.

Aims of premedication

- To reduce preoperative anxiety
- To reduce undesirable autonomic reflexes (salivation, bradycardia, etc.)
- To assist in smooth induction and maintenance of anaesthesia
- To prevent and treat pain
- To prevent postoperative nausea and vomiting
- To reduce the risk from acid aspiration.

Cricoid pressure

First described by Sellick in 1961. Traditional teaching is that 44 N force is required to occlude the oesophagus. This is the equivalent of the force required to produce pain when 'cricoid pressure' is applied to the bridge of the nose.

More than 20 N cricoid pressure is uncomfortable and causes retching, risking pulmonary aspiration or oesophageal rupture. More than 40 N cricoid pressure applied after loss of consciousness can obstruct the airway, prevent ventilation and cause difficulty with intubation.

Although suxamethonium fasciculations can increase gastric pressure, peak intragastric pressure rarely exceeds 25 mmHg. In 10 cadavers, 30 N pressure prevented regurgitation of gastric contents at 40 mmHg in all cases. Additionally, reduction in upper oesophageal sphincter tone occurs before consciousness is lost.

Cricoid pressure should therefore be applied before loss of consciousness. Recent recommendations suggest 10 N (1 kg) pressure when the patient is awake, increasing to 30 N following loss of consciousness.

Cricoid pressure impairs insertion of the laryngeal mask airway.

Nasogastric tubes should be in position before induction of anaesthesia to empty gastric contents and the lumen then left open to vent gastric contents. Their presence does not reduce the efficiency of cricoid pressure.

Prophylaxis of thromboembolic disease

Recognized by CEPOD reports as a common cause of postoperative morbidity and mortality. Incidence of postoperative deep venous thrombosis (DVT) varies from 18% post-hysterectomy to 75% post-repair of femoral neck fracture.

Several studies have shown that regional techniques reduce the incidence of postoperative DVT and pulmonary embolism. However, there is less evidence that overall outcome is affected. Regional techniques only appear to be effective in reducing DVT risk if the block involves both legs. Thoracic epidurals for abdominal surgery do not reduce the incidence of DVTs. Mechanisms of action may include increased lower limb blood flow through vasodilation, reduced blood viscosity through vasodilation and fluid preload, and less suppression of fibrinolysis compared with GA.

Hormone replacement therapy and low-dose oestrogen/progesterone oral contraceptives do not appear to increase the risk of DVT.

Recent THRIFT (Thromboembolic Risk Factors Consensus) study and CEPOD reports recommend that prophylaxis is given to most surgical patients. Low dose heparin (5000 units b.d.) does not increase the risk of bleeding, and reduces the risk of DVT by 66% and the risk of PE by 50%.

Low-molecular-weight heparins have a greater anti-Xa activity, which makes them more effective at preventing thrombin formation. There may be an increased risk of spinal haematoma in patients with epidurals.

Risk factors for deep venous thrombosis

Low-risk patients

- <40 years without additional risk factors
- Minor surgery (<30 min).

Moderate-risk patients

- >40 years
- Major surgery (>30 min)
- Immobilized medical patients with active disease.

High-risk patients

- Previous DVT/PE
- Major surgery for malignant disease
- Orthopaedic surgery to lower limbs
- Stroke, heart failure and acute MI.

Eye injuries after non-ocular surgery

In a study of 60965 patients (Roth et al 1996), eye injuries occurred in 0.06%. The commonest injury was corneal abrasion. This is usually due to the failure of the eyelids to close during anaesthesia with an associated reduction in tear production. Other common injuries include conjunctivitis, chemical injury and direct trauma. Risk factors are long surgical procedures, lateral positioning during surgery, operation to the head or neck and general anaesthesia.

Human immunodeficiency virus

First reported in homosexual men in New York in 1981. The HIV virus was first identified as the causative agent in 1983. The virus is a retrovirus which targets the T-helper lymphocyte and impairs the immune response to antigens.

There were 15712 cases reported in the UK by 1991, but the number now probably exceeds 50000. About 10% of cases are thought to result from heterosexual transmission. HIV virus is present in all body fluids, but is particularly high in blood, semen, pericardial fluid, amniotic fluid and cerebrospinal fluid. Most transmission occurs through blood, sexual contact and vertically through placental transfer to the fetus.

The disease progresses through three stages:

1. *Seroconversion illness.* Initial infection from the virus may result in a flu-like illness with fever, lymphadenopathy, arthralgia and sore throat. May not progress further for several years.
2. *Persistent generalized lymphadenopathy.* Defined as enlarged nodes at least 1 cm in diameter in more than one extrainguinal site, persisting for at least 3 months in the absence of any other illness or cause.
3. *Acquired immunodeficiency syndrome.* Characterized by tumours (Kaposi's sarcoma, non-Hodgkin's lymphoma, squamous cell carcinoma) and opportunistic infections (*Pneumocystis*, cytomegalovirus, herpes simplex, *Cryptococcus*).

Patients infected with the HIV virus present several anaesthetic problems:

- side-effects of drugs used in the treatment of AIDS
- patients presenting with respiratory failure
- risk of transmission of the HIV virus.

Drug side-effects

Nucleoside analogues

Zidovudine (AZT). This drug acts as a false transmitter for reverse transcriptase, inhibiting the incorporation of HIV DNA into the host cell genome. It may delay progression of the disease. Inhibition of DNA polymerase results in a megaloblastic anaemia and neutropenia, made worse by B_{12} or folate deficiency. Other side-effects of relevance to anaesthesia include convulsions, myopathy, impaired liver function and lactic acidosis.

Didanosine (DDI). Used as an alternative to AZT. May cause impaired liver function, diarrhoea, peripheral neuropathy and convulsions.

Protease inhibitors

Ritonavir, indinavir. These drugs inhibit the cytochrome P_{450} enzyme system. They increase plasma concentrations of benzodiazepines and cisapride. Ritonavir contains 43% alcohol, so its administration with disulfiram and metronidazole should be avoided.

Antibiotics

Co-trimoxazole (high dose). A mixture of trimethoprim and sulphamethoxazole for the prophylaxis and treatment of *Pneumocystis carinii*. May cause megaloblastic anaemia, leucopenia, thrombocytopenia and impaired liver function.

Antiviral agents

Ganciclovir. More active than aciclovir against cytomegalovirus. Causes anaemia, leucopenia and thrombocytopenia. Also arrhythmias, hypertension, hypotension and hypoglycaemia.

Respiratory failure

AIDS often presents with opportunistic respiratory infections, usually due to *Pneumocystis carinii*. Respiratory failure is common and requires the decision as to the appropriateness of ventilatory support. Early studies showed that the outcome from mechanical ventilation was universally poor, with mortality rates approaching 100%. Recent studies, however, have shown survival rates following mechanical ventilation as high as 36–54% although the median survival of patients weaned from ventilation was less than 1 year. Recurrence of *Pneumocystis carinii* infection or symptoms for more than 4 weeks are particularly poor prognostic indicators.

Anaesthetists infected with HIV

The General Medical Council (1988) advise that any anaesthetist who thinks that he or she may be infected with the HIV virus must seek appropriate counselling and treatment. Anaesthetists infected with HIV risk infecting patients following blood-to-blood contact. The Department of Health (1993) has defined procedures that place patients at risk as:

"surgical entry into tissues, cavities or organs, or repair of major traumatic injuries, cardiac catheterization and angiography, vaginal and Caesarian deliveries; the manipulation, cutting or removal of any oral or perioral tissues... during which bleeding may occur."

Therefore an anaesthetist who is HIV-positive should not carry out procedures which involve opening the patient's skin or tissues.

Concern has been expressed by the Association of Anaesthetists (1988) that HIV encephalopathy may impair the physical and mental skills of an anaesthetist. However, encephalopathy usually presents late in the course of the illness, by which time the patient is too ill to work. Encephalopathy should be detected early if the patient is under regular medical care.

Needlestick injury

- 0.3% risk of seroconversion if patient is HIV-positive
- 3% risk of seroconversion if patient is hepatitis C-positive
- 30% risk of seroconversion if patient is hepatitis B e antigen-positive.

Protection

- Avoid re-sheathing needles
- Use sharps bins
- Wear protective clothing
- Staff with open skin lesions should avoid patient contact
- Use of ventilation devices to avoid mouth-to-mouth ventilation
- Employers must have an exposure protection plan.

GUIDELINES ON POST-EXPOSURE PROPHYLAXIS (PEP) FOR HEALTHCARE WORKERS OCCUPATIONALLY EXPOSED TO HIV
Department of Health 1997

The risk of acquiring HIV following needlestick injury is about 3 per 1000 injuries. Risk factors include deep injury, hollow bore needles, blood from terminally ill HIV patients, and needles that have been in arteries or veins. This risk can be reduced if zidovudine is taken prophylactically as soon as possible after exposure.

Risk assessment

PEP should be considered whenever there has been exposure to material known to be infected with HIV. The three types of exposure in healthcare settings known to be associated with significant risk are:

- Percutaneous injury (needles, instruments, bone fragments)
- Exposure of broken skin (abrasions, cuts, eczema, etc.)
- Exposure of mucous membranes, including the eye.

Choice of PEP drugs

The currently recommended drug regimen is:
zidovudine 200 mg t.d.s. + lamivudine 150 mg b.d. + indinavir 800 mg t.d.s.

Any drug regimen must take into account whether the healthcare worker is allergic to any of these drugs; is pregnant; whether there would be an interaction with any other medication; and whether the virus might be resistant to any of the medication. Expert advice must be sought.

Making PEP available

PEP should be commenced as soon as possible after the incident, and ideally within the hour. Therefore, in a high-risk situation, it might be appropriate to give the initial doses immediately, pending full discussion and risk assessment later.

HIV AND OTHER BLOOD BORNE VIRUSES
Association of Anaesthetists of Great Britain and Ireland 1992

Risk of transmission of hepatitis B (HBV), human immunodeficiency virus (HIV) and HTLV-1 (causes T-cell leukaemia and adult tropical spastic paraparesis).

Epidemiology

A total of 15712 cases of HIV had been reported in the UK by June 1991, of which 1489 probably acquired the infection through heterosexual intercourse. The actual number of HIV-positive people is probably 50000. There are 2000 clinical cases of HBV but many more have asymptomatic infections; 1:500 adults in the UK are HBV carriers.

Transmission and occupational exposure

HIV is mostly transmitted by blood, sexual contacts and from mother to fetus (blood, vaginal delivery and breast milk).

- *High-risk fluids* – amniotic fluid, pericardial and pleural fluid, CSF, peritoneal fluid, semen and vaginal secretions
- *Low-risk fluids* – faeces, nasal secretions, sputum, saliva, sweat, urine and vomit.

HBV present in virtually all human fluids, particularly blood, semen and vaginal secretions.

Transmission of both HIV and HBV usually follows needlestick injury. HIV has been transmitted by infected blood on broken skin and mucous membranes. HBV transmission occurs more readily.

Screening

Screening for HIV does not reduce the risks of occupational transmission. Window period of 3 months before antibodies appear. Patient consent must be obtained before HIV testing.

Precautions against infection

Use mask, gloves and eye protection during invasive procedures. Needles must not be re-sheathed but placed into a sharps container. Cover all open skin lesions with waterproof plaster. Non-autoclavable equipment should be cleaned with 2% glutaraldehyde.

Resuscitation and intensive care

No reports of HIV or HBV infection from basic life support but still a risk so use protective devices. Relatives of organ donors should be counselled about HIV testing.

Protection against HBV

All anaesthetists should be immunized against HBV, with boosters at 3–5 years.

Post-exposure management

Following inoculation injury, encourage wound to bleed and wash with soap and water. Irrigate splashes on mucous membranes with copious volumes of water. Designate a person to contact following exposure. Early treatment with HBV immunoglobulin, AZT, antibiotics or anti-tetanus immunization as deemed necessary.

Anaesthetists with HIV infection

In 1988, the GMC set out the duties of doctors infected with HIV. Doctors must seek appropriate advice and modify their clinical practice accordingly. Similar guidelines apply for HBV-infected staff.

BLOOD-BORNE VIRUSES AND ANAESTHESIA – AN UPDATE
Association of Anaesthetists of Great Britain and Ireland 1996

Anaesthesia and exposure-prone procedures

Exposure-prone procedures (replacing the term 'invasive procedures') are:

"Those procedures where there is a risk that injury to the health worker may result in the exposure of the patient's open tissues to the blood of the worker. These procedures include those where the worker's gloved hand may be in contact with sharp instruments, needle tips or sharp tissues (spicules of bone or teeth) inside a patient's open body cavity, wound or confined anatomical space where the finger tips may not be visible at all times."

The report recommended that:
- although anaesthetists put their fingers into patients' mouths, anaesthesia should not be regarded as an exposure-prone specialty
- it should be mandatory for anaesthetists to wear surgical gloves when carrying out procedures which involve putting their hands into patients' mouths.

Transmission of hepatitis C virus (HCV) via the anaesthetic breathing system

A case report from Australia suggests that several patients may have become infected with HCV by cross-infection from a breathing system. The Council recommends that:

- either an appropriate filter should be placed between the patient and the breathing system, a new filter being used for each patient, or that a new breathing system be used for each patient
- where expired gas sampling is used, the sample should be taken from the breathing system side of the filter
- in paediatric practice, where the use of a filter would increase dead space and/or resistance unacceptably, filters should not be used but the breathing system should be changed between patients.

Hepatitis C virus (HCV)

Discovered in 1989 as the causative agent of non-A, non-B hepatitis. Single strand RNA virus.

European prevalence is 0.3–1.2%; highest in Japan, Middle East and the Mediterranean. Most transmission is via i.v. drug abuse; also tattoos, sexual transmission and needlestick injury. Patient-to-patient transmission has been documented in chronic haemodialysis patients and via heat-and-moisture exchange filters.

Following acute HCV infection, a lag period of 2–3 months occurs before anti-HCV is detected in serum. Acute illness often progresses to chronic disease. Recombinant α-interferon normalizes liver function tests and renders serum free from HCV RNA in these patients.

Bibliography

Association of Anaesthetists of Great Britain and Ireland: *HIV and other blood-borne viruses*, 1992. Reproduced with the kind permission of the Association of anaesthetists of Great Britain and Ireland.

Association of Anaesthetists of Great Britain and Ireland: *Blood-borne viruses and anaesthesia – an update*, 1996. Reproduced with the kind permission of the Association of anaesthetists of Great Britain and Ireland.

Department of Health: *Guidelines on post-exposure prophylaxis for health care workers occupationally exposed to HIV (Professional Letter: PL/CO(97)1)*, Wetherby, (West Yorkshire), 1997, Department of Health.

General Medical Council: *HIV infection and AIDS: the ethical considerations*, London, 1988, GMC.

Jackson SH, Cheung EC: Hepatitis B and hepatitis C: occupational considerations for the anesthesiologist, *Anesthesiol Clin North America* 22:355–357, 2004.

Leelanukrom R: Anaesthetic considerations of the HIV-infected patients, *Curr Opin Anaesth* 22:412–418, 2009.

White E, Crosse MM: The aetiology and prevention of perioperative corneal abrasions, *Anaesthesia* 53:157–161, 1998.

DISEASES OF IMPORTANCE TO ANAESTHESIA

Congenital syndromes

Down's syndrome (trisomy 21)

Incidence of 1:700 live births, increasing with maternal age; 50% have congenital heart disease. Defects include (in order of decreasing frequency) complete AV canal, VSD, PDA and tetralogy of Fallot (VSD, overriding aorta, pulmonary stenosis, left ventricular hypertrophy). Down's is associated with large protruding tongue, small mandible, mental retardation, epilepsy, duodenal obstruction, hypothyroidism and impaired immune system. Institutionalized patients have a higher incidence of hepatitis B. About 20% have atlantoaxial instability (poor muscle tone, ligamentous laxity and abnormal odontoid peg). Obstructive sleep apnoea and respiratory complications are common.

Anaesthetic problems include difficult intubation, requirement for a smaller endotracheal tube size than expected, cervical spine instability and a higher incidence of postoperative atelectasis and pulmonary oedema.

Pierre–Robin syndrome

Rare congenital syndrome with severe micrognathia and posterior prolapse of the tongue. Causes airway obstruction, which is worse in the supine position; improved by placing the child prone. If severe, may require tongue to be sutured to the lower gum. Can progress to cor pulmonale. Associated with problems feeding, and a risk of aspiration. Difficult intubation.

Marfan's syndrome

Autosomal dominant condition affecting connective tissue, causing ocular, skeletal and cardiac abnormalities. Premature death is common.

CVS lesions present in 50% by 22 years. Associated with ascending aortic aneurysm, aortic regurgitation, mitral regurgitation, myocardial infarction and myocardial fibrosis; also long thin extremities, high arched palate, upward lens displacement, spontaneous pneumothorax and scoliosis.

Anaesthetic problems include difficult intubation, cardiac and respiratory complications and joint dislocation.

Haemoglobinopathies

Sickle cell disease

Autosomal dominant inheritance. Affects people of African, Mediterranean, Indian, Caribbean and Middle Eastern descent. Found in 10% of black people in the UK.

The condition is due to substitution of glutamine by valine on position 6 of the β-chain of haemoglobin A to form HbS. Causes polymerization of deoxygenated haemoglobin at low $P_a o_2$ with alteration of the discoid cell to a rigid sickle shape. These abnormal cells increase blood viscosity and sludge in the microvascular circulation. Infarcts cause symptoms and signs of the disease. Sickling is precipitated by dehydration, acidosis, fever and hypoxia.

The *heterozygous form*, HbAS (sickle trait), has normal life expectancy with haemoglobin >11 g/dL, no clinical symptoms or signs and sickling only if P_aO_2 <2.5 kPa. Hb does not fall below 11.0.

The *homozygous form*, HbSS, usually presents by 6 months when HbF is replaced by HbS. Deoxygenation of HbS results in polymerization to form insoluble globin polymers. Associated with chronic anaemia, painful sickle crises, pulmonary thromboembolism, pulmonary, renal and bone infarcts, gallstones, priapism, TIAs and strokes. Splenic sequestration results in splenomegaly in infants, but multiple infarcts cause autosplenectomy by adulthood. Parvovirus causes aplastic crises. Target cells on blood film. HbSS sickles at P_aO_2 <5.0 kPa.

Haemoglobin S may combine with other haemoglobins, e.g. HbC, to give HbSC or with β-thalassaemia haemoglobin.

Diagnosis. Sickledex test causes sickling when affected erythrocytes are exposed to sodium metabisulphite. Unlike electrophoresis, it does not distinguish between homozygous and heterozygous conditions.

Anaesthetic considerations. Consider exchange transfusion if HbA <40%, aiming to reduce HbS to <25%. Postoperative mortality is about 5%. Patients are not suitable for day-case surgery. Impaired renal concentrating ability.

Reduce risk of sickling by:

- keeping well oxygenated
- good analgesia
- avoiding tourniquets, which induce sickling
- keeping warm
- keeping well hydrated
- prophylactic antibiotics.

A SICKLE CRISIS?
A Report of the National Confidential Enquiry into Patient Outcome and Death 2008

Principal recommendations

- A multidisciplinary and multi-agency approach is needed in the ongoing pain management of patients with sickle cell disease – essentially this takes place outside hospitals for the majority of patients.
- Cause of death in sickle cell disease patients must be better evaluated, whether by clinicians reviewing the records and writing a death certificate.
- All staff should be aware that people with sickle cell disease are subject to the diseases that other patients suffer from as well. If there

is uncertainty as to whether the problem is sickle cell related, advice should be sought from an experienced clinician.

- All sickle cell disease patients should have a carefully maintained fluid balance chart for the duration of their admission.
- Patients with sickle cell disease or beta thalassaemia major should be managed by, or have access to, clinicians with experience of haemoglobinopathy management.
- Healthcare centres responsible for the management of patients with haemoglobinopathies should have access to protocols/guidelines from their regional specialist centre.

Porphyria

Autosomal dominant metabolic disorder of porphyrin synthesis. Porphyrins are tetrapyrrole rings involved in the synthesis of haemoglobin, myoglobin and cytochromes. There are two types of porphyria:

- erythropoietic – anaemia and liver disease only
- hepatic – potentially fatal.

Increased production of aminolaevulinic acid (ALA) and porphobilinogen (PBG), together with their reduced metabolism by porphobilinogen deaminase, causes symptoms:

$$\uparrow \delta \text{ ALA synthetase} \rightarrow \uparrow \text{ ALA} \rightarrow \downarrow \text{ activity of porphobilinogen}$$
$$\text{triggered by drugs} \qquad \uparrow \text{ PBG} \qquad \text{deaminase}$$

Acute intermittent porphyria (hepatic) is the commonest form, presenting as hypertension (36%), tachycardia (80%) and abdominal pain (95%) due to autonomic neuropathy; also peripheral neuropathy (30%), bulbar palsy (30%), convulsions (20%) and mental confusion (55%). Urine turns red after standing in sunlight. Underlying defect is decreased activity of porphobilinogen deaminase.

Acute episodes are precipitated by:

- infection, starvation and dehydration
- steroids, barbiturates, etomidate
- alcohol
- oral contraceptive pill
- cimetidine, erythromycin, sulphonamides
- prochlorperazine, metoclopramide.

Safe drugs

- Volatile agents and nitrous oxide
- Propofol, midazolam, diazepam

- Morphine, codeine, alfentanil, fentanyl
- Lidocaine, bupivacaine
- All muscle relaxants, including suxamethonium
- Anticholinergics, anticholinesterases.

Treatment. Identify and remove the cause if possible. Ensure adequate hydration and correct any electrolyte imbalance. Hypertension and tachycardia respond well to β-blockers. Treat generalized convulsions with diazepam. Ensure adequate analgesia with opioids. Specific treatment involves infusion of heme arginate, which directly increases negative feedback to ALA synthetase.

General anaesthesia. Best avoided, by using regional techniques, but document any peripheral neuropathy first. Total dose of drug administered and duration of anaesthetic influences the probability of triggering a porphyric crisis. Postoperatively, good analgesia avoids the stress of pain triggering an acute attack. Monitor postoperatively for 5 days since onset may be delayed.

Haemophilia

Haemophilia A. Sex-linked recessive inherited condition with reduced levels of factor VIII. Males are affected, females are carriers. Spontaneous bleeding, mostly into joints with ankylosis and permanent joint deformities. Prolonged partial thromboplastin time (intrinsic pathway) with normal whole blood clotting time and normal bleeding time. Diagnose by factor VIII:C assay.

Haemophiliacs treated with factor VIII before it was available in its sterilized freeze-dried form may be carriers of hepatitis B, C or HIV. Avoid regional anaesthesia. Care is needed during laryngoscopy and intubation. Titrate factor VIII replacement against blood levels of factor VIII and nature of operation. Mild haemophiliacs may manage with an infusion of i.v. desmopressin. Avoid i.m. injections. NSAIDs may cause persistent bleeding.

Haemophilia B (Christmas disease). Sex-linked recessive inherited condition with reduced levels of factor IX. Coagulation tests are similar to those of haemophilia A with reduced factor IX assay. Treat with factor IX. Desmopressin is ineffective.

Von Willebrand's disease. Usually autosomal dominant. Abnormal production of von Willebrand factor which acts as a carrier molecule for FVIII and is also involved in platelet adhesion. Prolonged bleeding time in the presence of a normal platelet count. Responds to DDAVP and FVIII if severe.

Bibliography

A Sickle Crisis? A report of the National Confidential Enquiry into Patient Outcome and Death, 2008. www.ncepod.org.uk/2008sc.htm.

Firth PG: Anaesthesia for peculiar cells – a century of sickle cell disease, *Br J Anaesth* 95:287–299, 2005.

James MF, Hift RJ: Porphyrias, *Br J Anaesth* 85:143–153, 2000.
Martlew VJ: Peri-operative management of patients with coagulation disorders, *Br J Anaesth* 85:446–455, 2000.

Other conditions

Ankylosing spondylitis

An inflammatory condition of unknown aetiology, characterized by high ESR, fever, weight loss and anaemia. Causes progressive fibrosis, ossification and ankylosis of sacroiliac joints and spine. 50% have extra-articular involvement.

Difficult intubation may occur as a result of limited cervical spine movement and ankylosis of temporomandibular joint, limiting mouth opening in >10% patients. Cricoarytenoid arthritis presents as dyspnoea and hoarseness. Cardiovascular complications include aortic incompetence, mitral valve disease and conduction defects. Thoracic spine involvement limits chest expansion and is associated with pulmonary fibrosis.

Rheumatoid arthritis

An autoimmune disease of unknown aetiology. Affects females much more than males. Primarily affects joints but 50% have extra-articular involvement.

Cervical instability (atlantoaxial and subaxial subluxation) presenting as sensory symptoms, weakness, flexor spasms and urinary incontinence; 25% of patients are asymptomatic. Cricoarytenoid involvement may result in upper airway obstruction. Assess cervical spine with lateral X-rays in flexion and extension. Distance >3 mm between odontoid peg and posterior border of the anterior arch of the atlas suggests subluxation. Subluxation may necessitate awake fibreoptic intubation. Temporomandibular joint involvement may limit mouth opening.

Lung involvement includes generalized fibrosis with a restrictive defect, rheumatoid nodules and pleural effusions. Perform preoperative pulmonary function tests and arterial blood gases if necessary.

Cardiac involvement includes pericarditis, endocarditis and left ventricular failure. Renal failure is common due to vasculitis, amyloidosis and drug toxicity. Chronic anaemia results from anaemia of chronic disease, upper GI bleeding from NSAIDs, bone marrow suppression from gold and penicillamine and haemolytic anaemia.

Mucopolysaccharidoses (Hurler's, Hunter's syndromes)

A group of inherited connective tissue disorders. Enzyme defects result in the accumulation of intermediate products of degradation of mucopolysaccharides. Characterized by dwarfism, cardiac failure, abnormal airway anatomy, respiratory failure, hepatosplenomegaly and skeletal abnormalities. Associated with prolonged recovery from anaesthesia, with breath holding, bronchospasm and respiratory failure.

Glycogen storage diseases (von Gierke's, Pompe's, McArdle's, Thompson's diseases)

A group of genetic diseases with defects in enzymes controlling glycogen metabolism, causing muscle and liver disease. Cramps, stiffness, muscle weakness and muscle pains. Hypertrophic cardiomyopathy (Pompe's) and hypoglycaemia (von Gierke's). Avoid shivering, tourniquets and suxamethonium, all of which cause muscle damage. Avoid hypoglycaemia. Risk of post-operative respiratory failure.

Von Recklinghausen's neurofibromatosis

Autosomal dominant condition characterized by multiple neurofibromata and pigmented skin patches (café-au-lait spots). Airway difficulties due to upper airway neurofibromas. Kyphoscoliosis, undiagnosed associated malignancies, e.g. phaeochromocytoma, fibrosing alveolitis, renal artery stenosis and hypertension. Abnormal sensitivity to muscle relaxants.

Bibliography

Simpson KH, Ellis FR: Inherited metabolic diseases and anaesthesia. In: Nimmo WS, Rowbotham DJ, Smith G, editors: *Anaesthesia*, ed 2, Oxford, 1994, Blackwell Scientific Publications, pp 1113–1129.

INFECTION CONTROL

GUIDELINES – INFECTION CONTROL IN ANAESTHESIA
Association of Anaesthetists of Great Britain and Ireland 2008

Healthcare organizations now have a legal responsibility to implement changes to reduce healthcare associated infections (HCAIs). The Health Act 2006 provided the Healthcare Commission with statutory powers to enforce compliance with the Code of Practice for the Prevention and Control of Healthcare Associated Infection (The Code). The Code provides a framework for NHS bodies to plan and implement structures and systems aimed at prevention of HCAIs. The Code sets out criteria that mandate NHS bodies, including Acute Trusts, and which ensure that patients are cared for in a clean environment. Anaesthetists should be in the forefront of ensuring that their patients are cared for in the safest possible environment. Further advice can be obtained from the Department of Health website: www.clean-safe-care.nhs.uk.

Summary

1. A named consultant in each department of anaesthesia should liaise with Trust Infection Control Teams and Occupational Health Departments to ensure that relevant specialist standards are established and monitored in all areas of anaesthetic practice.

2. Precautions against the transmission of infection between patient and anaesthetist or between patients should be a routine part of anaesthetic practice. In particular, anaesthetists must ensure that hand hygiene becomes an indispensable part of their clinical culture.
3. Anaesthetists must comply with local theatre infection control policies including the safe use and disposal of sharps.
4. Anaesthetic equipment is a potential vector for transmission of disease. Policies should be documented to ensure that nationally recommended decontamination practices are followed and audited for all re-usable anaesthetic equipment.
5. Single use equipment should be utilized where appropriate but a sterile supplies department (SSD) should process reusable items.
6. An effective, new bacterial/viral breathing circuit filter should be used for every patient and a local policy developed for the re-use of breathing circuits in line with manufacturer's instructions. The AAGBI recommends that anaesthetic departments should consider changing anaesthetic circuits on a daily basis in line with daily cleaning protocols.
7. Appropriate infection control precautions should be established for each anaesthetic procedure, to include maximal barrier precautions for the insertion of central venous catheters, spinal and epidural procedures and any invasive procedures in high risk patients.

Bibliography

Association of Anaesthetists of Great Britain and Ireland: Infection control in anaesthesia, *Anaesthesia* 63:1027–1036, 2008.

MECHANISMS OF ANAESTHESIA

General anaesthetic agents are not related to any specific group of compounds, but depend more upon the solubility characteristics of the molecule. Although these agents have a selective effect on CNS function, at high doses, all organ systems are affected.

Meyer–Overton theory

States that MAC × solubility = K (Fig. 6.8).

May provide some evidence that the site of action of the volatile agents is at a hydrophobic site, i.e. lipids within the cell membrane. However, many discrepancies have led to a move away from this theory.

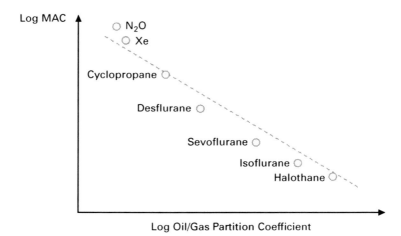

Figure 6.8 Meyer–Overton theory.

Hydrate hypothesis (Pauling and Miller 1961)

The fact that the brain consists of 78% water led to the suggestion that anaesthetics act on hydrophobic molecules. However, there is poor correlation between anaesthetic potency and water solubility. This theory also predicted that two anaesthetic agents would have a synergistic effect, but volatile agents appear only to have an additive effect (Fig. 6.9).

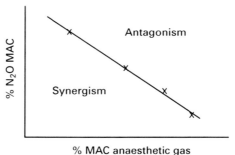

Figure 6.9 Hydrate hypothesis.

Clathrate hypothesis

This evolved from the hydrate hypothesis to suggest that anaesthetic molecules are trapped within a sphere of water molecules. These hydrates may then act to decrease nerve conduction or stiffen lipid membranes and occlude ion channels. Little evidence now exists for this theory.

Critical volume hypothesis (Lever 1971)

This followed on from pressure reversal studies to suggest that when cell membranes are expanded to a critical volume, cellular function is impaired. High pressures then reverse the expansion to restore normal cellular function. A 0.4% volume increase at the critical site correlates with onset of anaesthesia.

Evidence for critical volume comes from studies of pressure reversal. Light from luminous bacteria is dimmed by anaesthetic agents but returns to normal under high pressures (Johnson in 1940). Tadpoles stop swimming in an anaesthetic solution, but resume swimming as the hydrostatic pressure is increased (Johnson and Flagler in 1950). However, experiments to very high pressures with tadpoles show a loss of correlation of anaesthesia with pressure.

Multisite expansion hypothesis (Halsey 1979)

This hypothesis proposed that although anaesthetic agents expand the membrane at critical sites, the actual sites involved may vary between anaesthetic agents and have a finite size and limited capacity for the anaesthetic. Expansion at these sites may act to impair ion channel function and thus electrical activity of the cell membrane. Correctly predicts the non-additive potencies of i.v. anaesthetic agents.

Molecular site of action

Lipids. Anaesthetic agents may change the fluidity of the lipid membrane, thereby altering the function of membrane proteins contained within it.

Proteins. Anaesthetic agents may directly block ion channels or alter the ability of protein molecules to change their shape.

Cellular site of action

Synapses and axons. Local anaesthetics may act on axonal membranes to block ion channels. General anaesthetics act at synapses to reduce transmitter release and alter the interaction of the neurotransmitter with receptor. GAs may also affect presynaptic calcium channels, reducing the axonal calcium necessary for binding vesicles of neurotransmitter to the presynaptic membrane.

Higher neuronal circuits

GA may cause loss of consciousness by blocking the reticular formation processing of sensory input to the cortex (corticothalamic-reticular loop). Central noradrenaline release by some anaesthetic agents (e.g. ketamine, nitrous oxide, xenon) may also be associated with anaesthesia.

Studies in isolated spinal cord suggest that anaesthetics may also inhibit excitatory receptors (NMDA, neuronal nicotinic, $5HT_3$) and stimulate inhibitory receptors (glycine, $GABA_A$).

Nitric oxide

It is suggested that nitric oxide (NO) inhibition may be an important mechanism of action of some general anaesthetic agents. NO is involved in central nociceptive pathways and maintaining wakefulness. NO synthase inhibitors cause a dose-dependent reduction in MAC for volatile agents and impair the righting reflex in mice, suggesting that the effects involve higher integrative neuronal processes rather than analgesia alone.

Bibliography

Hameroff SR: The entwined mysteries of anesthesia and consciousness, *Anesthesiology* 105:400–412, 2006.

Hemmings HC: Sodium channels and the synaptic mechanisms of inhaled anaesthetics, *Br J Anaesth* 103:61–69, 2009.

Sonner JM, Antognini JF, Dutton RC, et al: Inhaled anesthetics and immobility: mechanisms, mysteries and minimum alveolar anesthetic concentration, *Anesth Anal* 97:718–740, 2003.

Weir CJ: The molecular mechanisms of general anaesthesia: dissecting the $GABA_A$ receptor, *Contin Edu Anaesth, Crit Care Pain* 6:49–53, 2006.

ORGAN DONATION AND TRANSPLANTATION

Diagnosis of brainstem death

A CODE OF PRACTICE FOR THE DIAGNOSIS OF BRAINSTEM DEATH
Department of Health 1998

Definition

Irreversible loss of capacity for consciousness combined with irreversible capacity to breathe; 50% of cases are due to trauma, 30% to subarachnoid haemorrhage.

Brainstem testing

Preconditions

1. No doubt that the patient's condition is due to irremediable brain damage of known aetiology
2. The patient is deeply unconscious, but not due to depressant drugs, hypothermia or reversible circulatory, metabolic or endocrine disturbances
3. The patient is being maintained on a ventilator because spontaneous respiration is inadequate or has ceased.

Diagnosis of brainstem death

All brainstem reflexes must be absent, i.e.:

- Pupils fixed, dilated and unresponsive
- No corneal reflex
- No vestibulo-ocular reflexes to >50 mL iced water (must view eardrums first)
- No cranial motor response to pain. No limb response to supraorbital pressure
- No gag or cough reflex
- No spontaneous ventilation on disconnection from ventilator. Give 100% O_2 for 10 min, then disconnect and give 6 L O_2/min via tracheal catheter during which time observe for respiratory effort. Allow $P_a co_2$ to rise >6.65 kPa before cessation of test. (Alternatively, ventilate with 100% O_2 for 10 min, then 5% CO_2 in oxygen for 5 min.)

Repetition of testing

Diagnosis should be made by at least two doctors (of whom at least one should be a consultant) registered for more than 5 years who are competent in this field and are not members of the transplant team.

Two sets of tests should be carried out, either separately or together. Timing between the two tests should be adequate for the reassurance of all those directly concerned. Legal time of death is the time of the first set of tests.

Management

Relatives, partners and carers must be kept fully informed.

Maintenance of treatment to sustain normal physiological parameters is allowed after diagnosis of brainstem death in order to maintain the condition of the organs. Elective ventilation solely to preserve organ function is unlawful.

Persistent vegetative state

Characterized by cortical damage with an intact brainstem.

Management of patients for organ donation

GUIDELINES FOR THE MANAGEMENT OF POTENTIAL ORGAN AND TISSUE DONORS
Department of Health 1998

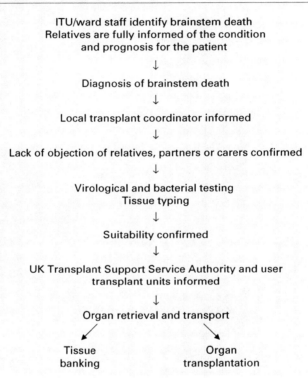

ITU/ward staff identify brainstem death
Relatives are fully informed of the condition
and prognosis for the patient
↓
Diagnosis of brainstem death
↓
Local transplant coordinator informed
↓
Lack of objection of relatives, partners or carers confirmed
↓
Virological and bacterial testing
Tissue typing
↓
Suitability confirmed
↓
UK Transplant Support Service Authority and user
transplant units informed
↓
Organ retrieval and transport

Tissue
banking

Organ
transplantation

It is important to maintain normal physiological parameters to prevent end-organ damage. As many as 20% of hearts from otherwise suitable patients are lost to donation through poor management. Sympathetic storm may occur as ICP rises, causing brainstem ischaemia (tachycardia, hypertension, neurogenic pulmonary oedema), which if untreated will cause end organ damage. As vasomotor centres in the brainstem die, endogenous sympathetic activity is lost and the patient develops a relative vasodilatory hypovolaemia and hypotension. Brainstem death also results in endocrine failure (diabetes insipidus, cortisol deficiency, hypothyroidism) and impaired thermoregulation.

Preoperative

Regular physiotherapy and careful fluid balance avoid deterioration in lung function. Maintain core temperature above 35°C with warming blanket and fluid warmer. Check electrolytes, full blood count, blood gases and urine/

plasma osmolality. Right subclavian artery and left brachiocephalic vein are divided early in the operation, so place a left radial arterial cannula and right central venous cannula. Fluid replacement with colloid is recommended to reduce tissue oedema caused with crystalloids.

Operative

Record ECG, central and venous pressure and core temperature. Maintain with O_2:N_2O mixture to provide adequate S_aO_2. Pancuronium prevents spinal reflexes causing muscular contraction. Severe hypertension may require treatment with isoflurane/sevoflurane or sodium nitroprusside. Cephalosporin and methylprednisolone are generally requested by transplant team. Anticipate large volume losses.

For multiple organ donation, the thorax and abdomen are opened by a longitudinal incision from the suprasternal notch to the umbilicus. The liver and kidneys are mobilized, during which compression of the inferior vena cava may cause hypotension. The patient is then anticoagulated with heparin (3 mg.kg^{-1}) and the thorax opened. Ensure each tidal breath is adequate to inflate all lobes of the lungs if lung harvest is being performed. Thoracic organs are then removed prior to removal of abdominal organs.

Management of recipients for renal transplantation

(See also 'Anaesthesia and renal failure' section in Ch. 4.)

Preoperative

Optimize fluid balance and consider preoperative dialysis. Aim to normalize electrolytes, particularly K$^+$. Use in-line leucocyte filter if blood transfusion is required. Avoid veins on forearms.

Anaesthesia preparation

ECG (CM5), invasive BP, pulse oximetry, CVP, urinary catheter, regular blood glucose. Avoid Hartmann's as this contains K$^+$.

Induction

Thiopentone, etomidate, midazolam and propofol are all suitable; 5–7 µg.kg^{-1} fentanyl on induction provides good perioperative analgesia and reduces the hypertension from the pressor response. Remifentanil is particularly suitable in these patients. Neuromuscular blockade with suxamethonium (if K$^+$ <5.0) if rapid sequence induction is required, followed by atracurium or cis-atracurium. High-dose methylprednisolone given at induction for renal transplantation may cause circulatory collapse, arrhythmias and cardiac arrest.

Maintenance

Patients with chronic renal failure (CRF) are acidotic, so avoid spontaneous respiration. Isoflurane has least metabolism to F$^-$ and minimal nephrotoxicity. N_2O is safe. Keep warm and well hydrated, particularly when clamp is removed (CVP above normal). Replace fluid loss with salt-containing solutions. Aim for normotension.

Other

Prior to removal of arterial clamp and reperfusion of transplant kidney, give mannitol $0.5\,g.kg^{-1}$, furosemide 250 mg (omit if live, related donor) and dopamine $3\,\mu g.kg^{-1}$ per min.

Postoperative

Usually extubated immediately postoperatively. Monitor CVP and renal function. Consider early postoperative dialysis if there is poor graft function. Fentanyl PCA provides good postoperative analgesia. Immunosuppression for transplantation is associated with increased infection risk. Currently 5-year organ survival is 60%.

Management of recipients for cardiac/lung transplantation

Survival rates are improving as follows:

- heart – 75–80% at 5 years
- lung – 65% at 1 year
- heart–lung – 55–60% at 1 year.

Similar anaesthetic technique to that for cardiac surgery.
  Specific problems with management include:

- No SNS-mediated tachycardia, making atropine ineffective; use isoprenaline
- No ANS response to hypovolaemia, with exaggerated responses to both hypovolaemia and decreased SVR
- Delayed response to circulating catecholamines (5–6 min)
- Arrhythmias (mostly ventricular) common for 6 months post-transplant
- No cough reflex following stimulation distal to bronchial anastomosis and no lung lymphatic drainage.

Anaesthesia for non-cardiac surgery after heart/lung transplant

Main problems are:

- Donor coronary artery disease – immunologically mediated. Presents as impaired LV function and arrhythmias. Maintain coronary perfusion pressure during surgery.
- Immunosuppression, resulting in increased infection risk. Ensure CMV-negative recipients only receive CMV-negative blood products.
- Cardiac denervation altering effects of sympathomimetic and anticholinergic drugs

General anaesthesia with i.v. induction, opioid, neuromuscular blocker and volatile agent with intubation and ventilation is suitable for most patients. Maintain adequate preload to minimize haemodynamic instability. Spinal and epidural techniques may cause exaggerated hypotensive responses. All cannulae should be placed using an aseptic technique and bacterial filters used on all intravenous lines. Avoid excessive airway pressures stretching suture lines in patients following lung transplant. Also avoid fluid overload in these patients because of impaired pulmonary lymphatic drainage. Use appropriate antibiotics. Prophylaxis. Regular physiotherapy and postural drainage postoperatively.

Bibliography

Baez B, Castillo M: Anesthetic considerations for lung transplantation, *Semin Cardiothorac Vasc Anesth* 12:122–127, 2008.

Blasco LM, Parameshwar J, Vuylsteke A: Anaesthesia for noncardiac surgery in the heart transplant recipient, *Curr Opin Anaesth* 22:109–113, 2009.

Colson P: Renal disease and transplantation, *Curr Opin Anaesth* 11:345–348, 1998.

Department of Health: *A code of practice for the diagnosis of brain stem death, including guidelines for the identification and management of potential organ and tissue donors*, London, 1998, Department of Health. www.dh.gov.uk/en/ Publicationsandstatistics/Publications/PublicationsPolicyAndGuidance/ DH_4009696.

Edgar P, Bullock R, Bonner S: Management of the potential heart-beating organ donor, *BJA CEPD Rev* 4:86–90, 2004.

Jennett B: Brain stem death defines death in law, *BMJ* 318:1755, 1999.

Morgan-Hughes NJ, Hood G: Anaesthesia for a patient with a cardiac transplant, *BJA CEPD Rev* 2:74–78, 2002.

Ozier Y, Klinck JR: Anesthetic management of hepatic transplantation, *Curr Opin Anaesth* 21:391–400, 2008.

Pallis C, Harley DH: *ABC of brainstem death*, London, 1996, BMJ Publishing.

Ramakrishna H, Jaroszewski DE, Arabia FA: Adult cardiac transplantation: a review of perioperative management (part I), *Ann Card Anaesth* 12:71–78, 2009.

Ramakrishna H, Jaroszewski DE, Arabia FA: Adult cardiac transplantation: a review of perioperative management (part II), *Ann Card Anaesth* 12:155–165, 2009.

SarinKapoor H, Kaur R, Kaur H: Anaesthesia for renal transplant surgery, *Acta Anaesth Scand* 51:1354–1367, 2007.

Patient safety

NATIONAL PATIENT SAFETY AGENCY
Never Events, February 2009

Never events are serious, largely preventable patient safety incidents that should not occur if the available preventative measures have been implemented.

1. Wrong site surgery
2. Retained instrument post-operation
3. Wrong route administration of chemotherapy
4. Misplaced naso or orogastric tube not detected prior to use
5. Inpatient suicide using non-collapsible rails
6. Escape from within the secure perimeter of medium or high secure mental health services by patients who are transferred prisoners
7. In-hospital maternal death from post-partum haemorrhage after elective caesarean section
8. Intravenous administration of mis-selected concentrated potassium chloride

SURGICAL SAFETY CHECKLIST
World Health Organization, January 2009

WHO Surgical Safety Checklist
(adapted for England and Wales)

SIGN IN (To be read out loud)

Before induction of anaesthesia

Has the patient confirmed his/her identity, site, procedure and consent?
☐ Yes

Is the surgical site marked?
☐ Yes

Is the anaesthesia machine and medication check complete?
☐ Yes

Does the patient have a:
Known allergy
☐ No
☐ Yes

Difficult airway/aspiration risk?
☐ No
☐ Yes, and equipment/assistance available

Risk of >500ml blood loss (7ml/kg in children)?
☐ No
☐ Yes, and adequate IV access/fluids planned

Name
Signature of
Registered Practitioner

Patient Details

Last name:
First name:
Date of birth:
NHS Number:
Procedure:
If the NHS Number is not immediately available, a temporary number ?????

TIME OUT (To be read out loud)

Before start of surgical intervention for example, skin incision

Have all team members introduced themselves by name and role?
☐ Yes

Surgeon, Anaesthetist and Registered Practitioner verbally confirms:
☐ What is the patient's name?
☐ What procedure, site and position are planned?

Anticipated critical events
Surgeon:
☐ How much blood loss is anticipated?
☐ Are there any specific equipment requirements or special investigations?
☐ Are there any critical or unexpected steps you want the team to know about?

Anaesthetist:
☐ Are there any patient specific concerns?
☐ What is the patient's ASA grade?
☐ What monitoring equipment and other specific levels of support are required, for example blood?

Nurse/ODP:
☐ Has the sterility of the instrumentation been confirmed (including indicator results)?
☐ Are there any equipment issues or concerns?

Has the surgical site infection (SSI) bundle been undertaken?
☐ Yes/not applicable
  • Antibiotic prophylaxis within the last 60 minutes
  • Patient warming
  • Hair removal
  • Glycaemic control

Has VTE prophylaxis been undertaken?
☐ Yes/not applicable

Is essential imaging displayed?
☐ Yes/not applicable

Name
Signature of
Registered Practitioner

SIGN OUT (To be read out loud)

Before any member of the team leaves the operating room

Registered Practitioner verbally confirms with the team:
☐ Has the name of the procedure been recorded?
☐ Has it been confirmed that instruments, swabs and sharps counts are complete (or not applicable)?
☐ Have the specimens been labeled (including patient name)?
☐ Have any equipment problems been identified that need to be addressed?

Surgeon, Anaesthetist and Registered Practitioner
☐ What are the key concerns for recovery and management of this patient

Name
Signature of
Registered Practitioner

This checklist contains the core content for England and Wales

www.npsa.nhs.uk/nrls

Figure 6.10 WHO surgical safety. (World Health Organisation, 2009.)

POST-ANAESTHETIC RECOVERY

Management of patients in the recovery room

Patients must be observed on a one-to-one basis by an anaesthetist, recovery nurse or other properly trained member of staff until they have regained airway control and cardiovascular stability and are able to communicate.

The frequency of observations will depend on the stage of recovery, nature of surgery and clinical condition of the patient. It should not be influenced by staffing levels. The following information should be recorded:

- Level of consciousness
- SaO_2 and oxygen administration
- Blood pressure
- Respiratory rate
- Heart rate and rhythm
- Pain intensity, e.g. verbal rating scale (none, mild, moderate, severe)
- Drugs administered
- Other parameters, e.g. temperature, urinary output, central venous pressure, surgical drainage.

Discharge from the recovery room

The following criteria must be fulfilled:

- The patient is fully conscious and able to maintain a clear airway.
- Respiration and oxygenation are satisfactory.

POST-ANAESTHETIC RECOVERY
Association of Anaesthetists of Great Britain and Ireland 2002

Key recommendations

1. After general, epidural or spinal anaesthesia, all patients should be recovered in a specially designated area which complies with the standards and recommendations described in this document.
2. The anaesthetist must formally hand over care of a patient to a recovery room nurse or other appropriately trained member of staff.
3. Agreed criteria for discharge of patients from the recovery room to the ward should be in place in all units.
4. An effective emergency call system must be in place in every recovery room.
5. No fewer than two staff should be present when there is a patient in the recovery room who does not fulfil the criteria for discharge to the ward.
6. All specialist recovery staff should be appropriately trained, ideally to a nationally recognized standard.

7. All patients must be observed on a one-to-one basis by an anaesthetist, recovery nurse or other appropriately trained member of staff until they have regained airway control and cardiovascular stability and are able to communicate.
8. The removal of tracheal tubes from patients in the recovery room is the responsibility of the anaesthetist.
9. There should be a specially designated area for the recovery of children.
10. All standards and recommendations described in this document should be applied to all recovery areas where anaesthesia is administered including obstetric, cardiology, X-ray, dental and psychiatric units and community hospitals.
11. Patient dignity and privacy should be considered at all times.
12. When critically ill patients are managed in the recovery room because of bed shortages, the primary responsibility for the patient lies with the critical care team. The standard of nursing and medical care should be equal to that within the critical care unit.
13. Audit and critical incident systems should be in place in all recovery rooms.

- The cardiovascular system is stable. The specific values of pulse and blood pressure should approximate to normal pre-operative values or be at an acceptable level commensurate with the planned postoperative care.
- Pain and emesis should be controlled and suitable analgesic and anti-emetic regimens prescribed.
- Temperature should be within acceptable limits.
- Oxygen and intravenous therapy, if appropriate, should be prescribed.

Bibliography

Association of Anaesthetists of Great Britain and Ireland: *Post-anaesthetic recovery*, London, 2002. Reproduced with the kind permission of the Association of anaesthetists of Great Britain and Ireland.
National Patient Safety Agency 2009 Never Events: www.nrls.npsa.nhs.uk/resources/collections/never-events.
WHO Surgical safety checklist (adapted for England and Wales). 2009: http://www.safesurg.org/uploads/1/0/9/0/1090835/npsa_checklist.pdf.

POSTOPERATIVE NAUSEA AND VOMITING (PONV)

Physiology

The vomiting centre is situated in the reticular formation of the medulla within the blood–brain barrier. The chemoreceptor trigger zone is situated in the area postrema on the floor of the IV ventricle and receives input from many afferents (Fig. 6.11).

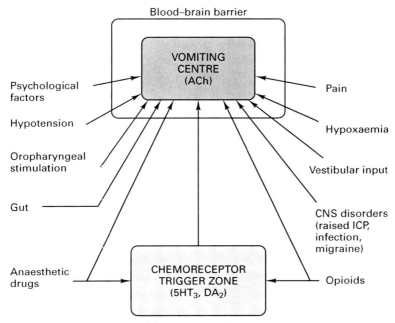

Figure 6.11 Afferent pathways of the vomiting reflex.

Vomiting reflex

Activated by the vomiting centre via the glossopharyngeal, hypoglossal, trigeminal, accessory and spinal nerves. Abdominal muscles contract against a closed glottis to raise intra-abdominal pressure. The lower oesophageal sphincter then relaxes and the pyloric sphincter contracts to expel the gastric contents.

One-third of all surgical patients experience nausea and vomiting, which may last for up to 24h postoperatively. Until recently, it has been an underestimated problem which is becoming more relevant with the rapid growth of day-case surgery.

Effects of PONV

- Wound pain
- Distress and exhaustion
- Commonest cause of patient dissatisfaction with surgery
- Dehydration and electrolyte imbalance
- Breakdown of surgical wound
- Prevents administration of oral medication and nutrition

- Risk of aspiration if impaired upper airway reflexes
- Delays mobilization and prolongs stay in hospital
- Increases need for extra nursing
- Admission of day-case patient.

Risk factors for PONV

- Female
- Obese
- Young age
- Past history of PONV
- History of motion sickness or migraine
- Prolonged starvation or recent oral intake.

Surgery associated with PONV

- GI surgery due to bowel manipulation
- ENT surgery with pharyngeal or middle ear stimulation
- Eye surgery involving extraocular muscles
- Gynaecological surgery
- Orthopaedic surgery
- Emergency surgery.

Perioperative drugs causing PONV

- Volatile agents: enflurane and halothane > isoflurane
- N_2O distends bowel
- Thiopentone, etomidate and methohexitone (propofol may have intrinsic antiemetic properties due to $5HT_3$ antagonism)
- Hypotension from regional techniques (duration > degree of hypotension)
- All opioids
- Anticholinergics.

Prevention

- Adequate but not prolonged fasting
- Avoid postoperative movement, e.g. bumpy trolleys
- Avoid excessive pharyngeal stimulation, e.g. suctioning
- Avoid gastric inflation
- Gentle handling of bowel because 5HT stored in enterochromaffin cells of the GI tract is released in response to surgical manipulation
- Ensure adequate oxygenation, analgesia, hydration and blood pressure.

Treatment

Use antiemetic prophylaxis in high-risk patients. (Low-dose droperidol 0.005 mg/kg may be more effective than high dose.)

Use drug appropriate to neurotransmitter: anticholinergic for vagally mediated vomiting, e.g. hyoscine; antidopaminergic for opioid-mediated vomiting, e.g. phenothiazines, butyrophenones. Ondansetron ($5HT_3$ antagonist) may be useful in chemotherapy-induced vomiting and vomiting resistant to conventional drugs where it is more effective than metoclopramide or droperidol.

Bibliography

Kenny GNC: Risk factors for postoperative nausea and vomiting, *Anaesthesia* 49(Suppl):6–10, 1994.

Naylor RJ, Inall FC: The physiology and pharmacology of postoperative nausea and vomiting, *Anaesthesia* 49(Suppl):2–5, 1994.

Kranke P, Schuster F, Eberhart LH: Recent advances, trends and economic considerations in the risk assessment, prevention and treatment of postoperative nausea and vomiting, *Expert Opin Pharmacother* 8:3217–3235, 2007.

PREOPERATIVE ASSESSMENT

Definition. Preoperative assessment establishes that the patient is fully informed and wishes to undergo the procedure. It ensures that the patient is fit for the surgery and anaesthetic. It minimizes the risk of late cancellations by ensuring that all essential resources and discharge requirements are identified.

Poor/no preoperative assessment is responsible for 50% of all day-case surgery cancellations. Work by the Modernisation Agency's Preoperative Assessment Project has shown that implementing preoperative assessment can decrease the number of patients who did not attend (DNAs).

Preoperative assessment should:

- Confirm that the patient wishes to have the operation and ensure that they have given informed written consent.
- Assess the patient's suitability and fitness for surgery and anaesthesia, including the risks of the combined effects of surgery and anaesthesia.
- Ensure the patient fully understands the proposed procedure and has had the opportunity for discussion.
- Provide information about the preoperative process, e.g. changes to preoperative medication, fasting instructions, etc., including any measures to improve the outcome of the surgery, e.g. weight loss, stopping smoking, etc.
- Ensure adequate arrangements are in place for post-discharge care.

Investigations

Blanket routine preoperative investigations are inefficient, expensive and unnecessary. Medical and anaesthetic problems are identified more efficiently by the taking of a history and by the physical examination of patients. No investigations are required prior to minor surgery in otherwise healthy patients.

- An ECG should be performed on every patient with a cardiac or related history but is not indicated for asymptomatic males <40 years or asymptomatic females <50 years.
- Hb is only required if the history indicates the Hb may be low or where it is anticipated there may be significant blood loss at surgery.
- Routine biochemistry is indicated only in those patients whose history or current medication makes it necessary.
- Routine chest X-ray is not indicated.

Fasting guidelines (AAGBI 2001)

- For safety reasons, patients should not eat or drink prior to anaesthesia. The AAGBI recommends the minimum fasting periods based on the American Society of Anaesthesiologists (ASA) guidelines:
  - 6h for solid food, infant formula, or other milk
  - 4h for breast milk
  - 2h for clear non-particulate and non-carbonated fluids.
- Each NHS Trust should have agreed written policies.
- The following patients should not be left for long periods without hydration, and may require intravenous fluids prior to surgery:
  - Elderly patients
  - Patients who have undergone bowel preparation
  - Sick patients
  - Children
  - Breast-feeding mothers.

PREOPERATIVE ASSESSMENT. THE ROLE OF THE ANAESTHETIST
Association of Anaesthetists of Great Britain and Ireland 2001

Summary

1. The anaesthetist is uniquely qualified to assess anaesthetic risk.
2. The anaesthetist is responsible for deciding whether a patient is fit for anaesthesia.
3. All patients must be seen by an anaesthetist before undergoing an operation that requires the services of an anaesthetist.
4. The aim in assessing patients before anaesthesia and surgery is to improve outcome.
5. The provision of a preoperative screening and assessment service improves efficiency and enhances patient care.

6. Nursing and other trained staff play an essential role when, working to agreed protocols, they screen patients for fitness for anaesthesia and surgery.
7. Access to an anaesthetist by pre-assessment personnel is essential.
8. Anaesthetic preoperative assessment clinics provide the opportunity for anaesthetists to see those patients who have been identified by screening and assessment as presenting potential anaesthetic problems.
9. The anaesthetic preoperative assessment clinic must involve consultant anaesthetist presence which is recognized as a fixed commitment within a job plan.
10. Blanket routine preoperative investigations are inefficient, expensive and unnecessary.

Bibliography

Association of Anaesthetists of Great Britain and Ireland: *Preoperative assessment, The role of the anaesthetist, 2001.* Reproduced with the kind permission of the Association of anaesthetists of Great Britain and Ireland.

Levy DM: Preoperative fasting – 60 years on from Mendelson, *Contin Edu Anaesth, Crit Care Pain* 6:215–218, 2006.

NHS Modernisation Agency: *National good practice guidance on pre-operative assessment for day surgery,* London, 2002, NHS.

NICE: *Preoperative tests – The use of routine preoperative tests for elective surgery,* London, 2003, National Institute of Clinical Excellence.

Royal College of Nursing: *Perioperative fasting in adults and children,* 2005. www.rcn. org.uk/publications/pdf/guidelines/perioperative_fasting_adults_children_full.pdf.

RESUSCITATION

The resuscitation guidelines are revised by the European Resuscitation Council every five years; the current version was published in 2010.

Adult basic life support guidelines

Basic life support is summarized in Figure 6.12a. The 2005 guidelines revised the compression:ventilation ratio to 30:2 following evidence that even short interruptions to external chest compression are disastrous for outcome. Compression-only CPR is acceptable if the rescuer is unwilling or unable to perform mouth-to-mouth ventilation.

Adult advanced life support guidelines (Fig. 6.12b)

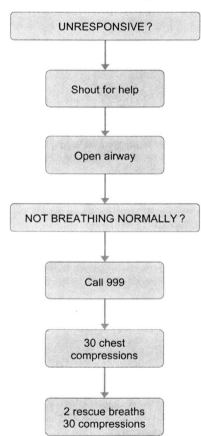

Figure 6.12 (A) Adult basic life support guidelines. (Resuscitation Council (UK) 2010 © RC(UK).)

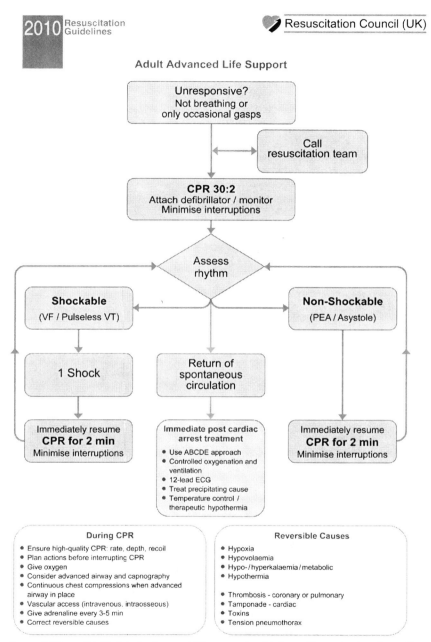

Adult Advanced Life Support

Unresponsive?
Not breathing or
only occasional gasps

Call
resuscitation team

CPR 30:2
Attach defibrillator / monitor
Minimise interruptions

Assess
rhythm

Shockable
(VF / Pulseless VT)

Non-Shockable
(PEA / Asystole)

1 Shock

Return of
spontaneous
circulation

Immediately resume
CPR for 2 min
Minimise interruptions

Immediate post cardiac
arrest treatment
• Use ABCDE approach
• Controlled oxygenation and
  ventilation
• 12-lead ECG
• Treat precipitating cause
• Temperature control /
  therapeutic hypothermia

Immediately resume
CPR for 2 min
Minimise interruptions

During CPR
• Ensure high-quality CPR: rate, depth, recoil
• Plan actions before interrupting CPR
• Give oxygen
• Consider advanced airway and capnography
• Continuous chest compressions when advanced
  airway in place
• Vascular access (intravenous, intraosseous)
• Give adrenaline every 3-5 min
• Correct reversible causes

Reversible Causes
• Hypoxia
• Hypovolaemia
• Hypo-/hyperkalaemia/metabolic
• Hypothermia

• Thrombosis - coronary or pulmonary
• Tamponade - cardiac
• Toxins
• Tension pneumothorax

Figure 6.12, cont'd (B) Adult advanced life support guidelines. (Resuscitation Council (UK) 2010 © RC(UK).)

Defibrillation

Biphasic waveforms (Fig. 6.13) have the following advantages over older monophasic waveforms (Fig. 6.14):

- Lower energy benefits – greater first shock efficacy at lower energy levels
- Biphasic defibrillators can alter the waveform to compensate for variations in transthoracic impedance.
- Less post-shock dysfunction – 90% less post-shock ST segment changes and fewer post-shock arrhythmias.

One paddle/pad should be placed below the right clavicle in the midclavicular line and the other over the lower left ribs in the mid/anterior axillary line (just outside the position of the normal cardiac apex).

Defibrillation strategy

Treat VF/pulseless VT with a single shock, followed by immediate resumption of CPR. Do not reassess the rhythm or feel for a pulse. After 2 min of CPR, check

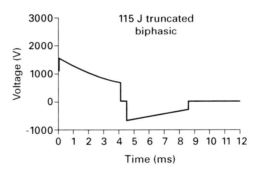

Figure 6.13 Biphasic waveform (biphasic truncated exponential).

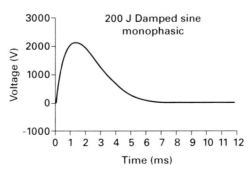

Figure 6.14 Monophasic waveform (damped sinusoidal).

the rhythm and give another shock (if indicated). If VF/pulseless VT occurs in the cardiac catheterisation laboratory or in the immediate post-operative period following cardiac surgery give up to three quick successive (stacked) shocks.

The initial shock energy level for biphasic defibrillators is 150–200 J. Give second and subsequent shocks at the same or higher levels. The shock energy level when using a monophasic defibrillator is 360 J for both the initial and subsequent shocks.

Drugs

Delivery of drugs via a tracheal tube is no longer recommended – if intravenous (IV) access cannot be achieved, give drugs by the intraosseous (IO) route. Drugs administered via peripheral veins or IO should be flushed with 20 ml of 0.9% saline.

Adrenaline (epinephrine)

The α-adrenergic effects of adrenaline cause vasoconstriction, which increases myocardial and cerebral perfusion pressure during cardiac arrest; however, there is no placebo-controlled study that shows that the routine use of any vasopressor at any stage during human cardiac arrest increases survival to hospital discharge. Despite the lack of human data the use of adrenaline is still recommended, based largely on experimental data.

When treating VF/VT cardiac arrest, adrenaline 1 mg is given once chest compressions have restarted after the third shock and then every 3–5 minutes (during alternate cycles of CPR). In the 2005 Guidelines, adrenaline was given just before third shock. This subtle change in the timing of adrenaline administration is to enable drug delivery to be separated totally from attempted defibrillation. In this way, it is hoped that shock delivery will be more efficient and will minimise the interruption in chest compressions. In patients in asystole or PEA, give adrenaline 1 mg IV immediately once IV/IO access is achieved.

Atropine

Atropine is no longer recommended for routine use in asystole or pulseless electrical activity.

Amiodarone

The use of amiodarone in shock-refractory VF improves survival to hospital admission compared with lidocaine. If VF/VT persists after three shocks, give amiodarone 300 mg by bolus injection after the third shock. A further dose of 150 mg may be given for recurrent or refractory VF/VT, followed by an infusion of 900 mg over 24 h. Lidocaine 1 mg.kg^{-1} may be used as an alternative if amiodarone is not available.

Bicarbonate

Although acidosis is known to depress myocardial contractility (pH <7.2), reduce tissue oxygen delivery and increase susceptibility to VF, there is no good evidence that correction of pH improves outcome of CPR.

Side-effects of bicarbonate include:

- increased osmolality through large sodium load
- increased $P_a co_2$ causing respiratory acidosis
- metabolic alkalosis
- paradoxical intracellular acidosis (limited evidence)
- decreased ionized Ca^{2+}
- impaired arterial oxygenation and reduced myocardial oxygen consumption
- increased risk of neonatal intraventricular haemorrhage.

Giving sodium bicarbonate routinely during cardiac arrest is not recommended. Give sodium bicarbonate (50 mmol) if cardiac arrest is associated with hyperkalaemia or tricyclic antidepressant overdose. Repeat the dose according to the clinical condition of the patient and the results of repeated blood gas analysis.

Magnesium

Give magnesium sulphate 8 mmol for refractory VF if there is any suspicion of hypomagnesaemia (e.g. patients on potassium-losing diuretics) or:

- ventricular tachyarrhythmias in the presence of possible hypomagnesaemia
- torsade de pointes
- digoxin toxicity.

Thrombolytics

The commonest cause of thromboembolic or mechanical circulatory obstruction is massive pulmonary embolus. If cardiac arrest is thought to be caused by pulmonary embolism, consider giving a thrombolytic drug immediately but be prepared to continue CPR for up to 90 min. Thrombolytics have been shown to be ineffective when given for cardiac arrest resulting from acute coronary artery thrombosis.

Post-resuscitation Care

A comprehensive, structured post-resuscitation treatment protocol may improve survival in cardiac arrest victims after ROSC. In particular:

- Unconscious adult patients with spontaneous circulation after out-of-hospital (all rhythms) cardiac arrest should be cooled to 32–34°C for 12–24 h. Mild hypothermia may also benefit unconscious patients with spontaneous circulation after cardiac arrest in hospital.
- Hyperoxaemia after ROSC is achieved may cause harm. Therefore titrate inspired O_2 to achieve a SaO_2 of 94–98%.
- Blood glucose values >10 mmol.l^{-1} should be treated, but hypoglycaemia must be avoided.

Resuscitation during pregnancy

- <25 weeks: as above
- 25–32 weeks: use wedge to relieve aortocaval compression
- >32 weeks: degree of aortocaval compression precludes effective CPR; therefore, perform immediate caesarean section whilst CPR is continued.

Guidelines for paediatric basic and advanced life support (Fig. 6.15a and b)

Causes of paediatric arrest are significantly different from those in adults. Cardiac arrest at birth is usually due to asphyxia; in infancy to respiratory illness or sepsis; and in later childhood to trauma.

Trained responders should give 15 compressions: 2 ventilations. (Lay people should use the 30:2 compression:ventilation ratio). Massage at the junction of middle/lower third sternum and compress the chest to a depth of at least 1/3 the AP diameter at a rate of 100–120 per minute.

Humidified oxygen with as high a F_iO_2 as possible should be used. (Once spontaneous circulation has been restored, O_2 should be titrated to limit the risk of hyperoxaemia.) Bag-mask ventilation is the preferred method for achieving airway control and ventilation. If this fails, a supraglottic airway device is an acceptable alternative. Once the airway is secured give 10 breaths/min.

Asystole is the commonest paediatric arrest arrhythmia and is usually preceded by an agonal bradycardia. VF occurs in only 6–9% of arrests, when shocks (all waveforms) should be given at 4 J.kg^{-1}. A standard AED can be used in children over 8 years. Purpose-made paediatric pads, or programmes which attenuate the energy output of an AED, are recommended for children between 1 and 8 years given after the third shock for shockable rhythms. The dose is repeated after the fifth shock, if still in VF/pulseless VT. Look for specific causes of VF, including congenital heart disease, hypothermia, tricyclic antidepressants and hyperkalaemia.

The initial dose of adrenaline is 10 μg.kg^{-1}. High-dose (100 μg.kg^{-1}) adrenaline may be considered for children where vasodilation may be significant, e.g. septic shock. Adrenaline is given after the third shock for shockable rhythms and then during every alternate cycle (i.e. every 3–5 minutes during CPR). Adrenaline is still initially given as soon as vascular access is available in the non-shockable side of the algorithm.

Hypernatraemia secondary to sodium bicarbonate administration greatly increases the risk of intracranial haemorrhage in neonates. The initial dose is 1 mmol.kg^{-1} given as a slow bolus before the second dose of adrenaline. Give further doses of bicarbonate according to arterial or mixed venous pH. Calcium (chloride or gluconate) should be given in a dose of 10–30 mg.kg^{-1}.

Hypoglycaemia is common in sick infants. Check glucose during resuscitation and treat hypoglycaemia with glucose 0.5 g.kg^{-1} as a 10% or 25% solution.

The commonest causes of electromechanical dissociation are hypovolaemia, cardiac tamponade and tension pneumothorax. Correct hypovolaemia with boluses of 20 mL.kg^{-1} crystalloid or colloid.

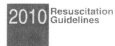 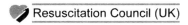

Paediatric Basic Life Support
(Healthcare professionals with a duty to respond)

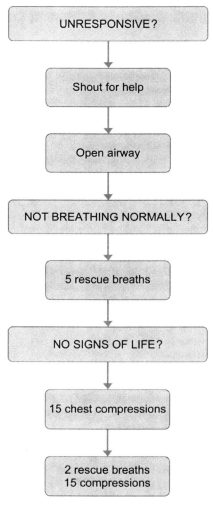

UNRESPONSIVE?

Shout for help

Open airway

NOT BREATHING NORMALLY?

5 rescue breaths

NO SIGNS OF LIFE?

15 chest compressions

2 rescue breaths
15 compressions

Call resuscitation team

Figure 6.15 (A) Paediatric basic life support guidelines. (Resuscitation Council (UK) 2010 © RC(UK).)

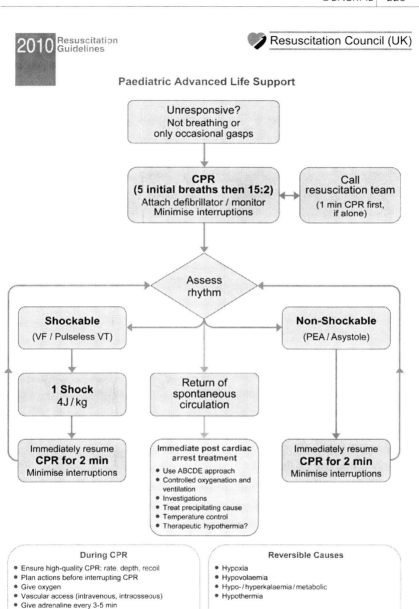

Figure 6.15, cont'd (B) Paediatric advanced life support guidelines. (Resuscitation Council (UK) 2010 © RC(UK).)

If venous access cannot be gained within 90 s, use an intraosseous needle which is suitable for all resuscitation drugs, colloid, crystalloid and blood. It also allows samples of marrow aspirate to be withdrawn for estimation of haemoglobin, venous pH and electrolytes.

Apgar scores

Table 6.5 Apgar scores

	0	1	2
Colour	Blue, pale	Body pink, extremities blue	All pink
Pulse	Absent	<100/min	>100/min
Reflex irritability	No response	Some motion	Cry
Muscle tone	Limp	Some flexion of extremities	Well flexed
Respiratory effort	Absent	Slow, irregular	Good strong cry

PAEDIATRIC RESUSCITATION DRUG DOSES

- Adrenaline $10\,\mu g.kg^{-1}$. Consider $100\,\mu g.kg^{-1}$ in septic shock
- Atropine $20\,\mu g.kg^{-1}$
- Sodium bicarbonate $1–2\,mmol.kg^{-1}$. Further doses should be titrated against blood gases
- Calcium chloride $0.2\,mL\,kg^{-1}$ of the 10% solution
- Amiodarone $5\,mg.kg^{-1}$
- Glucose $0.5\,g.kg^{-1}$
- Furosemide $1\,mg.kg^{-1}$
- Crystalloid $20\,mL.kg^{-1}$ if hypovolaemic. Repeat three times and then give $10\,mL.kg^{-1}$ blood if shock persists.

Guidelines for the management of peri-arrest arrhythmias (Fig. 6.16a,b)

The 2010 European Resuscitation Council guidelines cover the management of bradyarrhythmias, broad complex tachycardias and narrow complex tachycardias (supraventricular tachycardias, SVTs), including atrial fibrillation.

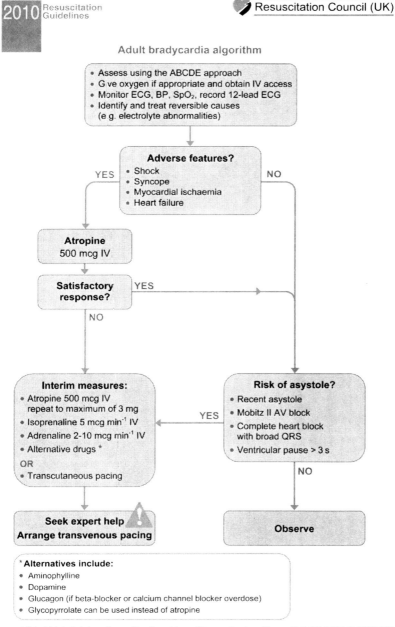

2010 Resuscitation Guidelines

Resuscitation Council (UK)

Adult bradycardia algorithm

- Assess using the ABCDE approach
- Give oxygen if appropriate and obtain IV access
- Monitor ECG, BP, SpO₂, record 12-lead ECG
- Identify and treat reversible causes
  (e.g. electrolyte abnormalities)

Adverse features?
- Shock
- Syncope
- Myocardial ischaemia
- Heart failure

YES

NO

Atropine
500 mcg IV

Satisfactory response?

YES

NO

Interim measures:
- Atropine 500 mcg IV
  repeat to maximum of 3 mg
- Isoprenaline 5 mcg min⁻¹ IV
- Adrenaline 2-10 mcg min⁻¹ IV
- Alternative drugs *

OR
- Transcutaneous pacing

Risk of asystole?
- Recent asystole
- Mobitz II AV block
- Complete heart block
  with broad QRS
- Ventricular pause > 3 s

YES

NO

Seek expert help
Arrange transvenous pacing

Observe

* **Alternatives include:**
- Aminophylline
- Dopamine
- Glucagon (if beta-blocker or calcium channel blocker overdose)
- Glycopyrrolate can be used instead of atropine

Figure 6.16 (A) Adult bradycardia algorithm. (Resuscitation Council (UK) 2010 © RC(UK).)

(Continued)

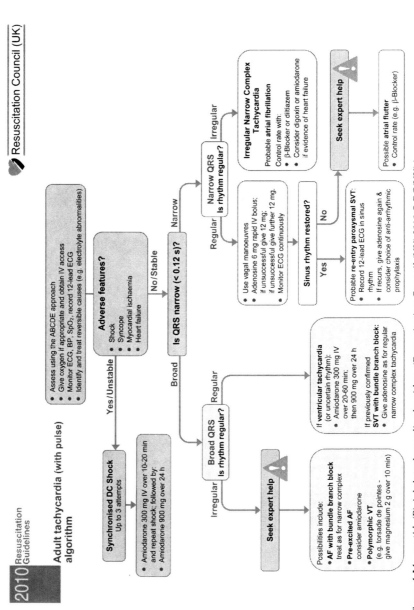

Figure 6.16, cont'd (B) Adult tachycardia algorithm. (Resuscitation Council (UK) 2010 © RC(UK).)

Physiology of circulation during closed chest massage

There are two theories of blood flow:

- *Cardiac pump theory.* Blood is ejected from the heart as it is squeezed between the sternum and spine. The aortic valve prevents retrograde flow.
- *Thoracic pump theory.* Cardiac massage raises intrathoracic pressure and forces blood out of the thorax. Venous valves and venous compression prevent retrograde flow.

Both mechanisms are probably involved. Adrenaline constricts vascular beds to direct most flow to the brain and heart, so although total cardiac output is 10–30%, brain and heart flows approach 50% of normal. All flows decrease rapidly with time.

Use of end-tidal CO_2 monitoring

CO_2 excretion during CPR is dependent upon cardiac output and not ventilation. A high correlation exists between $P_{ET}co_2$ and cardiac output, coronary perfusion pressure and survival from cardiac arrest. $P_{ET}co_2$ <10 mmHg during resuscitation is associated with an unsuccessful outcome. Monitoring $P_{ET}co_2$ during cardiac massage therefore provides feedback to optimize chest compression and may also give an early indication of operator fatigue. Current resuscitation guidelines encourage the use of end-tidal CO_2 monitoring both as a means of monitoring the effectiveness of CPR and for confirmation of correct tracheal tube placement.

Bibliography

Biarent D, Bingham R, Richmond S, et al: European Resuscitation Council guidelines for resuscitation. Section 6. Paediatric life support, *Resuscitation* 67:S97–S133, 2005.

Bouch DC, Thompson JP, Damian MS: Post-cardiac arrest management: more than global cooling? *Br J Anaesth* 100:591–594, 2008.

Deakin CD, Nolan JP, European Resuscitation Council: European Resuscitation Council guidelines for resuscitation. Section 3. Electrical therapies: automated external defibrillators, defibrillation, cardioversion and pacing, *Resuscitation* 67:S25–S37, 2005.

Handley AJ, Koster R, Monsieurs K, et al: European Resuscitation Council guidelines for resuscitation. Section 2. Adult basic life support and use of automated external defibrillators, *Resuscitation* 67:S7–S23, 2005.

Nolan JP, Deakin CD, Soar J, et al: European Resuscitation Council guidelines for resuscitation. Section 4. Adult advanced life support, *Resuscitation* 67:S39–S86, 2005.

STATISTICS

- Incidence = rate of occurrence of new cases
- Prevalence = total number of cases:
  - point prevalence – at a given moment in time
  - period prevalence – over a given period of time.

Normal (Gaussian) distribution

A sample of data may form a normal distribution curve which is bell-shaped and symmetrical about the mean value, e.g. height, weight, heart rate (Fig. 6.17).

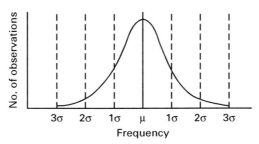

Figure 6.17 Normal (Gaussian) distribution curve. μ = mean; σ = standard deviation.

Mean, median and mode

- Mean = average of all values
- Median = the value above and below which half the observations lie
- Mode = most frequently occurring value.

The mean, median and mode have identical values within normally distributed data (Fig. 6.18a).

Curves of normal distribution have symmetry about the mean. A curve that is not symmetrical is referred to as skewed. A curve is positively skewed if most data lie below the mean, and negatively skewed if most data lie above the mean. In a skewed distribution, mean, median and mode are not equal (Fig. 6.18b,c). The amount of skewness is given by the following equation:

$$\text{Skewness} = \frac{\sum (x - \bar{x})^3}{N(SD^3)}$$

where:
x = observed mean
$\bar{x}$ = expected mean
n = number of observations
$n - 1$ = degrees of freedom (N).

A result of zero indicates a completely symmetrical distribution; positive values indicate positively skewed distribution and vice versa. Strongly skewed data must be examined using non-parametric tests.

Variance, standard deviation and standard error

The variance of a sample is a measure of the scatter about the sample mean:

$$\text{Variance} = \frac{\sum (x - \bar{x})^3}{n - 1}$$

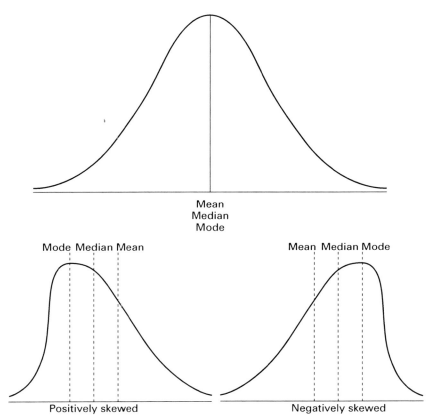

Figure 6.18 Mean, median and mode: (A) normal distribution; (B) positively skewed distribution; (C) negatively skewed distribution.

Variance is derived from a 'squared' equation, so to return to a measure of scatter about the mean that fits with original data, the square root of the variance is used. This is the standard deviation (SD):

$$SD(\sigma) = \sqrt{\text{variance}}$$

Therefore:

$$SD = \sqrt{\frac{\sum (x - \bar{x})^2}{n - 1}}$$

Standard error (SE) is the standard deviation of the population mean:

$$SE = \sqrt{\frac{\text{variance}}{n}} \text{ or } \frac{SD}{\sqrt{n}}$$

Standard error of the mean (SEM)

Describes the deviation of the sample mean from the estimated population mean:

$$SE_m = \sqrt{\frac{variance_m}{n}} \text{ or } \frac{SD_m}{\sqrt{n}}$$

Confidence intervals

Confidence limits express a range of values within which the true mean is likely to lie. The 95% confidence limits are given as the mean value ± 1.96 times the standard error, i.e. there is a 95% chance that the true population mean will lie within the calculated range. The limits either side of the mean are the 'confidence limits' and the interval between them is the 'confidence interval' (CI).

For example, if the 95% confidence interval for percentage improvement between two groups following a given treatment is 15–35%, there is a 95% chance that the true difference lies between these two values.

Statistical tests (Tables 6.6, 6.7)

Parametric tests

Used for data fitting a normal distribution curve and for comparison of the sample mean with the population mean:

- *t-test* – Used to compare data from different groups (Student's *t*-test) or paired samples (paired *t*-test)
- *Analysis of variance* (ANOVA) – similar to *t*-test but for three or more sample groups. Assesses whether the variability in group means is greater than that expected by chance.

Table 6.6 Statistical tests for comparing two or more groups

Data type	Statistical test				
	t-test	Mann–Whitney	Analysis of variance	Kruskal–Wallis	χ^2 test
Normal distribution		×		×	×
Non-parametric distribution	×		×		×
Binary	×	×	×	×	

Table 6.7 Statistical tests for one or paired samples

Data type	Statistical test		
	t-test	Wilcoxon	McNemar
Normal distribution		×	×
Non-parametric distribution	×		×
Binary	×	×	

Non-parametric tests

Used for data not fitting, or assumed not to fit, a normal distribution, e.g. number of times patient pregnant, number of visits to GP/year, binomial data (true/false, heads/tails, etc.).

Chi-squared test

$$\chi^2 = \sum \frac{(O - E)^2}{E}$$

where:
O = observed frequencies
E = expected frequencies.

(O – E) is squared because some of the values will be negative. This value is then divided by the expected number (E) and the sum of these values is calculated to give χ^2. The probability of the observed difference occurring by chance is then calculated from χ^2 tables.

Ranking tests

- Fisher's exact test
- Wilcoxon's signed rank test.

Ranking tests involve placing the data from both groups in an ascending/descending order. Numerical values are then assigned to each of the numbers of data and the sum of these numerical values calculated for each group. Probabilities are then calculated from tables.

Significance values

Expressed as *p*-values, e.g. $p = 0.01$ means 1 chance in 100 that the results occurred by chance:

- $p > 0.05$ is taken as non-significant
- $p < 0.05$ and > 0.01 are significant
- $p < 0.01$ is highly significant.

Linear correlation and linear regression

Observation of a scattergram may suggest some form of correlation between two variables (Fig. 6.19).

The best-fit straight line is calculated for the data (Fig. 6.20). The position of the best-fit straight line is adjusted to minimize the sum of the distances d1–d4 so that Σd is a minimum.

The best-fit line is given by the equation:

$$y = m\,x + C$$

where:
x = independent variable
y = dependent variable
m = slope of the straight line
C = a constant.

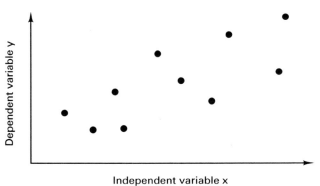

Figure 6.19 Scattergram of x against y.

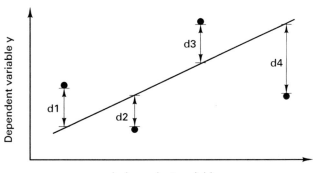

Figure 6.20 Linear regression for scattergram data.

Multiple linear regression is designed to establish any relationships when several variables are present within the same set of data.

Correlation coefficient

The correlation coefficient, r, is an indication of how close the points lie to the best-fit line. As the data lie closer to the best-fit line, r tends towards 1.0 (Fig. 6.21).

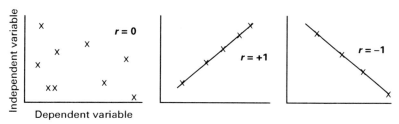

Figure 6.21 Correlation coefficients.

Bland–Altman plot

When comparing unrelated data, e.g. height versus weight, correlation coefficient is appropriate. When comparing related data (e.g. different methods of measuring the same variable), a Bland–Altman plot is more appropriate. The mean of each individual data pair is shown on the x-axis and the difference between each data pair on the y-axis. An example is given in Figure 6.22.

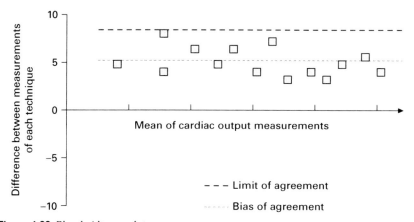

Figure 6.22 Bland–Altman plot.

Sensitivity and specificity

Sensitivity is a measure of the ability of a test to correctly select patients with a condition from an affected population, i.e. true positives:

$$\text{Sensitivity} = \frac{\text{number tested as positive}}{\text{total with condition}}$$

Specificity is a measure of the ability of a test to correctly select patients without the condition from an unaffected population, i.e. true negatives:

$$\text{Specificity} = \frac{\text{number tested as negative}}{\text{total without condition}}$$

Sample size

Studies must be of sufficient size to be able to detect a difference between the study populations. Failure to show a difference between groups is only of significance if the sample size was adequate. Sample size can be calculated by equations but nomograms are easier for most studies. The power of a study is the chance of showing a difference between study populations if one exists, e.g. a study with a power of 0.80 has an 80% chance of detecting a difference if one exists.

Type I error occurs when a difference is found statistically where none actually exists. There is always a random chance of making a type I error.

Type II error occurs when inadequate sample size results in no difference being shown between two comparative groups.

Types of clinical studies

Retrospective

- *Cross-sectional study.* Examine either a random sample or all subjects in a well-defined study population in order to obtain the answer to a specific question, e.g. prevalence of a disease.
- *Case-controlled study.* Specific disease or condition matched to a control group. Pairings then compared for risk factors, e.g. smokers versus non-smokers with lung cancer.

Prospective

- *Observational cohort study* Two or more groups followed up for a specific period of time, comparing exposure to a specific substance/drug with development of a specific illness.
- *Randomized and non-randomized (cohort) interventional controlled trials* evaluate an intervention rather than observing groups over time. Aim to reduce systematic bias (a variable that distorts comparisons between groups). The comparative groups should only be different in terms of the intervention applied or the causative agent.

Systematic trials

Systematic review is the formal process of identification, appraisal and evaluation of research studies using strict criteria in order to review a specific issue.

Meta-analysis

A statistical integration of a number of studies which individually are either too small or give conflicting results. Identical methodologies are not needed, but the studies must be sufficiently similar to ensure that the pooled data arise from reasonably homogenous study groups.

Bibliography

Gardner MJ, Altman DG: *Statistics with confidence*, London, 1989, British Medical Association.

McCluskey A, Lalkhen AG: Statistics I: data and correlations, *Contin Edu Anaesth, Crit Care Pain* 7:95–99, 2007.

McCluskey A, Lalkhen AG: Statistics II: Central tendency and spread of data, *Contin Edu Anaesth, Crit Care Pain* 7:127–130, 2007.

McCluskey A, Lalkhen AG: Statistics III: Probability and statistical tests, *Contin Edu Anaesth, Crit Care Pain* 7:167–170, 2007.

McCluskey A, Lalkhen AG: Statistics IV: Interpreting the results of statistical tests, *Contin Edu Anaesth, Crit Care Pain* 7:208–212, 2007.

McCluskey A, Lalkhen AG: Statistics V: Introduction to clinical trials and systematic reviews, *Contin Edu Anaesth, Crit Care Pain* 8:143–146, 2007.

Swinscow TDV: *Statistics at square one*, ed 8, London, 1983, British Medical Association.

TRAUMA MANAGEMENT

A Royal College of Surgeons Working Party (RCS 1988) highlighted serious deficiencies in trauma patient management.

A Major Trauma Outcome Study (MTOS) was published in 1992 with similar conclusions:

- worse outcome when comparing 6111 UK patients with USA data
- 21% patients with major trauma took >1 h to reach hospital
- SHO in charge of resuscitation for 57% patients with major trauma.

Trunkey described a trimodal pattern of death seen after major trauma (Fig. 6.23). The first peak comprises patients with serious, generally non-survivable injuries. The second peak comprises patients with life-threatening injuries in whom prompt, appropriate treatment may be life-saving. It is these patients to which the Advanced Trauma Life Support (ATLS) protocol is directed. The third peak comprises patients who die several days/weeks later from sepsis or multiple organ failure.

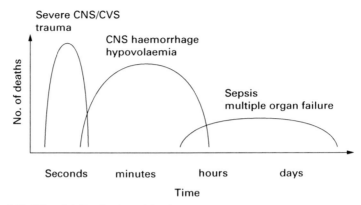

Figure 6.23 Trimodal distribution of death.

Advanced Trauma Life Support

- Introduced from the USA in 1988
- Some controversial aspects, e.g. no anaesthetic input to first edition, nasal versus oral intubation, colloids versus crystalloids
- Introduced concept of trauma team
- Limited data to suggest any improvement in outcome following its introduction
- Focuses on 'golden hour'.

Primary survey

1. *Airway* with cervical spine control
   - Assess the airway for patency. Avoid neck extension/flexion if there is a risk of cervical spine injury.
   - Assume cervical spine injury in multisystem trauma and, in particular, in patients with impaired consciousness or blunt injury above the clavicle.
   - Stabilize the cervical spine with manual in-line stabilization or hard collar + head blocks.
2. *Breathing* with ventilatory support
   - Look, listen and feel
   - Tension pneumothorax, haemothorax or flail chest may require immediate treatment.
3. *Circulation* and haemorrhage control.

Pulses

- Radial – present if systolic BP >80 mmHg
- Femoral – present if systolic BP >70 mmHg
- Carotid – present if systolic BP >60 mmHg.

Classification of hypovolaemic shock

Table 6.8 Classification of hypovolaemic shock

	Class I	Class II	Class III	Class IV
% blood loss	<15	15–30	30–40	>40
Volume	<750	800–1500	1500–2000	>2000
Systolic	Normal	Normal	Reduced	Very low
Diastolic	Normal	Raised	Reduced	Very low
Pulse	Normal	>100/min	>120/min	>120/min
Capillary refill	Normal	>2 s	>2 s	Absent
Respiratory rate	Normal	Normal	>20/min	>20/min
Urine (mL/h)	>30	20–30	10–20	0–10
Mental state	Alert	Anxious	Drowsy	Confused

Intravenous access

- ATLS recommends insertion of two 14G cannulae.
- Remember flow ∝ r^4/l, so a small increase in cannula radius (r) results in large increase in flow. Doubling the length (l) of an infusion set halves the flow.
- Increasing evidence that attempting to establish normovolaemia *before* surgical haemostasis dislodges any blood clots and accelerates the rate of bleeding. Intravenous fluids at this stage also cause dilution of clotting factors and hypothermia, increasing overall morbidity and mortality.

Until haemostasis is secured, aim for systolic BP of 80 mmHg, which is thought to be adequate to perfuse vital organs.

4. **Disability** – a rapid assessment of neurological function
   - Assess GCS and pupils
   - Check cord function by observing arms and legs for spontaneous movement
   - A GCS <8 is associated with impaired gas exchange. Therefore consider intubating head-injured patients to reduce 2° injury.
5. **Exposure** – completely undress the patient, but prevent hypothermia
   - Hypothermia correlates with mortality.

Secondary survey

Involves a systematic head-to-toe survey:

- Head
- Maxillofacial

- Cervical spine and neck
- Chest
- Abdomen
- Perineum/rectum/vagina
- Musculoskeletal
- Neurological
- Do not forget to examine the back (log roll).

Fluids in resuscitation

Quantity of fluid

Concept of permissive hypotension to limit fluid resuscitation until surgical haemostasis is achieved. Increasing BP in a bleeding patient dislodges clots, accelerates bleeding, results in more i.v. fluid requirement, which further dilutes clotting factors and inevitably results in a cold acidotic patient. A systolic BP of 80 mmHg is adequate for vital organ perfusion until haemostasis is achieved. It may need to be higher in patients with raised ICP. Base deficit and lactate better endpoints than BP.

Type of fluid

The recently completed safe versus albumin fluid evaluation (SAFE) trial in Australia showed no difference in outcomes among ICU patients receiving crystalloid vs colloid (albumin) as their primary resuscitative fluid.

Hypertonic saline is effective in restoring blood volume through hypertonic recruitment of interstitial and intracellular fluid. Although small clinical studies and animal studies have shown benefit, recent meta-analysis has failed to demonstrate any improvement in morbidity or mortality.

HEAD INJURY: TRIAGE, ASSESSMENT, INVESTIGATION AND EARLY MANAGEMENT OF HEAD INJURY IN INFANTS, CHILDREN AND ADULTS

National Institute for Health and Clinical Excellence, September 2007

Investigation for injuries to the cervical spine

Which investigation?

- **In most circumstances, plain radiographs are the initial investigation of choice to detect cervical spine injuries – three views of sufficient quality for reliable interpretation (two views for children under 10 years of age).**
- CT imaging is recommended in some circumstances.

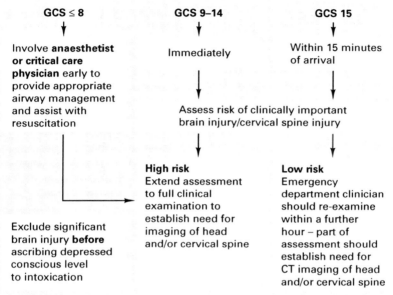

Figure 6.24 Assessment in emergency department. (National Institute of Health and Clinical Excellence.)

- CT imaging is recommended in some circumstances.
- Children under 10 have increased risk from irradiation, so restrict CT imaging of cervical spine to children with indicators of more serious injury, in circumstances such as:
  - severe head injury (GCS ≤8)
  - strong suspicion of injury despite normal plain films
  - plain films are inadequate.

As a minimum, CT imaging should cover any areas of concern or uncertainty on plain film or clinical grounds.

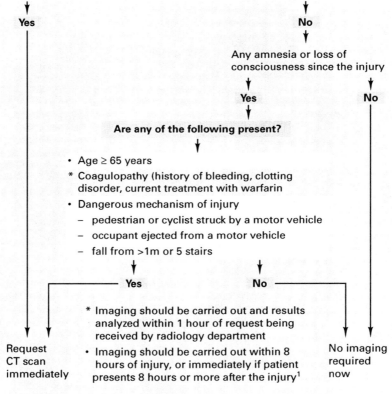

Are any of the following present?

* GCS <13 when first assessed in emergency department
* GCS <15 when assessed in emergency department 2 hours after the injury
* Suspected open or depressed skull fracture
* Sign of fracture at skull base (haemotympanum, 'panda' eyes, cerebrospinal fluid leakage from ears or nose, Battle's sign)
* Post-traumatic seizure
* Focal neurological deficit
* >1 episode of vomiting
• Amnesia of events >30 minutes before impact

Yes   No

Any amnesia or loss of consciousness since the injury

Yes   No

Are any of the following present?

• Age ≥ 65 years
* Coagulopathy (history of bleeding, clotting disorder, current treatment with warfarin)
• Dangerous mechanism of injury
  − pedestrian or cyclist struck by a motor vehicle
  − occupant ejected from a motor vehicle
  − fall from >1m or 5 stairs

Yes   No

* Imaging should be carried out and results analyzed within 1 hour of request being received by radiology department
• Imaging should be carried out within 8 hours of injury, or immediately if patient presents 8 hours or more after the injury[1]

Request CT scan immediately

No imaging required now

[1] If patient presents out of hours and is ≥65, has amnesia for events more than 30 minutes before impact or there was a dangerous mechanism of injury, it is acceptable to admit for overnight observation, with CT imaging the next morning, **unless CT result is required within 1 hour because of the presence of additional clinical finding listed above**

Figure 6.25 Selection of adults for CT scanning of the head. (National Institute of Health and Clinical Excellence.)

Are any of the following present?

Check both lists

- Patient cannot actively rotate neck to 45 degrees to left and right (if safe to assess the range of movement in the neck)[2]
- Not safe to assess range of movement in the neck[2]
- Neck pain or midline tenderness plus:
  - age≥ 65 years, or
  - dangerous mechanism of injury[3]
- Definitive diagnosis of cervical spine injury required urgently (for example, prior to surgery)

- GCS < 13 on initial assessment
- Has been intubated
- Plain film series technically inadequate (for example, desired view unavailable), suspicious or definitely abnormal
- Continued clinical suspicion of injury despite normal X-ray
- Patient is being scanned for multi-region trauma

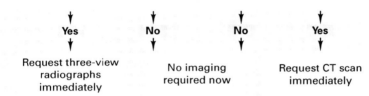

Yes	No	No	Yes
Request three-view radiographs immediately	No imaging required now		Request CT scan immediately

[2] Safe assessment can be carried out if patient: was involved in a simple rear-end motor vehicle collision; is comfortable in a sitting position in the emergency department; has been ambulatory at any time since injury and there is no midline cervical spine tenderness; or if the patient presents with delayed onset of neck pain.

[3] Dangerous mechanism of injury: fall from >1m or 5 stairs; axial load to head – for example, diving; high-speed motor vehicle collision; rollover motor accident; ejection from a motor vehicle; accident involving motorized recreational vehicles; bicycle collision.

Figure 6.26 Selection of adults and children (age 10+) for imaging of the cervical spine. (National Institute of Health and Clinical Excellence.)

When to involve the neurosurgeon

- Discuss the care of all patients with new, surgically significant abnormalities on imaging with a neurosurgeon (definition of 'surgically significant' to be developed by local neurosurgical unit and agreed with referring hospitals).
- Regardless of imaging, other reasons for discussing a patient's care plan with a neurosurgeon include:
  - persisting coma (GCS ≤8) after initial resuscitation
  - unexplained confusion for more than 4 h
  - deterioration in GCS after admission (pay greater attention to motor response deterioration)
  - progressive focal neurological signs
  - seizure without full recovery
  - definite or suspected penetrating injury
  - cerebrospinal fluid leak.

Transfer from secondary setting to neuroscience unit

Follow local guidelines on patient transfer and transfer of responsibility for patient care – these should be drawn up by the referring hospital trusts, neuroscience unit and local ambulance service. They should recognize that transfer would benefit all patients with serious head injuries (GCS ≤8), irrespective of the need for neurosurgery, but if transfer of those who do not require neurosurgery is not possible, ongoing liaison with the neuroscience unit over clinical management is essential.

- For emergency transfers, the patient should be accompanied by a doctor with appropriate training and experience and an adequately trained assistant.
- A child or infant should be accompanied by staff experienced in the transfer of critically ill children.
- The transfer team should be provided with a means of communicating with their base hospital and the neurosurgical unit during the transfer (a portable phone may be suitable providing it is not used within 1 m of medical equipment prone to electrical interference, such as infusion pumps).
- *The multiply injured patient*: consider the possibility of occult extracranial injuries, and do not transfer to a service unable to deal with other aspects of trauma.

Medical care during transfer

- *In all circumstances*: complete initial resuscitation and stabilization of the patient and establish comprehensive monitoring before transfer to avoid complications during the journey.
- *Patient persistently hypotensive despite resuscitation*: do not transport until the cause of hypotension has been identified and the patient stabilized.

Figure 6.27 Neurosurgical involvement.

Table 6.9 Intubation and ventilation

Circumstances	Action
Coma – GCS ≤8 (use paediatric scale for children)	Intubate and ventilate immediately
Loss of protective laryngeal reflexes	
Ventilatory insufficiency:	
hypoxaemia (P_aO_2 <13 kPa on oxygen)	
hypercarbia (P_aCO_2 >6 kPa)	
Spontaneous hyperventilation causing P_aCO_2 <4 kPa	
Irregular respirations	
Significantly deteriorating conscious level (1 or more points on motor score), even if not coma	Intubate and ventilate before the journey starts
Unstable fractures of the facial skeleton	
Copious bleeding into mouth	
Seizures	
Ventilate an intubated patient with muscle relaxation and appropriate short-acting sedation and analgesia	
Aim for:	
P_aO_2 >13 kPa	
P_aCO_2 4.5–5.0 kPa	
If clinical or radiological evidence of raised intracranial pressure, more aggressive hyperventilation is justified	
Increase the inspired oxygen concentration if hyperventilation is used	
Adult: maintain mean arterial pressure at ≥80 mmHg by infusing fluid and vasopressors as indicated	
Child: maintain blood pressure at level appropriate for age	

GUIDELINES FOR THE MANAGEMENT OF SEVERE TRAUMATIC BRAIN INJURY
Brain Trauma Foundation 2007

Recommendations

Blood pressure and oxygenation

A significant proportion of patients with traumatic brain injury (TBI) have hypotension and/or hypoxaemia, which increases morbidity and mortality. Hypotension (systolic BP <90 mmHg) and hypoxaemia (P_aO_2 <60 mmHg) must be avoided, or corrected immediately.

Hyperosmolar therapy

Mannitol is effective in lowering ICP in the management of TBI. The evidence for the use of hypertonic saline is not sufficient to make specific recommendations.

Prophylactic hypothermia

Some studies have shown that hypothermia may increase the chance of patients recovering from severe TBI to a Glasgow Outcome Score of 4 or 5. Hypothermia may have to be maintained for >48 h.

Deep vein thrombosis prophylaxis

Graduated compression stockings and low dose heparin reduce the risk of DVT, but the optimal dosing regimen and optimal time to start this therapy is unknown.

Intracranial pressure monitoring

The use of ICP monitoring in patients with severe TBI allows appropriate management of raised ICP, which is associated with improved outcome. Raised ICP pressure >20–25 mmHg requires treatment.

Cerebral perfusion thresholds

The optimal cerebral perfusion pressure (CPP) is unknown. Cerebral ischaemia generally occurs below 50–60 mmHg. A minimum of 60 mmHg is therefore recommended. No evidence that the use of pressors and volume expansion to drive CPP above 70 mmHg is beneficial.

Anaesthetics, analgesics and sedation

Barbiturates have been shown to control elevated ICP, but no evidence for any improvement in long-term survival. Important to avoid hypotension caused by many of these drugs.

Nutrition

Patients with severe TBI lose weight at a rate of 15% per week. Weight loss of >30% is associated with increased mortality in TBI patients. The optimal feeding regimen has not been established, but full feeding should be instigated by day 7.

Anti-seizure prophylaxis

Routine seizure prophylaxis is not indicated in patients >1 week post-injury.

Hyperventilation

Although hyperventilation may reduce raised ICP, it may also reduce cerebral blood flow to cause ischaemia. No good evidence to support hyperventilation following TBI.

Steroids

There is good evidence that high dose steroids worsen outcome in TBI and should therefore be avoided.

TRAUMA: WHO CARES?
A Report of the National Confidential Enquiry into Patient Outcome and Death 2007

Summary

Road trauma accounts for over one-third of all deaths due to injury. In 2001–2003, there were (on average) 3460 traffic-related fatalities per annum in Great Britain. The incidence of severe trauma, defined as an Injury Severity Score (ISS) ≥16, is estimated to be four per million per week. Given that the UK population in mid-2003 was in the region of 59.5 million, there are approximately 240 severely injured patients in the UK each week.

Recommendations

Organizational data

There is a need for designated Level 1 trauma centres and a verification process needs to be developed to quality assure the delivery of trauma care (as has been developed in USA by American College of Surgeons).

Prehospital care

All agencies involved in trauma management, including emergency medical services, should be integrated into the clinical governance programmes of a regional trauma service.

Hospital reception

Trusts should ensure that a trauma team is available 24 h a day, 7 days a week. This is an essential part of an organized trauma response system.

A consultant must be the team leader for the management of the severely injured patient. There should be no reason for this not to happen during the normal working week.

Trusts and consultants should work together to provide job plans that will lead to better consultant presence in the emergency department at all times to provide more uniform consultant leadership for all severely injured patients.

Airway and breathing

The current structure of prehospital management is insufficient to meet the needs of the severely injured patient. There is a high incidence of failed intubation and a high incidence of patients arriving at hospital with a partially or completely obstructed airway. Change is urgently required to provide a system that reliably provides a clear airway with good oxygenation and control of ventilation. This may be through the provision of personnel with the ability to provide anaesthesia and intubation in the prehospital phase or the use of alternative airway devices.

Management of circulation

Trauma laparotomy is potentially extremely challenging and requires consultant presence within the operating theatre.

If CT scanning is to be performed, all necessary images should be obtained at the same time. Routine use of 'top to toe' scanning is recommended in the adult trauma patient if no indication for immediate intervention exists.

Head injury management

Patients with severe head injury should have a CT head scan of the head performed as soon as possible after admission and within 1 hour of arrival at hospital.

All patients with severe head injury should be transferred to a neurosurgical/critical care centre, irrespective of the requirement for surgical intervention.

Paediatric care

Each receiving unit should have up-to-date guidelines for children, which recognize the paediatric skills available on site and their limitations and include agreed guidelines for communication and transfer with specialized paediatric services within the local clinical network.

Transfers

There should be standardized transfer documentation of the patients' details, injuries, results of investigations and management with records kept at the dispatching and receiving hospitals. Published guidelines must be adhered to and audits performed of the transfers and protocols.

Incidence of trauma and organization of trauma services

Given the relatively low incidence of severe trauma in the UK, it is unlikely that each individual hospital can deliver optimum care to this challenging group of patients. Regional planning for the effective delivery of trauma services is therefore essential.

Bibliography

Brain Trauma Foundation: Guidelines for the management of severe traumatic brain injury, 2007. www.braintrauma.org/site/PageServer?pagename=Guidelines.

Bratton SL, Chestnut RM, Ghajar J, et al; Brain Trauma Foundation; American Association of Neurological Surgeons; Congress of Neurological Surgeons; Joint Section on Neurotrauma and Critical Care, AANS/CNS: Guidelines for the management of severe traumatic brain injury, *J Neurotrauma* 24(Suppl 1):S37–S44, 2007.

Brussel T: Anaesthetic considerations for acute spinal cord injury, *Curr Opin Anaesth* 11:467–472, 1998.

Dutton RP: Fluid management for trauma; where are we now? *Contin Edu Anaesth, Crit Care Pain* 6:144–147, 2006.

Meyer P-G: Paediatric trauma and resuscitation, *Curr Opin Anaesth* 11:285–288, 1998.

National Confidential Enquiry into Patient Outcome and Death: Trauma: who cares? 2007, http://www.ncepod.org.uk/2007t.htm.

NICE: Head injury: Triage, assessment, investigation and early management of head injury in infants, children and adults, *NICE Clinical Guideline* 56, September 2007. www.nice.org.uk/nicemedia/pdf/CG56QuickRedGuide.pdf.

Nolan JP, Parr MJA: Aspects of resuscitation in trauma, *Br J Anaesth* 79:226–240, 1997.

Royal College of Surgeons of England: Report of the Working Party on the Management of Patients with Major Injuries, London, 1988, RCS.

Shaz BH, Dente CJ, Harris RS, et al: Transfusion management of trauma patients, *Anesth Analg* 108:1760–1768, 2009.

Strandvik GF: Hypertonic saline in critical care: a review of the literature and guidelines for the use in hypotensive states and raised intracranial pressure, *Anaesthesia* 64:990–999, 2009.

Intensive care

ACUTE RESPIRATORY DISTRESS SYNDROME (ARDS)

First described in Denver, Colorado, in 1967 by Ashbaugh. North American–European consensus group has changed the definition to *'acute'* (as opposed to 'adult') respiratory distress syndrome, since the syndrome can occur in children. It is often the pulmonary component of the systemic inflammatory response syndrome (SIRS) and is characterized by severe hypoxia refractory to oxygen, low compliance, high airway pressure, bilateral diffuse alveolar infiltrates and microscopic atelectasis. It has an annual incidence of about 3.5:100000.

Causes

Table 7.1 Causes of ARDS

Direct injury	Indirect injury
Pulmonary contusion	Septicaemia
Gastric aspiration	Major trauma
Fat and amniotic fluid embolus	Cardiopulmonary bypass
Infection	Massive blood transfusion
Cytotoxic drugs	Prolonged hypotension
Smoke inhalation	Hepatic and renal failure
Oxygen toxicity	Disseminated intravascular coagulation

Pathophysiology

Activated neutrophils adhere to endothelial cells and release inflammatory mediators, including oxygen-free radicals and proteases, to cause lung damage. Direct lung damage or endotoxins alone are sufficient to damage endothelial cells with cytokine release and an inflammatory cascade (Fig. 7.1).

Endothelial damage results in increased capillary permeability and formation of protein-rich alveolar exudate rich in neutrophils. Type I alveolar cells

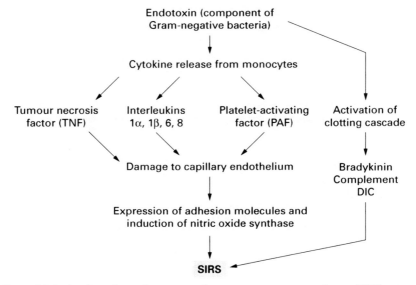

Figure 7.1 Pathophysiology of systemic inflammatory response syndrome (SIRS).

are damaged and type II cells proliferate. As the disease progresses, fibro-blast infiltration and collagen proliferation cause microvascular obliteration and widespread fibrosis. Areas of lung involvement are not fixed but shift to dependent areas. Within areas of reduced lung volume, some alveoli remain open and capable of gas exchange, whereas others are filled with alveolar exudate.

IPPV may cause damage more through excess volume ('volutrauma') than through pressure itself. The significance of oxygen toxicity is controversial.

Treatment

Treat underlying cause

Ensure adequate resuscitation. Guided by invasive pulmonary artery pressure monitoring to prevent multiple organ failure. Aim for the lowest PCWP pro-ducing an adequate cardiac output to prevent high levels of lung water, which are associated with a poor outcome.

Ventilatory support. Standard tidal volumes of $10-12\,mL.kg^{-1}$ are inappro-priate in the presence of reduced functional lung volume and cause a signifi-cant increase in airway pressure. $F_iO_2 > 0.6$ may cause oxygen toxicity and does little to improve oxygenation in the presence of large shunts.

ARDS Network study showed benefit from a ventilation strategy aiming for tidal volume 6 mL.kg^{-1}, respiratory rate 6–35 min^{-1}, I:E ratio 1:1–1:3, plateau airway pressure <30 cmH$_2$O, increased PEEP if high F_iO_2, PaO_2 7.3–10.7 kPa and permissive hypercapnia.

PEEP may avoid cyclic closure/reopening of atelectatic alveolar units, but it has been suggested that PEEP only fails to recruit units filled with alveolar exudate and overdistends open alveoli causing further damage. ARDS Network ALVEOLI study recent failed to show any difference between high PEEP/low F_iO_2 versus low PEEP/high F_iO_2.

Other methods of improving oxygenation

- Patients with ARDS have profound pulmonary vasoconstriction and ↑ PAP due to loss of endothelium-derived relaxing factor (EDRF). Nitric oxide (NO) can selectively vasodilate the pulmonary vascular bed at <40 ppm, improving V/Q and arterial oxygenation. Long-term benefits have not been proven.
- Prone ventilation recruits dorsal alveoli and may improve gas exchange.
- Artificial surfactant is of benefit in neonates with idiopathic respiratory distress syndrome but results in adults with ARDS are disappointing.
- Extracorporeal membrane oxygenation (ECMO) and intravascular oxygenation (IVOX) have produced poor results.

Reduce oedema formation. Decreasing hydrostatic pressure, increasing colloid osmotic pressure and reducing capillary leak with NSAIDs all show disappointing results.

Cardiovascular support. Naturally occurring nitric oxide causes systemic vasodilatation seen with SIRS. Preliminary studies show vasodilatation may be reduced by inhibitors of nitric oxide synthetase.

Gut-derived endotoxin. May initiate and maintain SIRS. Gut failure may be reduced by early parenteral feeding with glutamine-rich substrates. Selective decontamination of the gut may reduce the incidence of nosocomial pneumonia.

Anti-inflammatory mediators. Platelet-activating factor (PAF) antagonists, IL-1 and IL-6 antagonists and tumour necrosis factor antagonists are experimental but may have a role to play in terminating the inflammatory cascade.

Corticosteroids may reduce production of inflammatory mediators but increase risk of infection. May benefit some patients in the fibroproliferative stage of the disease with no associated infection. Overall benefit is unclear.

Secondary infection. High risk of secondary infection reduced with prophylactic antibiotics.

Outcome. In early reports, ARDS was associated with a 60% mortality, but recent studies have documented mortality rates of 34–36%. In survivors, pulmonary dysfunction is rare, consisting principally of mild lung restriction, but progressive pulmonary fibrosis has been reported.

ACUTELY ILL PATIENTS IN HOSPITAL: RECOGNITION OF AND RESPONSE TO ACUTE ILLNESS IN ADULTS IN HOSPITAL

National Institute for Clinical Excellence 2007

Guidance

Adult patients in acute hospital settings, including patients in the emergency department for whom a clinical decision to admit has been made, should have:

- physiological observations recorded at the time of their admission or initial assessment
- a clear written monitoring plan that specifies which physiological observations should be recorded and how often. The plan should take account of the:
  - patient's diagnosis
  - presence of comorbidities
  - agreed treatment plan.

Physiological observations should be recorded and acted upon by staff who have been trained to undertake these procedures and understand their clinical relevance.

Physiological track and trigger systems should be used to monitor all adult patients in acute hospital settings.

- Physiological observations should be monitored at least every 12 h, unless a decision has been made at a senior level to increase or decrease this frequency for an individual patient.
- The frequency of monitoring should increase if abnormal physiology is detected, as outlined in the recommendation on graded response strategy.

Staff caring for patients in acute hospital settings should have competencies in monitoring, measurement, interpretation and prompt response to the acutely ill patient appropriate to the level of care they are providing. Education and training should be provided to ensure staff have these competencies, and they should be assessed to ensure they can demonstrate them.

A graded response strategy for patients identified as being at risk of clinical deterioration should be agreed and delivered locally. It should consist of the following three levels.

- Low-score group:
  - Increased frequency of observations and the nurse in charge alerted.
- Medium-score group:
  - Urgent call to team with primary medical responsibility for the patient.
  - Simultaneous call to personnel with core competencies for acute illness. These competencies can be delivered by a variety of models at a local level, such as a critical care outreach team, a hospital-at-night team or a specialist trainee in an acute medical or surgical specialty.

- High-score group:
  - Emergency call to team with critical care competencies and diagnostic skills. The team should include a medical practitioner skilled in the assessment of the critically ill patient, who possesses advanced airway management and resuscitation skills. There should be an immediate response.
- If the team caring for the patient considers that admission to a critical care area is clinically indicated, then the decision to admit should involve both the consultant caring for the patient on the ward and the consultant in critical care.

After the decision to transfer a patient from a critical care area to the general ward has been made, he or she should be transferred as early as possible during the day. Transfer from critical care areas to the general ward between 22.00 and 07.00 should be avoided whenever possible, and should be documented as an adverse incident if it occurs.

The critical care area transferring team and the receiving ward team should take shared responsibility for the care of the patient being transferred. They should jointly ensure:

- there is continuity of care through a formal structured handover of care from critical care area staff to ward staff (including both medical and nursing staff), supported by a written plan
- that the receiving ward, with support from critical care if required, can deliver the agreed plan. The formal structured handover of care should include:
  - a summary of critical care stay, including diagnosis and treatment
  - a monitoring and investigation plan
  - a plan for ongoing treatment, including drugs and therapies, nutrition plan, infection status and any agreed limitations of treatment
  - physical and rehabilitation needs
  - psychological and emotional needs
  - specific communication or language needs.

Bibliography

Chan KP, Stewart TE, Mehta S: High-frequency oscillatory ventilation for adult patients with ARDS, *Chest* 131:1907–1916, 2007.

Dernaika TA, Keddissi JI, Kinasewitz GT: Update on ARDS: beyond the low tidal volume, *Am J Med Sci* 337:360–367, 2009.

Malarkkan N, Snook NJ, Lumb AB: New aspects of ventilation in acute lung injury, *Anaesthesia* 58:647–667, 2003.

McLuckie A: High-frequency oscillation in acute respiratory distress syndrome (ARDS), *Br J Anaesth* 93:322–323, 2004.

Moloney ED, Griffiths MJD: Protective ventilation of patients with acute respiratory distress syndrome, *Br J Anaesth* 92:261–270, 2004.

NICE: Quick reference guide. Acutely ill patients in hospital, *NICE clinical guideline* 50:2007. www.nice.org.uk/nicemedia/pdf/CG50QuickRefGuide.pdf.

Rouby J-J, Consstantin J-M, Girardi CR, et al: Mechanical ventilation in patients with acute respiratory distress syndrome, *Anesthesiology* 101:228–234, 2004.

CARDIOVASCULAR SYSTEM

Inotropes

If shock persists despite adequate volume replacement and vital organ perfusion is jeopardized, inotropic drugs may be required to improve blood pressure and cardiac output (Table 7.2).

Table 7.2 Receptor actions of inotropes

	α_1	α_2	β_1	β_2	DA_1	DA_2
Adrenaline						
Low dose	+	±	+	+	0	0
Moderate dose	++	+	++	+	0	0
High dose	++++	+++	+++	+++	0	0
Noradrenaline	+++	+++	++	0	0	0
Isoprenaline	0	0	+++	+++	0	0
Dopamine						
Low dose	±	+	±	0	++	+
Moderate dose	++	+	++	+	++	+
High dose	+++	+	+++	++	+++	+
Dopexamine	0	0	+	+++	++	+
Dobutamine	±	0	++	+	0	0

Cardiogenic shock. Characterized by low cardiac output, high filling pressures and increased systemic vascular resistance (SVR). Inodilators (dobutamine, enoximone, milrinone, dopexamine) improve cardiac contractility and decrease SVR. Specific vasodilators (nitroprusside, GTN) may reduce afterload further, increasing stroke volume and decreasing cardiac work by decreasing systolic wall tension.

Septic shock. Characterized by high cardiac output (if hypovolaemia corrected) and decreased SVR. Vasoconstrictors (noradrenaline) reduce SVR. Dobutamine or adrenaline may be required to improve myocardial contractility.

Adrenergic receptor function

Arterioles and veins contain α_1 and α_2 receptors which cause vasoconstriction. Vessels in skeletal muscle are rich in β_2 receptors which cause vasodilation. Myocardium is rich in β_1 and β_2 receptors which are pro-chronotropic and pro-inotropic.

α_1 receptors activate phospholipase C which cleaves phosphoinositol 4,5-biphosphate (PIP$_2$) to diacylglycerol (DAG) and inositol triphosphate (IP$_3$). DAG activates protein kinase C to release arachidonic acid which increases cGMP synthesis (Fig. 7.2). Activation of β_1, β_2 and dopamine (D$_1$) receptors triggers the conversion of ATP to cAMP, activating protein kinase C and triggering protein phosphorylation which causes tachycardia and increases contractility (Fig. 7.3).

Pulmonary artery catheters

Although a recent meta-analysis concluded that PAC did not affect mortality, intensive care unit or hospital length of stay, analysis of the National Trauma Data Bank in 2006 (53312 patients) has demonstrated improved outcomes when used for major trauma. Although there is limited evidence to show improved outcome with PAC use, the general consensus is that their use in appropriate patients by clinicians skilled in their insertion and data interpretation is of benefit.

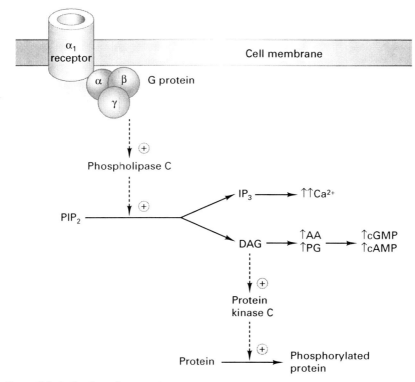

Figure 7.2 Activation of α_1 receptors.

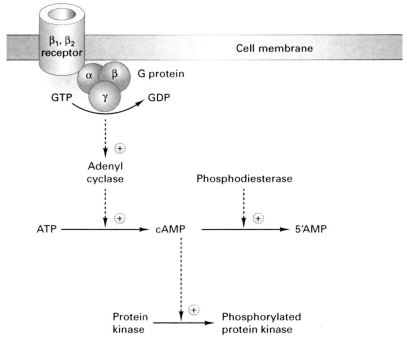

Figure 7.3 Activation of β_1, β_2 receptors.

Indications

- Haemodynamic instability with unknown diagnosis
- Major trauma – as a guide to volume replacement and haemodynamic support
- Myocardial infarction – to differentiate hypovolaemia from cardiogenic shock
- Pulmonary oedema – to differentiate cardiogenic from non-cardiogenic causes
- Hypotension when right atrial pressure may not equal that of the left atrium, e.g. right heart failure, chronic obstructive airway disease, pulmonary hypertension
- Pre-eclampsia with hypertension, oliguria and pulmonary oedema
- High-risk surgical patients
- Pulmonary embolism to assist in diagnosis and guide haemodynamic support.

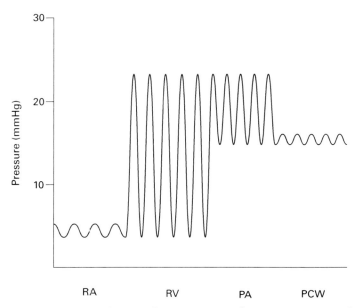

Figure 7.4 Pressure changes during pulmonary artery catheter insertion. RA, right atrium; RV, right ventricle; PA, pulmonary artery; PCW, pulmonary capillary wedge.

Pressure changes during PAC insertion (Fig. 7.4)

Place catheter so that it does not wedge until at least 1.2 mL air is in the balloon (1.5 mL max.). Greatest degree of accuracy if tip of catheter is placed in West's zone III. Zone I tends to measure airway pressure, particularly with hypovolaemia. Measure wedge from 'a' wave at end of expiration.

Complications

Table 7.3 Complications of pulmonary artery catheter insertion

Associated with insertion	Associated with catheter presence
Pneumothorax/haemothorax	Infection of catheter or site
Haematoma	Pulmonary thrombosis/infarct
Cardiac arrhythmias	Cardiac arrhythmias
Arterial puncture	Valve damage/endocarditis
Pulmonary artery perforation	Pulmonary artery erosion
Catheter knotting	Thrombocytopenia
Cardiac valve damage	

Cardiac output monitoring

Invasive techniques

- **Intermittent thermodilution.** Change in temperature of blood following injection of iced saline. Calculated from the Stuart–Hamilton equation:

$$CO = \frac{VI(BT - IT)}{(BT_0 - BT)}$$

where:
CO = cardiac output
VI = volume of injectate
BT = blood temperature after injection
BT_0 = blood (pulmonary artery) temperature before injection
IT = injectate temperature.

- **Continuous thermodilution.** Change in temperature of blood warmed by heating coil on pulmonary artery catheter. Calculated from a modified Stuart–Hamilton equation.
- **Indocyanine green dilution** (historical)

$$CO = \frac{\text{milligrams of dye injected} \times 60}{\text{Average concentration of dye in blood for the duration of the curve} \times \text{duration of the curve}}$$

- **Fick calculated cardiac output**

$$CO = \frac{O_2 \text{ consumption}}{\text{arteriovenous } O_2 \text{ content difference}}$$

- **Pulse contour cardiac output (PiCCO).** Calculates cardiac output continuously from pulse contour analysis of the aortic waveform via an arterial catheter. Requires central venous access to perform a thermodilution cardiac output measurement for calibration (analysed by a thermistor present in the arterial catheter tip).
- **Combined lithium dilution and pulse contour analysis (LiDCO).** Uses lithium dilution curve for initial calibration followed by a pulse contour algorithm to determine beat-to-beat stroke volume from a mathematical analysis of the peripheral arterial waveform.

Non-invasive techniques

- **Transthoracic/oesophageal Doppler ultrasonography.** Measurement of aortic cross-sectional area and blood flow velocity allows calculation of cardiac output. Acceleration and peak velocity indicate myocardial performance, while flow time is related to circulating volume and peripheral resistance.

- *Transthoracic impedance*. Can be measured across externally applied electrodes. Small changes in impedance (<1Ω) occur with the cardiac cycle as the blood volume in the heart increases during diastole and decreases during systole. Rate of change of impedance can be used to estimate cardiac output.
- *Pulse contour analysis*. Analyses the arterial waveform to calculate cardiac output by using an estimated compliance of the arterial tree to calculate the stroke volume needed to increase the blood pressure by a given amount. Accuracy limited by non-linear vascular compliance, damped waveforms and aortic wall pathology.

Transoesophageal echocardiography (TOE)

Increasing use in critical care. Uses the physical principle that sound is reflected from tissue interfaces. Piezoelectric crystals transmit and receive acoustic signals to build a two-dimensional image. TOE provides better cardiac views than transthoracic echocardiography, particularly of valves, contractility and filling status.

TOE is of particular use in the assessment of:

- left ventricular systolic function
- left ventricular filling
- wall motion abnormalities
- cardiac tamponade
- valve function
- chest trauma (limited views of ascending aorta).

TOE has shown a poor relationship between PCWP and left ventricular end-diastolic volume, particularly in septic patients and those on high doses of inotropes. In these patients, mean pulmonary capillary pressure may be a more accurate measure.

Bibliography

American Society of Anesthesiologists Task Force on Pulmonary Artery Catheterization: Practice guidelines for pulmonary artery catheterization, *Anesthesiology* 99:988–1014, 2003.

Antonelli M, Levy M, Andrews PJ, et al: Hemodynamic monitoring in shock and implications for management. International Consensus Conference, *Intensive Care Med* 33:575–590, 2007.

Dawson S, Jhanji S, Pears JRM: Cardiac output monitoring: basic science and clinical application, *Anaesthesia* 63:172–181, 2008.

Jhanji S, Dawson J, Pearse RM: Cardiac output monitoring: basic science and clinical application, *Anaesthesia* 63:172–181, 2008.

Klein AA, Snell A, Nashef SA, et al: The impact of intra-operative transoesophageal echocardiography on cardiac surgical practice, *Anaesthesia* 64:947–952, 2009.

Moppett I, Shajar M: Transoesophageal echocardiography, *BJA CEPD Rev* 1:72–75, 2001.
Van Lieshout JJ, Wesseling KH: Continuous cardiac output by pulse contour analysis? *Br J Anaesth* 86:467–469, 2001.

FLUID AND ELECTROLYTE BALANCE

The neonate has a greater proportion of body water and in a different distribution than the adult (Fig. 7.5). More fluid is distributed within the extracellular compartment (interstitial and plasma volume) compared with the adult, resulting in a larger volume of distribution for water-soluble drugs. A large proportion of interstitial fluid is excreted within the first few weeks after birth and adult levels are attained by adolescence.

A 70 kg male has about 42 kg of water distributed through three body compartments.

- extracellular fluid – 20% (plasma volume 4%, interstitial fluid 16%)
- intracellular fluid – 40%

$$= 60\% = 42\,L$$

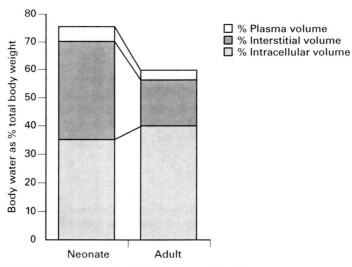

Figure 7.5 Body water distribution in the neonate and adult.

Plasma volume expansion is least effective with fluids that are distributed throughout all body compartments and most effective with those that remain within the intravascular compartment. Therefore:

- 1000 mL 5% dextrose (plasma, interstitial and intracellular compartments) expands plasma by $1000 \times 4/60 = 67\,mL$

- 1000 mL normal saline (plasma and interstitial compartments) expands plasma by 1000 × 4/20 = 200 mL
- 1000 mL colloid (plasma only) expands plasma by 1000 × 4/4 = 1000 mL.

Starling equation

$$Q = K[(Pc - P_i) - \sigma(\pi_c - \pi_i)]$$

where:
Q = fluid flux out of capillary bed
K = capillary filtration coefficient (permeability of membrane to water)
P_c = capillary hydrostatic pressure
P_i = interstitial hydrostatic pressure
σ = reflection coefficient of albumin (permeability of membrane to protein)
π_c = capillary colloid osmotic pressure
π_i = interstitial colloid osmotic pressure.
Osmolality is the number of osmotically active particles per kg of solvent:

$$= 2Na^+ + glucose / 18 + urea / 2.8$$

Homeostatic control

A rise in serum osmolality stimulates osmoreceptors in the anterior hypothalamus to release ADH from the supraoptic nuclei. ADH release is also stimulated by volume receptors in the left atrium and carotid sinus baroreceptors in response to hypovolaemia.

ADH increases permeability of the distal collecting ducts, resulting in more fluid reabsorption and a reduction in the osmolality of body fluids.

Aldosterone is produced by the adrenal cortex in response to ACTH, renin, hyponatraemia or hyperkalaemia. It acts on the distal tubules and collecting ducts to increase Na^+ resorption and K^+ excretion.

Renin is secreted by the juxtaglomerular apparatus in response to a fall in extracellular volume or BP and acts on angiotensinogen to form angiotensin I which is converted to angiotensin II by passage through the lungs. Vasoconstriction produced by angiotensin II produces a marked rise in both systolic and diastolic blood pressures.

Normal fluid requirements

Fluid and electrolyte requirements per 24 h

- Water: $35 \, mL.kg^{-1}$
- Na^+: $2 \, mmol.kg^{-1}$
- K^+: $1 \, mmol.kg^{-1}$

Loss

- Insensible loss (skin and lungs) 500–1000 mL.24 h^{-1}.
- Urine (minimum) 300 mL.24 h^{-1}.
- Faeces 500 mL.24 h^{-1}.

Assessment of hydration

Thirst, skin turgor (loss of turgor at >10% fluid deficit), hydration of mucous membranes, core–peripheral temperature gradient, pulse rate and volume, postural hypotension (>20% fluid deficit), urine output and osmolality and fluid balance.

Postoperative fluid requirements

Intravenous fluids administered perioperatively during minor gynaecological surgery reduce morbidity, particularly nausea and dizziness. However, blood coagulation appears to be accelerated by haemodilution with saline, and in patients undergoing elective abdominal surgery, the incidence of DVT was four times greater than in the fluid-restricted group (Janvrin et al 1980).

Despite this latter study, it is generally agreed that the advantages of perioperative fluids outweigh any disadvantages. Hartmann's 15 mL.kg^{-1}.h^{-1} has been suggested for major surgery; a rate shown to improve postoperative renal function. Septic patients or those with lung trauma have raised extravascular lung water, and lesser rates may be necessary to avoid pulmonary oedema. In addition, give blood to maintain Hb >8.5–9.0 g.dL^{-1}.

Surgical stress causes release of ADH, renin and aldosterone, resulting in sodium and water retention, potassium excretion and an inability to excrete a hypotonic urine. Postoperative catabolism increases the minimum metabolic demand for water from 20 to 30 mL.kg^{-1} per day, i.e. 2000 mL.day^{-1}. The addition of 100 g.day^{-1} of glucose reduces nitrogen loss by up to 60%. Therefore, give maintenance fluids of 2000 mL 5% dextrose.24 h^{-1} postoperatively with 30 mmol KCl added to each 1 L bag to provide daily K$^+$ requirements. Hidden losses are difficult to judge so titrate fluids according to urine output (>0.5 mL.kg^{-1}.h^{-1}). Sodium retention is greatly reduced by 48 h so then add Na$^+$ to maintenance fluids and reduce KCl supplements.

Albumin

Single polypeptide of 585 amino acids. Synthesized in the endoplasmic reticulum of hepatocytes at 9–12 g/day but can increase 2–3 times in states of maximum synthesis. Stimulus to production is colloid osmotic pressure, osmolality of the extravascular liver space, insulin, thyroxine and cortisol. Catabolized by vascular endothelium. 5% of albumin is removed from the intravascular space per hour. Clinical properties of albumin include:

- *Binding and transport* – strong negative charge binds Ca^{2+} (40%), Cu^{2+}, thyroxine, bilirubin and amino acids; also binds warfarin, phenytoin, NSAIDs and digoxin

- *Maintenance of colloid osmotic pressure* (COP) – contributes to 80% of COP
- *Free radical scavenging* – thiol groups scavenge reactive oxygen and nitrogen species
- *Platelet inhibition and antithrombotic effects*
- *Effects on vascular permeability* – may bind within the subendothelium to alter capillary membrane permeability.

Serum albumin decreases due to dilutional effects with crystalloid/colloid solutions, redistribution due to altered capillary permeability (five-fold increase during sepsis), decreased synthesis in septic patients, and increased loss from kidney or gut.

Correlation between COP and serum albumin is poor. Therefore, oedema associated with hypoalbuminaemia is not necessarily related and may be related more to lymphatic dysfunction. The acute-phase response is initially associated with a decrease in albumin synthesis, possibly due to IL-6-mediated inhibition of synthesis. A later hypermetabolic phase results in increased albumin synthesis.

Benefits of correcting hypoalbuminaemia are unclear. A prospective randomized study of 475 ICU patients comparing albumin and gelatin solutions failed to show any benefit (Stockwell et al 1992). In 70 children with burns, albumin supplementation failed to improve morbidity or mortality (Greenhalgh et al 1995). In septic patients, albumin infusions will only increase COP for a relatively short period. Increased capillary permeability results in >60% of albumin leaving the intravascular compartment within 4 h, potentially worsening oedema.

A controversial systematic review by the Cochrane Group of 23 randomized controlled trials found that the risk of death was 6% greater in the group treated with albumin compared with those receiving crystalloids or no treatment (Cochrane Injuries Group 1998). The Committee on Safety of Medicines now advises doctors to restrict the use of, and take special care when using, human albumin, but states that there is 'insufficient evidence of harm to warrant withdrawal of albumin'. Hypoalbuminaemia in itself is not an appropriate indication. Risks of hypervolaemia and cardiovascular overload warrant monitoring in patients receiving albumin.

Intravenous fluids
Crystalloids
0.9% normal saline (per 1000 mL)
- Sodium 150 mmol
- Chloride 150 mmol
- Osmolality 308.

RescueFlow is a hypertonic salt solution and is available as 6% dextran 70/7.5% sodium chloride. The hypertonic saline induces a rapid fluid shift from the intracellular to intravascular space; dextran then sustains volume expansion. This may be useful in patients predisposed to tissue oedema, e.g. severe burns, traumatic brain injuries.

Hartmann's (per 1000 mL)

- Sodium 131 mmol
- Chloride 111 mmol
- Lactate 29 mmol
- Potassium 5 mmol
- Calcium 2 mmol
- Osmolality 280.

Dextrose saline (per 1000 mL) (4% dextrose, 0.18% saline)

- Sodium 30 mmol
- Chloride 30 mmol
- Osmolality 300
- Calories 160 (40 g CHO).

5% Dextrose (per 1000 mL)

- Osmolality 278
- Calories 200 (50 g CHO).

Colloids

Gelofusine (per 1000 mL)

4% solution of succinylated gelatine in saline. $t_{1/2}$ is 2–4 h.

- Sodium 154 mmol
- Chloride 125 mmol
- Calcium 0.4 mmol
- Magnesium 0.4 mmol
- Gelatin 40 g with MW 30 000.

Haemaccel (per 1000 mL)

A 3.5% solution of polygeline in a mixed salt solution. It is cross-linked with urea, which may be released after hydrolysis, a potential problem in patients with renal failure. $t_{1/2}$ is 6 h.

- Sodium 145 mmol
- Chloride 145 mmol
- Potassium 5 mmol
- Calcium 6.25 mmol.

Starches

Amylopectin linked with hydroxyethyl groups in a glucose moiety making a polymer similar to glycogen. Large range of molecular weights.

Hespan is 6% hetastarch; $t_{1/2}$ 24 h because of the hydroxyethyl–glucose bond.

Voluven is similar to Hespan but with a lower molecular weight. Allergic reactions are less likely than with Voluven compared with other colloids.

Human albumin solution

Derived from human plasma by fractionation. Heat sterilized with minimal risk of infective transmission.

Colloid versus crystalloid controversy (Table 7.4)

There is some evidence to suggest that crystalloid resuscitation is associated with a lower mortality in trauma patients.

Table 7.4 Comparison of crystalloids and colloids

	Advantages	Disadvantages
Crystalloid	Cheap	Larger volumes needed
	Replaces extravascular loss	Small ↑ in plasma volume
	Increased GFR	Peripheral and pulmonary oedema
	Minimal effect on clot quality	
Colloid	Smaller volumes needed	Risk of anaphylaxis
	Prolonged ↑ in plasma volume	Relatively expensive
	Reduced peripheral oedema	Coagulopathy
		Poor clot quality

BRITISH CONSENSUS GUIDELINES ON INTRAVENOUS FLUID THERAPY FOR ADULT SURGICAL PATIENTS
Powell-Tuck et al 2008

Summary and recommendations

Food and fluids should be provided orally or enterally and i.v. infusions discontinued as soon as possible. The effects of surgical and metabolic stress on the renin-angiotensin–aldosterone system and on vasopressin should be understood. Nutrition should be assessed and cautiously maintained. The oedematous patient should be managed with particular care, in order to achieve successful negative sodium and water balance.

1. Because of the risk of inducing hyperchloraemic acidosis in routine practice, when crystalloid resuscitation or replacement is indicated, balanced salt solutions, e.g. Ringer's lactate/acetate or Hartmann's solution should replace 0.9% saline, except in cases of hypochloraemia, e.g. from vomiting or gastric drainage.

2. Solutions such as 4%/0.18% dextrose/saline and 5% dextrose are important sources of free water for maintenance, but should be used with caution as excessive amounts may cause dangerous hyponatraemia, especially in children and the elderly. These solutions are not appropriate for resuscitation or replacement therapy except in conditions of significant free water deficit, e.g. diabetes insipidus.

3. To meet maintenance requirements, adult patients should receive sodium 50–100 mmol/day, potassium 40–80 mmol/day in 1.5–2.5 L of water by the oral, enteral or parenteral route (or a combination of routes). Additional amounts should only be given to correct deficit or continuing losses. Careful monitoring should be undertaken using clinical examination, fluid balance charts, and regular weighing when possible.

Preoperative fluid management

4. In patients without disorders of gastric emptying undergoing elective surgery clear non-particulate oral fluids should not be withheld for more than 2 hours prior to the induction of anaesthesia.

5. In the absence of disorders of gastric emptying or diabetes, preoperative administration of carbohydrate rich beverages 2–3 h before induction of anaesthesia may improve patient well being and facilitate recovery from surgery. It should be considered in the routine preoperative preparation for elective surgery.

6. Routine use of preoperative mechanical bowel preparation is not beneficial and may complicate intra and postoperative management of fluid and electrolyte balance. Its use should therefore be avoided whenever possible.

7. Where mechanical bowel preparation is used, fluid and electrolyte derangements commonly occur and should be corrected by simultaneous intravenous fluid therapy with Hartmann's or Ringer–Lactate/acetate type solutions.

8. Excessive losses from gastric aspiration/vomiting should be treated preoperatively with an appropriate crystalloid solution which includes an appropriate potassium supplement. Hypochloraemia is an indication for the use of 0.9% saline, with sufficient additions of potassium and care not to produce sodium overload.

9. Losses from diarrhoea/ileostomy/small bowel fistula/ileus/obstruction should be replaced volume for volume with Hartmann's or Ringer-Lactate/acetate type solutions. Saline depletion, for example due to excessive diuretic exposure, is best managed with a balanced electrolyte solution such as Hartmann's.

10. In high-risk surgical patients, preoperative treatment with intravenous fluid and inotropes should be aimed at achieving predetermined goals for cardiac output and oxygen delivery as this may improve survival.

11. Although currently logistically difficult in many centres, preoperative or operative hypovolaemia should be diagnosed by flow-based measurements wherever possible. The clinical context should also be taken into account, as this will provide an important indication of whether hypovolaemia is possible or likely. When direct flow measurements are not possible, hypovolaemia will be diagnosed clinically on the basis of pulse, peripheral perfusion and capillary refill, venous (JVP/CVP) pressure and Glasgow Coma Scale, together with acid–base and lactate measurements. A low urine output can be misleading and needs to be interpreted in the context of the patient's cardiovascular parameters above.

12. Hypovolaemia due predominantly to blood loss should be treated with either a balanced crystalloid solution or a suitable colloid until packed red cells are available. Hypovolaemia due to severe inflammation such as infection, peritonitis, pancreatitis or burns should be treated with either a suitable colloid or a balanced crystalloid. In either clinical scenario, care must be taken to administer sufficient balanced crystalloid and colloid to normalize haemodynamic parameters and

13. Minimize overload. The ability of critically ill patients to excrete excess sodium and water is compromised, placing them at risk of severe interstitial oedema. The administration of large volumes of colloid without sufficient free water (e.g. 5% dextrose) may precipitate a hyperoncotic state.

14. When the diagnosis of hypovolaemia is in doubt and the CVP is not raised, the response to a bolus infusion of 200 mL of a suitable colloid or crystalloid should be tested. The response should be assessed using the patient's cardiac output and stroke volume measured by flow-based technology if available. Alternatively, the clinical response may be monitored by measurement/estimation of the pulse, capillary refill, CVP and blood pressure before and 15 min after receiving the infusion. This procedure should be repeated until there is no further increase in stroke volume and improvement in the clinical parameters.

Intraoperative fluid management

15. In patients undergoing some forms of orthopaedic and abdominal surgery, intraoperative treatment with intravenous fluid to achieve an optimal value of stroke volume should be used where possible as this may reduce postoperative complication rates and duration of hospital stay.

16. Patients undergoing non-elective major abdominal or orthopaedic surgery should receive intravenous fluid to achieve an optimal value of stroke volume during and for the first 8 hours after surgery. This may be supplemented by a low dose dopexamine infusion.

Postoperative fluid and nutritional management

17. Details of fluids administered must be clearly recorded and easily accessible.

18. When patients leave theatre for the ward, HDU or ICU their volume status should be assessed. The volume and type of fluids given

perioperatively should be reviewed and compared with fluid losses in theatre including urine and insensible losses.

19. In patients who are euvolaemic and haemodynamically stable a return to oral fluid administration should be achieved as soon as possible.

20. In patients requiring continuing i.v. maintenance fluids, these should be sodium poor and of low enough volume until the patient has returned their sodium and fluid balance over the perioperative period to zero. When this has been achieved the i.v. fluid volume and content should be those required for daily maintenance and replacement of any on-going additional losses.

21. The haemodynamic and fluid status of those patients who fail to excrete their perioperative sodium load, and especially whose urine sodium concentration is <20 mmol/L, should be reviewed.

22. In high-risk patients undergoing major abdominal surgery, postoperative treatment with intravenous fluid and low dose dopexamine should be considered, in order to achieve a predetermined value for systemic oxygen delivery, as this may reduce postoperative complication rates and duration of hospital stay.

23. In patients who are oedematous, hypovolaemia if present must be treated, followed by a gradual persistent negative sodium and water balance based on urine sodium concentration or excretion. Plasma potassium concentration should be monitored and where necessary potassium intake adjusted.

24. Nutritionally depleted patients need cautious refeeding orally, enterally or parenterally, with feeds supplemented in potassium, phosphate and thiamine. Generally, and particularly if oedema is present, these feeds should be reduced in water and sodium. Though refeeding syndrome is a risk, improved nutrition will help to restore normal partitioning of sodium, potassium and water between intra and extra-cellular spaces.

25. Surgical patients should be nutritionally screened, and NICE guidelines for perioperative nutritional support adhered to. Care should be taken to mitigate risks of the re-feeding syndrome.

Fluid management in acute kidney injury (AKI)

26. Based on current evidence, higher molecular weight hydroxyethyl starch (hetastarch and pentastarch MW ≥200 kDa) should be avoided in patients with severe sepsis due to an increased risk of AKI.

27. Higher molecular weight hydroxyethyl starch (hetastarch and pentastarch MW ≥200 kDa) should be avoided in brain-dead kidney donors due to reports of osmotic nephrosis-like lesions.

28. Balanced electrolyte solutions containing potassium can be used cautiously in patients with AKI closely monitored on HDU or ICU in preference to 0.9% saline. If free water is required, 5% dextrose or dextrose saline should be used. Patients developing hyperkalaemia or progressive AKI should be switched to non potassium containing crystalloid solutions such as 0.45% saline or 4%/0.18 dextrose/saline.

29. In patients with AKI, fluid balance must be closely observed and fluid overload avoided. In patients who show signs of refractory fluid overload, renal replacement therapy should be considered early to mobilize interstitial oedema and correct extracellular electrolyte and acid–base abnormalities.

30. Patients at risk of developing AKI secondary to rhabdomyolysis must receive aggressive fluid resuscitation with an isotonic crystalloid solution to correct hypovolaemia. There is insufficient evidence to recommend the specific composition of the crystalloid.

Bibliography

Boldt J: The balanced concept of fluid resuscitation, Br J Anaesth 99:312–315, 2007.

Chappell D, Hofmann-Kiefer K, Conzen P, et al: A rational approach to perioperative fluid management, Anesthesiology 109:723–740, 2008.

Choi PTL, Yip G, Quinonez LG, et al: Crystalloids vs colloids in fluid resuscitation: a systematic review, Crit Care Med 27:200–210, 1999.

Cochrane Injuries Group: Human albumin administration in critically injured patients: systematic review of randomised controlled trials, BMJ 317:235–240, 1998.

Greenhalgh DG, Housinger TA, Kagan RJ, et al: Maintenance of serum albumin levels in pediatric burn patients: a prospective, randomized trial, J Trauma 39:67–74, 1995.

Grocott MPW, Mythen M, Gan TJ: Perioperative fluid management and clinical outcome in adults, Anesth Analg 100:1093–1106, 2005.

Janvrin SB, Davies G, Greenhalgh RM: Postoperative deep vein thrombosis caused by intravenous fluids during surgery, Br J Surg 67:690–693, 1980.

Powell-Tuck J, Gosling P, Lobo DN, et al: British Consensus Guidelines on Intravenous Fluid Therapy for Adult Surgical Patients, 2008. www.ics.ac.uk/intensive_care_professional/standards_and_guidelines/british_consensus_guidelines_on_intravenous_fluid_therapy_for_adult_surgical_patients__giftasup__2008.

Rassam SS, Counsell DJ: Perioperative fluid therapy, Contin Edu Anaesth, Crit Care Pain 5:161–165, 2005.

Stockwell MA, Soni N, Riley B: Colloid solutions in the critically ill. A randomised comparison of albumin and polygeline. 1. Outcome and duration of stay in the intensive care unit, Anaesthesia 47:3–6, 1992.

Strandvik GF: Hypertonic saline in critical care: a review of the literature and guidelines for use in hypotensive states and raised intracranial pressure, Anaesthesia 64:990–1003, 2009.

METHICILLIN RESISTANT STAPHYLOCOCCUS AUREUS (MRSA)

Increasing resistance to penicillin-based antibiotics since their introduction in the 1950s. Due to ß-lactamase enzyme and penicillin binding protein. MRSA first recognized in Europe in the 1960s. Rates of infection greatest in ICU > surgical wards > general wards > community.

Routes of transmission are hands, environment and colonized patients. Control spread through hand washing, cleaning, screening of patients and eradication.

Risk factors for infection are:

- MRSA colonization (60% critically ill patients will develop infection).
- Length of ICU and hospital stay (odds ratio = 2.5 for hospital stay of >2 weeks).
- Severity of illness and intensity of care.
- Intravascular devices. Nine-fold increase in MRSA infection in patients with intravascular catheters.
- Antibiotic therapy – some studies have shown that number of antibiotics used and duration of therapy directly increases risk of MRSA infection.

Mandatory reporting of all MRSA bacteraemias to the Department of Health since 2001. Mortality greater with MRSA than methicillin-sensitive *Staph aureus* (MSSA). NCEPOD 2001 showed that 1.8% of surgical deaths were associated with MRSA infection.

Glycopeptides (vancomycin, teicoplanin) are still the mainstay of treatment. Vancomycin-resistant strains may be sensitive to linezolid and quinupristin/dalfopristin.

Bibliography

Hardy KJ, Hawkey PM, Gao F, et al: Methicillin resistant *Staphylococcus aureus* in the critically ill, *Br J Anaesth* 92:121–130, 2004.

NITRIC OXIDE

In 1987, nitric oxide (NO) was identified as an endothelium-derived relaxing factor. It is a free radical acting as a local transcellular messenger through binding to transition metals within enzymes such as guanylate cyclase. About 1 mM of endogenous nitric oxide is synthesized per day. The synthesis and actions of NO are shown in Figure 7.6. NO is involved in:

- regulation of smooth muscle tone
- antimicrobial defence by its free radical action
- platelet and neutrophil adherence and aggregation
- peripheral and central neurotransmission
- regulation of smooth muscle proliferation.

Cardiovascular effects

Endothelial nitric oxide synthase (NOS) produces nitric oxide in response to changes in blood velocity (shear stress). NO in turn causes smooth muscle relaxation by activating cGMP which modulates calcium concentration and therefore vascular smooth muscle cell tone to match blood vessel calibre to

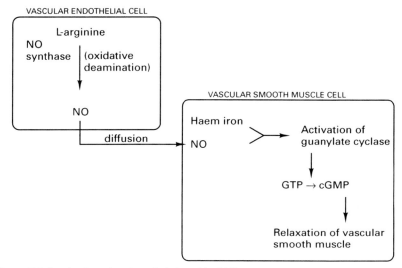

Figure 7.6 Synthesis and action of nitric oxide (NO).

flow. NO synthesis is also increased by acetylcholine, bradykinin, hypoxia and α-adrenergic stimulation, although the degree of vasodilation induced by these factors is uncertain. Excess NO produced in the presence of ischaemia may contribute to ischaemic damage through its free radical damage to myocardium. Inhibitors of NO synthesis may protect against myocardial reperfusion injury. Inadequate NO production increases platelet aggregation and adhesion.

Pharmacological nitrates (nitroprusside, isosorbide mononitrate, nitrites) are converted to NO within smooth muscle cells, increasing cGMP production. Sulphydryl (-SH) groups are required to form NO, but excessive nitrate therapy depletes –SH, leading to therapeutic tolerance.

Hypertension

Basal production of NO continuously vasodilates the peripheral circulation. Basal NO release is greater in arteries than in veins. Untreated hypertension in humans is associated with reduced NO synthesis. L-arginine supplementation alone does not restore NO levels to normal, suggesting that other mechanisms in addition to substrate depletion are involved. Excess end-products of glycosylation and oxidized lipoproteins in atherosclerosis have been proposed to inactivate nitric oxide synthetase.

Synthetic vasodilators

Organic nitrates such as GTN and nitroprusside undergo enzymatic reduction, releasing NO within vascular smooth muscles. Small vessels, e.g. coronary arteries, lack the capacity for this metabolism and only large capacitance vessels and coronary vessels >100 μm dilate in response to clinical doses of nitroglycerine. This selective vasodilation is less likely to cause coronary steal and contributes to the anti-anginal effects of nitrates. Tolerance to organic nitrates occurs due to a reduction in the biotransformation of the drug.

Respiratory effects

Normal pulmonary vascular tone is very low and exogenous NO has little effect on pulmonary vascular resistance. However, in disease states where pulmonary vascular tone is increased (pulmonary hypertension, ARDS, chronic respiratory failure), NO selectively vasodilates pulmonary vasculature around functioning alveolar units. This local vasodilation diverts blood towards functioning alveoli, reduces intrapulmonary shunting and may improve oxygenation. Significant systemic vasodilation does not occur because NO is rapidly inactivated by binding to haemoglobin.

Although NO improves arterial oxygen tension, no studies yet show improvement in mortality in adults with ARDS. Treatment of persistent pulmonary hypertension of the newborn appears promising and may avoid the need to use extracorporeal membrane oxygenation. In infants with hypoxic respiratory failure, NO appears as effective as ECMO in reducing mortality but is cheaper and simpler to use. Normal dose range is 0.5–20 ppm.

Neuronal NO

NO acts as a neurotransmitter in both the central and peripheral nervous systems, where its release is stimulated by excitatory amino acids. Neural functions of NO include peripheral non-adrenergic non-cholinergic transmission, neurotransmission in contractile and secretory tissue, synaptic plasticity, learning and memory.

Toxicity of NO

NO forms several toxic products, including nitrogen dioxide and nitric and nitrous acids. NO also reacts with free radicals to form peroxynitrite ($ONOO^{2-}$), which is highly cytotoxic. The clinical significance of these effects is uncertain. In the circulation, NO combines with iron to form methaemoglobin, which may be a problem with high levels of inhaled NO.

NO and sepsis

Inflammatory mediators such as TNF, cytokines and interferon induce nitric oxide synthase in endothelial cells, parenchymal cells and macrophages, increasing NO production. This may be the mechanism by which sepsis results in vasodilation. Some studies have shown that inhibition of NO synthesis with l-NMMA prevents these haemodynamic changes. Nitric oxide synthase inhibition may be a potential route for the treatment of sepsis. A large randomized controlled trial of a specific nitric oxide synthase antagonist in human septic shock was stopped because of an increased mortality rate in the treatment group and a large study of ketoconazole (which has anti-nitric oxide properties) showed no difference in mortality in ARDS.

Bibliography

Griffiths MJ, Evans TW: Inhaled nitric oxide therapy in adults, *N Engl J Med* 353:2683–2695, 2005.
Young D: Nitric oxide, *BJA CEPD Rev* 2:161–164, 2002.

NON-INVASIVE VENTILATION

Advantages

Avoids the morbidity associated with invasive ventilation (see Box 7.1).

Box 7.1　Morbidity associated with invasive ventilation

Insertion of tracheal tube
- Haemodynamic instability associated with anaesthetic induction.

Presence of tracheal tube
- Sedation in order to tolerate the tracheal tube
- Ventilator-associated pneumonia
- Cost
- Greater level of nursing care
- Sinusitis
- Inability to talk
- Inability to eat/drink.

Weaning
- Conversion of orotracheal tube to tracheostomy
- Tracheal stenosis
- Psychological dependence on invasive ventilatory support.

Post-extubation
- Tracheal stenosis
- Tracheal oedema causing airway obstruction.

Equipment

Requires ventilators that can deliver low resistance, high flow rates. Most popular machines deliver bilevel positive airway pressure (BiPAP). Simplest form is CPAP only. High levels of support are PEEP + pressure/volume support. Pressure-controlled modes have the advantage over volume-control in that they can compensate for air leaks. Three main types of mask:

- Nasal prongs
- Nasal mask
- Full face mask.

Indications (Box 7.2)

Main use is for management of exacerbation of COPD and acute cardiogenic pulmonary oedema where it reduces the need for tracheal intubation by 50–80% and reduces mortality by 50%. Also reduces ICU and hospital stay in these patients. Show to worsen morbidity when used as respiratory support for failed extubation.

Box 7.2   Indications for non-invasive ventilation

- Exacerbation of COPD
- Hypoxaemic respiratory failure
- Community-acquired pneumonia
- Nosocomial pneumonia
- Early ARDS
- Aspiration pneumonia
- Pulmonary oedema
- Asthma.

Bibliography

Caples SM, Gay PC: Noninvasive positive pressure ventilation in the intensive care unit, *Crit Care Med* 33:2651–2658, 2005.

Hill NS, Brennan J, Garpestad E, et al: Noninvasive ventilation in acute respiratory failure, *Crit Care Med* 35:2402–2407, 2007.

NUTRITION

Malnutrition

Malnutrition is common in hospital patients. Preoperative nutritional support can improve nutritional status but may only improve morbidity and mortality in severely malnourished patients. This support must be maintained for at least 7 days preoperatively to show any benefit. Prospective studies have demonstrated a benefit for postoperative nutritional support.

Assessment of malnutrition

- Weight loss >10%
- Skinfold thickness (lags behind nutritional status by 3–4 weeks)
  - arm muscle circumference decreased 20%
  - triceps skin fold thickness decreased 50%
- Hand grip tests – specific and reproducible measure
- Serum albumin <35 g/L, transferrin, total iron-binding capacity (TIBC), thyroxine-binding prealbumin
- Lymphocyte count <3.5
- Negative reaction to five skin antigens.

Effects of malnutrition

CVS. Decreased HR, CO and CVP

Respiratory. Decreased inspiratory force and FVC; weaning more difficult.

GI. Decreased gut motility, gut atrophy and increased gut permeability to intestinal bacteria.

Other. Decreased metabolic rate. Increased susceptibility to infection, poor wound healing, muscle weakness resulting in immobility, oedema and impaired organ function. Increased morbidity and mortality.

Starvation and stress result in different rates of malnutrition and changes in catabolic pathways (Table 7.5).

Table 7.5 Effect of starvation and stress on energy expenditure and malnutrition

	Starvation	Stress
Energy expenditure	+	+++
R:Q	0.7	0.8–0.85
Malnutrition	+	+++
Rate of malnutrition	+	+++

R:Q

$R:Q = CO_2 \text{ output} / O_2 \text{ consumption}$

- CHO = 1.0
- Protein = 0.83
- Fat = 0.71.

Nutritional support

Indications for nutritional support

- Albumin <30 g/L
- Marked weight loss, muscle wasting and oedema
- Dietary history showing decreased intake for >1 week
- Medical and surgical disorders likely to result in malnutrition
- Postoperative starvation for >10 days.

Composition

Optimal combination of water, carbohydrate, protein, fat, vitamins and trace elements. Calories as glucose or fat; protein as amino acids.

Calorie:nitrogen ratio of 200 calories:1 g N_2, decreasing to 100 calories:1 g N_2 in catabolic and septic patients.

Monitor electrolytes daily, monitor blood sugar every 48 h, monitor liver function tests weekly.

Caloric content

- CHO – 4 kcal/g
- Protein – 4 kcal/g
- Fat – 9 kcal/g.

Daily requirements (per 24 h)

- Calories – 30 kcal/kg
- Protein – 0.3 g N_2/kg (for burns = 0.5 g N_2/kg)
- Glucose – 2 g/kg
- Fat – 2 g/kg
- Water – 30 mL/kg
- Sodium – 1.2 mmol/kg
- Potassium – 0.8 mmol/kg.

The following are also required:

- *Glutamine*. Involved in repairing injured gut mucosa, generates substrate for renal ammonia production and supports lymphocyte proliferation. Supplementation decreases bacterial translocation, restores secretory IgA and improves N_2 balance.
- *Arginine*. Precursor for nitric oxide synthesis. Enhances wound healing and survival in animal models of sepsis.
- *Insulin*. Improves protein sparing and nitrogen balance.
- *Folic acid*.
- *Branch chain amino acids*. Encourage amino acid utilization and reduce oxidation.

Enteral feeding

Requires at least 25 cm ileum. Paralytic ileus only affects the stomach and colon. Small bowel motility and absorption often remain normal and therefore bowel sounds and flatus are not required to start enteral feeding. Early enteral feeding through a nasojejunal tube or feeding jejunostomy may prevent paralytic ileus.

Advantages of enteral over parenteral feeding

* Cheaper
* More efficient utilization of nutrients
* Stimulates intestinal blood flow
* Enteral feeding maintains GI mucosal barrier, preventing bacterial translocation and portal endotoxaemia. Bacterial translocation implicated in MODS
* Disuse atrophy of GI tract occurs rapidly without enteral feeding
* Postoperative enteral feeding reduces septic complications more than parenteral route
* Avoids complications of central venous cannula insertion
* Avoids TPN-induced immunosuppression
* Shorter hospital stay and greater survival compared with TPN in some studies.

Complications

* Infection – infusion phlebitis, mediastinitis
* Hyperglycaemia – requiring insulin
* Mineral deficiencies – especially zinc (poor wound healing), phosphate (muscle weakness)
* Thrombosis and embolism – reduced antithrombin III levels necessitate heparin
* Metabolic bone disease – osteomalacia, hypercalciuria
* Acid–base imbalance
* Hepatic dysfunction
* Fat overload.

Bibliography

Bistrian BR, McCowen KC: Nutritional and metabolic support in the adult intensive care unit: key controversies, *Crit Care Med* 34:1525–1531, 2006.

Napolitano L, Cresci G, Martindale RG, et al: Guidelines for the provision and assessment of nutrition support therapy in the adult critically ill patient: Society of Critical Care Medicine and American Society for Parenteral and Enteral Nutrition: Executive Summary, *Crit Care Med* 37:1757–1761, 2009.

OXYGEN TRANSPORT

Physiology

Oxygen cascade (PO_2) (kPa)

- Dry atmospheric gas 21.1
- Inspired tracheal gas 19.8
- Alveolar gas 14.7
- Arterial blood 13.3
- Mixed venous blood 5.3.

Table 7.6 Oxygen content of arterial and mixed venous blood

	Oxygen content (mL/dL)	
	Arterial	Mixed venous
Total	20.0	15.0
Attached to Hb	19.7	14.9
Dissolved	0.3	0.1
	2.0 (100% O_2)	
Saturation	97%	73%

Haemoglobin

- Complex compound of MW 64 500
- O_2-carrying capacity (Hufner's constant) = 1.39 mL.g^{-1}
- Because of impurities (e.g. methaemoglobin) = 1.34–1.36 mL.g^{-1}
- P_{50} (50% saturation)
  - adults: 3.5–3.9 kPa
  - fetus: 2.6 kPa.

Haemoglobin dissociation curve

Bohr effect. Increase H$^+$ shifts dissociation curve to right
2,3-DPG. Produced by glycolysis. Reduces O_2 affinity
Temperature. Pyrexia shifts dissociation curve to right.

Oxygen content

$$C_aO_2 = (1.3 \times Hb \times S_aO_2) + (0.003 \times P_aO_2)$$

where:
C_aO_2 = arterial oxygen content
$(1.3 \times Hb \times S_aO_2)$ – i.e. 1 g Hb, when completely saturated, binds 1.3 mL O_2
$(0.003 \times PaO_2)$ = amount of O_2 dissolved in plasma = 0.003 mL.mmHg^{-1}.

Oxygen delivery

$$DO_2 = \dot{Q} \times C_aO_2$$

where:
DO_2 = oxygen delivery
$\dot{Q}$ = cardiac output.

$$DO_2 = 3 \times (1.3 \times 14 \times 0.98) \times 10 (\times 10 \text{ converts volumes \% to mL/s})$$
$$= 540 \text{ mL.min}^{-1}.\text{m}^{-2}$$

Oxygen uptake

$$VO_2 = \dot{Q} \times (C_aO_2 - C_vO_2) \text{ (Fick equation)}$$

where:
VO_2 = oxygen uptake
C_vO_2 = venous oxygen content.

$$VO_2 = \dot{Q} \times (13 \times Hb) \times (S_aO_2 - S_vO_2)$$
$$= \dot{Q} \times (13 \times Hb) \times (0.97 \times 0.73)$$
$$= 130 \text{ mL / min per m}^2$$

Oxygen extraction ratio

The oxygen extraction ratio (O_2ER) is the fractional uptake of oxygen from the capillary bed.

$$O_2ER = VO_2 / DO_2 \times 100$$
$$= 130 / 540 \times 100$$
$$= 24\%$$

Normal response

Decreased blood flow results in increased O_2 extraction, i.e. drop in cardiac index is balanced by increased $(S_aO_2 - S_vO_2)$. Thus VO_2 remains unchanged.

All vascular beds can increase O_2 extraction if flow drops, *except* coronary circulation and diaphragm. Therefore it is necessary to maintain cardiac output in patients with coronary artery disease because DO_2 is flow dependent.

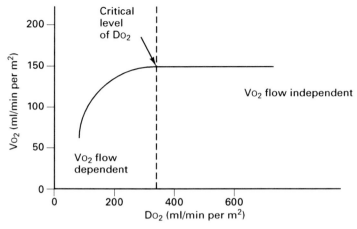

Figure 7.7 Oxygen delivery (Do_2) versus uptake (Vo_2) in critically ill patients.

Response in critically ill patients

Oxygen extraction from capillary beds may not increase where necessary and oxygen uptake (VO_2) becomes flow-dependent (Fig. 7.7). Therefore it is imperative to maintain cardiac output to maintain oxygen supply to the tissues.

Mixed venous oxygen

Under normal conditions, venous oxygen levels will vary directly with changes in cardiac output. This is the rationale for using mixed venous (pulmonary artery) oxygen saturation to monitor changes in cardiac output:

$$S_VO_2 = S_aO_2 - (VO_2 / \dot{Q} \times Hb \times 13)$$

Causes of low mixed venous oxygen

- Hypoxaemia
- Increased metabolic rate
- Low cardiac output
- Anaemia.

Causes of high mixed venous oxygen

- Decreased O_2 uptake, e.g. hypothermia, cell poisoning
- Left-to-right shunt
- Inappropriately high cardiac output, e.g. excessive use of inotropes/vasodilators.

S_vO_2 usually reflects cardiac output, but in seriously ill patients unable to mount a compensatory response to low blood flow, S_vO_2 will change little in response to changes in cardiac output. Thus, these patients show little correlation between venous oxygen and cardiac index.

Lactic acid

When the metabolic rate exceeds the rate of oxygen supply, tissues will switch to anaerobic metabolism and produce lactic acid. Therefore, the serum lactate concentration reflects the balance between VO_2 and the metabolic demand for oxygen.

Lactate is the end-product of anaerobic glycolysis, but it is also produced under normal aerobic conditions. The lactate anion is cleared by the liver and used for gluconeogenesis. Renal clearance becomes significant once levels reach 6–7 mEq/L. Hepatic failure probably contributes little to raised lactate levels in critically ill patients. A normal serum lactate does not exclude tissue ischaemia.

Raised lactate levels not associated with organ ischaemia are found with bacterial pneumonia, thiamine deficiency, generalized seizures, respiratory alkalosis and generalized trauma.

Bibliography

Morris CG, Low J: Metabolic acidosis in the critically ill: part 1. Classification and pathophysiology, *Anaesthesia* 63:294–301, 2008.
Morris CG, Low J: Metabolic acidosis in the critically ill: part 2. Causes and treatment, *Anaesthesia* 63:396–411, 2008.

RENAL REPLACEMENT THERAPY

In patients with severe acute renal failure, renal excretory function is lost. Resolution may take several weeks during which catabolism is marked, producing increased amounts of waste products. Requirements for intravascular space arise from intravenous drugs, fluids and feeding.

Renal replacement therapy therefore aims to remove excess water and remove unwanted solutes.

Normal kidney

- filters 180 L/day
- filters solutes weighing <60 000 Da
- reabsorbs 99% filtrate.

Urea is the waste product of protein metabolism (60 Da). Creatinine is the waste product of muscle metabolism (113 Da).

Immediate management of oliguria/acute renal failure

- Assess and treat any circulatory impairment
- Assess and treat any respiratory impairment

- Treat any acute manifestations if acute renal failure (salt and water retention, hypertension, hyperkalaemia, acidosis)
- Exclude urinary tract obstruction or infection
- Establish underlying cause and begin treatment as soon as possible
- Ensure patient is not taking nephrotoxic drugs.

Indications for dialysis

Absolute

- K^+ >6.5 mmol.L^{-1}
- Pulmonary oedema unresponsive to diuretics
- Uraemic encephalopathy/pericarditis/neuropathy.

Relative

- Urea >35 mmol.L^{-1}
- Creatinine >600 mmol.L^{-1}
- Oliguria (<5 mL.kg^{-1}.day^{-1})
- Metabolic acidosis (pH <7.2)
- To create intravascular volume for feeding, drugs, etc.
- Hyperpyrexia.

History

Intermittent haemofiltration was introduced in the 1950s and remained the only form of renal replacement therapy until the introduction of intermittent haemodialysis in 1967. Technical problems delayed the introduction of continuous techniques until the 1980s with continuous arteriovenous haemofiltration (CAVH) followed by continuous arteriovenous haemodiafiltration (CAVHD).

Filters

- Clear molecules <60 000 Da
- Filter surface area approx. 70 m^2
- Low resistance to enable high flow.

Principles

Water removal

Water is removed by a process called ultrafiltration. This process is similar to that performed by the glomerulus in the kidney. It requires a hydrostatic driving force to overcome oncotic pressure and move water across a semi-permeable membrane.

In the artificial kidney, this can be achieved by:

- applying a positive pressure (patient's blood pressure/pump pressure) across a semi-permeable membrane
- using a hyperosmolar solution (e.g. peritoneal dialysis)
- applying a negative pressure to the dialysate side of the membrane (e.g. haemodialysis).

Solute removal

This can be achieved by either diffusion or ultrafiltration.

Diffusion across a semi-permeable membrane. This is movement of solutes across a semi-permeable membrane from an area of high concentration to one of low concentration. A concentration gradient is therefore always necessary for diffusion to occur. Molecules of a smaller MW will move across the membrane more readily than those with a larger MW (Fig. 7.8). A semi-permeable membrane has a defined pore size; any molecule exceeding this will not be able to pass through.

This is the principle utilized for dialysis.

Ultrafiltration (convective transport) is the bulk movement of water molecules containing permeable solutes through a semi-permeable membrane (Fig. 7.9). Water molecules are small and can pass through all semi-permeable membranes. The driving force for ultrafiltration can be either an osmotic

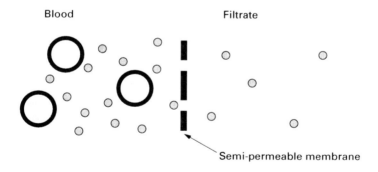

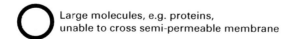

Figure 7.8 Diffusion across a semi-permeable membrane.

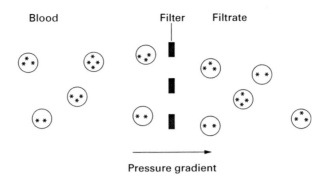

Figure 7.9 Ultrafiltration through a semi-permeable membrane.

gradient or hydrostatic pressure. Haemofiltration is based on the principle of ultrafiltration.

The volume of filtrate removed can be in excess of 2 L/h, and to maintain CVS stability, fluid must be replaced concurrently. The fluid used as replacement should be isotonic and should aim to replace the solutes lost as filtrate that would otherwise be selectively reabsorbed by the 'normal' kidney.

Types of filtration circuit

Continuous arteriovenous haemofiltration (CAVH) (Fig. 7.10a)

Blood flows from an artery (A) into the filter to produce an ultrafiltrate before return to the body via a vein (V). Used as an intermittent technique, this was the earliest method of renal replacement therapy. A systolic BP >90 mmHg is adequate for a driving pressure.

Continuous venovenous haemofiltration (CVVH) (Fig. 7.10b)

A similar technique to CAVH, except that because venous pressure is inadequate to overcome resistance of a filter and circuit tubing, a roller pump is used to generate a perfusing pressure. This is a commonly used technique in ITU patients.

Continuous arteriovenous haemodiafiltration (CAVHD) (Fig. 7.10c)

The circuit is the same as that for CAVH, but ultrafiltrate is added as a countercurrent across the membrane to generate diffusive and convective clearance. This produces an ultradiafiltrate (UDF).

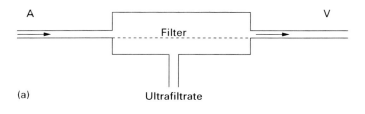

(a)

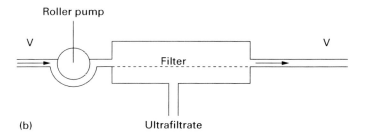

(b)

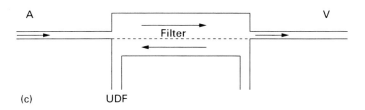

(c)

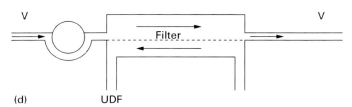

(d)

Figure 7.10 Types of filtration circuit. (A) Continuous arteriovenous haemofiltration (CAVH). (B) Continuous venovenous haemofiltration (CVVH). (C) Continuous arteriovenous haemodiafiltration (CAVHD). (D) Continuous venovenous haemodiafiltration (CVVHD).

Continuous venovenous haemodiafiltration (CVVHD) (Fig. 7.10d)

This is the same circuit as for CVVH but with the addition of dialysate to increase clearance of waste products.

Factors affecting the efficacy of haemofiltration

- Driving pressure
- Blood flow rate
- Haematocrit
- Oncotic pressure (glucose, protein)
- Arterial/venous access/flow
- Height of filter in relation to:
  - heart (CAVH)
  - filtrate collection bag
- Countercurrent dialysis
- Filter surface area.

Filtration may be increased by:

- improving arterial flow from access site
- CVVH – increasing pump speed (normal range 150–250 mL/min)
- CAVH – increasing cardiac output
- adding suction to filter
- increasing anticoagulation
- changing filter if volumes are poor.

Intermittent versus continuous filtration

Fluid removal in intermittent dialysis has to occur over a short period of time, but if it is too rapid or too large a volume, hypotension will result. A longer duration of dialysis at a lesser ultrafiltration rate is more appropriate for ITU patients, who are often haemodynamically unstable.

Intermittent dialysis is less effective than continuous dialysis because waste products and water in the interstitial compartment do not have time to equilibrate with blood. Following a short period of dialysis, urea and creatinine levels are initially low, but will rise relatively quickly as these waste products equilibrate with the lower levels in the blood.

Intermittent, large-volume dialysis also risks a disequilibrium syndrome in which a relatively high intracellular concentration of urea and creatinine following dialysis causes an osmotic effect, drawing water into cells.

Techniques using dialysate fluid reduce the chance of electrolyte imbalance as serum electrolyte levels equilibrate with the dialysate fluid; for example, if the dialysate fluid's K^+ is 4.6 mmol.L^{-1} and the serum K^+ falls below that level, K^+ will diffuse across the membrane until the level reaches $4.6\,mmol.L^{-1}$. Equally, the reverse would happen if the patient's level was greater than that of the dialysate.

Replacement fluids

Bicarbonate ions are lost by filtration, resulting in a metabolic acidosis unless replaced.

Bicarbonate ions are not present in most replacement solutions because:

- bicarbonate ions are converted to carbonates which dissociate, with resultant loss of CO_2 by diffusion through the container wall
- mixtures of bicarbonate and calcium precipitate to form calcium carbonate.

Lactate is used as a bicarbonate substitute, but depends upon adequate hepatic metabolism to convert it to new bicarbonate ions via the TCA cycle. In patients with hepatic dysfunction or lactic acidosis, bicarbonate containing replacement fluid (without calcium) or lactate-free replacement fluid (where sodium bicarbonate is infused independently of the circuit) must be used as an alternative.

Vascular access

- Arterial
  - large-bore single-lumen catheter
  - cutdown and direct arterial cannulation
  - exiting AV shunt (Cimino) fistula.
- Venous
  - double-lumen catheter
  - large-bore single-lumen catheter.

Anticoagulation

Contact of blood with plastic surfaces and filter activates clotting cascade. Anticoagulation is therefore required to prevent thrombus deposition in the circuit. Usually with heparin ($5–10\,u.kg^{-1}$, aiming to keep APTR 2.0–2.5. Prostacyclin ($2.5–10\,ng.kg^{-1}.min^{-1}$) may be used as an alternative to prevent heparin-induced thrombocytopenia, but it can cause hypotension.

Many ITU patients have coagulopathies and do not require further anticoagulation.

Potential problems

- Arterial/venous access
- Infection

- Bleeding
- Heat loss
- Emboli – air/thrombus
- Disconnection
- Intravascular fluid depletion
- Drug/colloid clearance.

Drug clearance

The effect of renal failure and renal replacement therapy on drug levels is variable and difficult to predict. Many factors affect drug levels in these patients, such as whether the drug is normally eliminated entirely or partly by renal excretion and the effect of plasma protein levels (often low) on drug binding. For many drugs with minor or no side-effects, no modification to dose is required. For more toxic drugs with a low therapeutic index, monitoring of drug levels is required. The loading dose should be the same as that used in a patient with normal renal function, but subsequent doses should be given according to drug levels. It is important to try to avoid nephrotoxic drugs in patients with renal failure, or if they are used, care should be taken to prevent doses reaching nephrotoxic levels.

Elimination of aminoglycosides, vancomycin, aminophylline and digoxin is greatly reduced in patients with renal failure; they require dosing based on drug levels to prevent toxicity.

Bibliography

Hall NA, Fox AJ: Renal replacement therapies in critical care, *Contin Edu Anaesth, Crit Care Pain* 6:197–202, 2006.
Joannidis M: Continuous renal replacement therapy in sepsis and multisystem organ failure, *Semin Dial* 22:160–164, 2009.
Mallick NP, Gokal R: Haemodialysis, *Lancet* 353:737–742, 1999.
Short A, Cumming A: ABC of intensive care. Renal support, *BMJ* 319:41–44, 1999.

SCORING SYSTEMS

Problems of predictive scoring systems

Physiological reserve. Prior health is an important predictor of outcome in acute illness. Best correlation with age.

Selection bias. Errors in predictive power if patients used to create the database are different to those being evaluated.

Lead-time bias. Patients delayed in their arrival to ITU may fare worse than those admitted earlier, despite having the same disease.

APACHE (acute physiology and chronic health evaluation)

Designed to predict outcome in groups of ITU patients, such as risk of death, ICU length of stay, type and amount of therapy, and nursing intensity. Standardized mortality rate (actual versus predicted mortality rate) can also be used to assess unit performance. Daily APACHE risk predictions are a precise measure of the patient's condition and may aid in patient treatment decisions. An increasing score is associated with increasing risk of death.

APACHE I was developed in 1981 based on 34 variables, age and previous health. Criticisms that it considered unmeasured variables as normal and that it involved too many variables led to the development of APACHE II in 1985.

APACHE II was simplified to 12 physiological variables, age and chronic health evaluation and one of 34 admission diagnoses. Its main criticisms are failure to compensate for lead-time bias and the ability to select only one diagnostic criterion. This led to poor performance when applied to trauma victims, patients receiving TPN, severely ill postoperative patients, patients with myocardial infarction and those with congestive cardiac failure.

APACHE III was developed in 1991 and is based on multiple regression values from a database of approximately 300 000 patients. The APACHE III system consists of three scores:

- age – maximum score 24 points
- chronic health evaluation – maximum score 23 points
- acute physiology score – 17 variables using the worst value in 24 h, giving a maximum score of 252 points. The variables are:

Mean blood pressure	Respiratory rate	Temperature
Pulse	Glasgow Coma Scale	Urine output
Haematocrit	White cell count	Blood pH
PaO_2	P_aCO_2	Serum sodium
Serum albumin	Serum bilirubin	Serum glucose
Serum creatinine	Blood urea nitrogen	

The total APACHE score is then determined by the total of the above three categories multiplied by a specific weight for one of 78 diagnostic categories. APACHE III also allows estimation of length of ICU stay, amount and type of therapy required and the intensity of nursing care.

APACHE IV was developed in 2006 because the accuracy of APACHE III changed significantly over the last decade. Reasons for this include inadequate diagnostic data, unreliable Glasgow Coma Scale score assessment, international and regional differences, differing selection for and timing of ICU admission, changes in the effectiveness of therapy over time, care before and after ICU admission and the frequency of early discharge to skilled nursing facilities. Main changes are improving the accuracy of physiologic risk by rescaling PaO_2/F_iO_2 and GCS variables, increasing the precision of disease labeling, use of more advanced statistical methods, and adjusting for the prognostic impact of patient location before ICU admission.

TISS (therapeutic intervention scoring system)

Scores the severity of illness by analysing degree of nursing care required in a 24-h period. Each therapeutic intervention is scored from 1 to 4, e.g. PA catheter monitoring, transfusion of blood products, inotropic support etc. Total score is used to calculate severity of illness, required staff:patient ratio and costs of patient care.

Mortality probability model (MPM)

Predicts probability of hospital mortality on admission to ITU before treatment is commenced (MPM_0) and after 24 h of treatment (MPM_{24}). MPM_0 is based on 13 variables, with MPM_{24} based on seven of these variables plus another eight to allow assessment of the effects of ICU treatment. It does not require a diagnosis. Now revised to the MPM II model following analysis of 12 610 patients treated in 139 ICUs in 12 countries. MPM II coefficients have been developed for patients at 48 and 72 h. These have shown that if a patient's physiological condition is remaining static, the patient is actually deteriorating with a decreasing chance of survival.

Simplified acute physiology score (SAPS)

SAPS II is based on 12 997 patients from 137 European centres. It uses 12 physiological variables, age, type of admission and three underlying disease variables. SAPS III is a supplement to the SAPS II scoring system. The risk of death is estimated without having to specify an underlying diagnosis.

The severity scores all show very good discriminatory values with area under the curve (ROC) ranging between 0.80 and 0.90.

Bibliography

Beck DH, Taylor BL, Millar B, et al: Prediction of outcome from intensive care: a prospective cohort study comparing Acute Physiology and Chronic Health Evaluation II and III prognostic systems in a United Kingdom intensive care unit, *Crit Care Med* 25:9–15, 1997.

Bouch DC, Thompson JP: Severity scoring systems in the critically ill, *Contin Edu Anaesth, Crit Care Pain* 8:181–185, 2008.

Le Gall JR, Lemeshow S, Saulnier F: A new simplified acute physiology score (SAPS II) based on a European/North American multicenter study, *JAMA* 270:2957–2963, 1993.

Lemeshow S, Teres D, Klar J, et al: Mortality probability models (MPM II) based on an international cohort of intensive care unit patients, *JAMA* 270: 2478–2486, 1993.

Zimmerman JE, Kramer AA, McNair DS, et al: Acute physiology and chronic health evaluation (APACHE) IV: hospital mortality assessment for today's critically ill patients, *Crit Care Med* 34:1297–1310, 2006.

SEDATION

Aims

- To reduce awareness and stress of the patient in intensive care
- To facilitate treatment, e.g. ventilation and weaning, physiotherapy
- To reduce awareness during invasive or painful procedures
- To aid management of acute confusional and withdrawal states.

Consider whether better analgesia would reduce sedation requirements, the effects of disease pathology on pharmacokinetics and unwanted side-effects of the sedative drugs. Sedative drugs must have a short half-life, enabling rapid reversal to assess the patient.

Side-effects of sedation

- Impaired respiratory effort, if excessive
- Accumulation of active metabolites in hepatic/renal failure
- Altered sleep patterns may paradoxically produce sleep deprivation
- Paralytic ileus
- Withdrawal symptoms when the drug is stopped.

Sedative drugs

Opioids. Dependence does not occur when used for short-term pain relief. Morphine and pethidine result in accumulation of metabolites (morphine 6-glucuronide and norpethidine, respectively). Remifentanil shown to shorten duration of mechanical ventilation and shorten time to ICU discharge compared with other opioids.

Beware of side-effects, particularly respiratory depression, decreased cough reflex, gastric stasis and hypotension.

Benzodiazepines. Cause anxiolysis, sleep, amnesia and muscle relaxation. Diazepam is unsuitable because of accumulation of long-acting metabolites (desmethyldiazepam). Midazolam has a shorter duration of action and is metabolized to inactive metabolites. Accumulation of midazolam and opioids may result in prolonged sedation on cessation of the infusion.

Propofol. Approved for sedation of ITU patients. Propofol allows regular waking of the patient to assess neurological status. If the patient is well filled and the infusion rate titrated carefully, hypotension is not usually a problem. Propofol has also been shown to decrease O_2 requirements and decrease requirements for vasodilators in hypertensive patients. Also used on ITU for patient-controlled sedation. Propofol infusion for sedation at 25–75 µg/kg per min.

Ketamine. May be useful for bronchodilator properties in sedation of asthmatics and analgesic properties for sedation of burns patients. Fewer hallucinations if combined with benzodiazepine infusion.

Volatile agents. Isoflurane has been studied as a sedative agent but it is expensive, requires low flow circle systems and scavenging.

Clonidine. Clonidine is particularly useful in agitated patients. It acts via stimulation of α_2-receptors in the lateral reticular nucleus of the medulla, resulting in reduced sympathetic outflow, to cause profound analgesia and sedation without respiratory depression.

Assessing sedation

Scoring systems, e.g. Ramsay sedation score

1. Patient anxious, restless or agitated
2. Patient cooperative, orientated and calm
3. Patient responds to commands only
4. Brisk response
5. Sluggish response
6. No response.

Plasma drug concentrations. But interpatient variation in pharmacodynamics and it does not take into account levels of active metabolites.

EEG. Difficult to interpret and correlates poorly with depth of sedation. Different drugs alter the EEG in different ways.

Lower oesophageal contractility. Wide variation between patients and between drugs.

Evoked responses. Lack of agent specificity.

Sinus arrhythmia. Reflects autonomic activity. Being investigated as a monitor of depth of sedation.

Bibliography

Rowe K, Fletcher S: Sedation in the intensive care unit, *Contin Edu Anaesth, Crit Care Pain* 8:50–55, 2008.

SEPSIS

Infection resulting in a systemic inflammatory response and organ failure (*severe sepsis*) is present in 27% of ICU admissions in the UK. Of these, approx 50% die during their hospital stay.

The Surviving Sepsis Campaign is a collaboration between the European Society of Intensive Care Medicine, the Society of Critical Care Medicine and the International Sepsis Forum, which published evidence-based guidelines for the management of severe sepsis. The campaign uses two care bundles; a resuscitation bundle and a management bundle. Strongly supported by the UK Department of Health, listing the campaign as one of the '10 High Impact Changes for Service Improvement and Delivery'. Although controversial, early evidence suggests that the care bundles have led to a halving in hospital mortality.

SURVIVING SEPSIS CAMPAIGN – SEPSIS CARE BUNDLES
Fletcher and Quinn 2006

Sepsis resuscitation bundle (to be achieved within 6 h of presentation)

- Measure serum lactate
- Obtain blood cultures prior to antibiotic administration
- If hypotensive, or lactate >4 mmol.L^{-1}, give an initial minimum of 20 mL. kg^{-1} crystalloid or colloid and apply vasopressor for hypotension not responding to initial fluid resuscitation
- In the event of persistent hypotension despite fluid resuscitation and/or lactate >4 mmol.L^{-1}, achieve a central venous pressure of >8 mmHg and a central venous blood oxygen saturation >70%.

Sepsis management bundle (to be achieved within 24 h of presentation)

- Consider low dose steroids
- Consider Drotrecogin alfa (activated protein C)
- Maintain blood glucose between lower limit of normal and 8.3 mmol.L^{-1}
- Maintain inspiratory plateau pressure <30 cmH$_2$O for mechanically ventilated patients.

Bibliography

Dellinger RP, Levy MM, Carlet JM, et al: Surviving Sepsis Campaign: international guidelines for management of severe sepsis and septic shock, 2008, *Crit Care Med* 36:296–327, 2008.

Fletcher SJ, Quinn AC: The surviving sepsis campaign and sepsis care bundles: substance or sophistry? *Anaesthesia* 61:313–315, 2006.

SYSTEMIC INFLAMMATORY RESPONSE SYNDROME

The systemic inflammatory response syndrome (SIRS) and multiple organ dysfunction syndrome (MODS) are terms aimed at facilitating standardization of terminology for research into critically ill patients. The systemic inflammatory response is triggered by sepsis, burns, trauma or hypovolaemia, and may be driven by bacterial and endotoxin translocation across an ischaemic, damaged gut (Fig. 7.11).

SIRS is defined as the presence of two or more of the following:

- Temperature >38°C or <36°C
- Heart rate >90/min
- Tachypnoea >20/min
- Leucocytosis <4 × 10^9/L or >12 × 10^9/L.

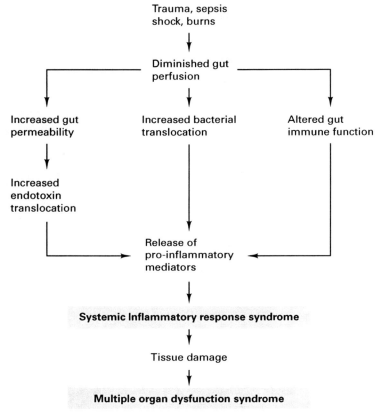

Figure 7.11 Pathophysiology of systemic inflammatory response syndrome (SIRS) and multiple organ dysfunction syndrome (MODS).

Inflammatory mediators include:

- Stress hormones: steroids, catecholamines, insulin, glucagon, growth hormone
- Arachidonic acid derivatives: interleukins, prostaglandins, thromboxanes, leukotrienes
- Histamine, serotonin, neuropeptides, myocardial depressant factor
- Macrophage-derived growth factor, platelet-activating factor.

Multiple organ dysfunction syndrome (MODS) frequently develops in previously healthy patients following resuscitation from the initial insult. It is commonly associated with sepsis, trauma, ARDS and acute renal failure. Pathophysiology involves tissue hypoperfusion with a failure of O_2 supply, intense inflammatory mediator activity, tissue catabolism, activation of leucocytes, macrophages and platelets and ischaemia-reperfusion injury. If the resulting cellular dysfunction is of sufficient magnitude, cell death occurs.

MODS develops as a progressive deterioration of two or more organ systems, usually cardiovascular, respiratory, renal, hepatic, gastrointestinal or haematological, to a state in which the organ cannot maintain homeostasis without intervention. Risk factors for the development of MODS include the severity of pathology at the time of ITU admission, presence of sepsis at the time of ITU admission and age.

Bibliography

El-Menyar AA, Davidson BL: Clinical implications of cytokines in the critical-care unit, *Expert Rev Cardiovasc Ther* 7:835–845, 2009.

Marik PE: Total splanchnic resuscitation, SIRS, and MODS, *Crit Care Med* 27:257, 1998.

Muckart DJ, Bhagwanjee S: American College of Chest Physicians/Society of Critical Care Medicine Consensus Conference definitions of the systemic inflammatory response syndrome and allied disorders in relation to critically injured patients, *Crit Care Med* 25:1789–1795, 1997.

Webster NR, Galley HF: Immunomodulation in the critically ill, *Br J Anaesth* 103:70–81, 2009.

8 Obstetrics

ANAESTHESIA FOR NON-OBSTETRIC SURGERY DURING PREGNANCY

A total of 1% of patients require GA during pregnancy. In the first trimester, there is a risk of organogenesis; in the third trimester there is a risk of premature labour. Therefore, the second trimester is the safest.

In descending order of preference:

- spinal: method of choice
- epidural: higher doses of LA required and block less effective
- other regional blocks
- combined epidural and GA: lower doses of inhalational agents and narcotics, good postoperative analgesia and can avoid N_2O
- GA (NB delayed gastric emptying present from first trimester onwards).

Known teratogenic drugs in humans

- tetracycline: bone defects, dental enamel staining
- warfarin: bone malformations
- alcohol: craniofacial abnormalities
- thalidomide: limb abnormalities
- synthetic progestogens: masculinization of female genitalia
- cocaine
- ACE inhibitors
- possibly diazepam.

Anaesthetic management of LSCS

AAGBI and the Obstetric Anaesthetist's Association have together recommended a decision-to-delivery interval of $\leq 30\,min$. Some 78% LSCS in the UK are performed under a regional rather than general anaesthetic.

REGIONAL ANAESTHESIA

Epidurals give excellent/satisfactory analgesia in 91% of mothers. Increased use of regional techniques probably accounts for the continuing reduction in maternal mortality by avoiding risks of failed intubation and aspiration. Comparative Obstetric Mobile Epidural Trial (COMET) 2001 showed that women requesting analgesia for pain relief were more likely to require instrumental delivery if receiving 0.25% bupivacaine boluses rather than low dose bupivacaine infusion or combined spinal/epidural, but no significant difference in LSCS rates between groups (Table 8.1).

Table 8.1 Advantages and disadvantages of epidural anaesthesia

Advantages	Disadvantages
Maternal participation at delivery	May take too long to perform if there is fetal distress
Avoids risk of failed intubation	Hypotension
Reduced risk of aspiration	Risk of patchy, incomplete block
Avoids morbidity from GA drugs	Backache
Avoids risk of awareness	Urinary retention
Earlier breast-feeding	
Good postoperative analgesia	
Less postnatal depression	

Indications for epidural

- Slow or painful labour
- Pregnancy-induced hypertension
- Cardiac or respiratory disease
- Premature or high risk fetus
- Multiple pregnancy
- Breech delivery
- Trial of labour.

Pain pathways (Fig. 8.1)

First stage
- pain due to cervical dilatation and uterine contractions
- pain transmitted via uterine sympathetic nerves to T_{10}–T_{12}
- some transmission via tubo-ovarian vessels.

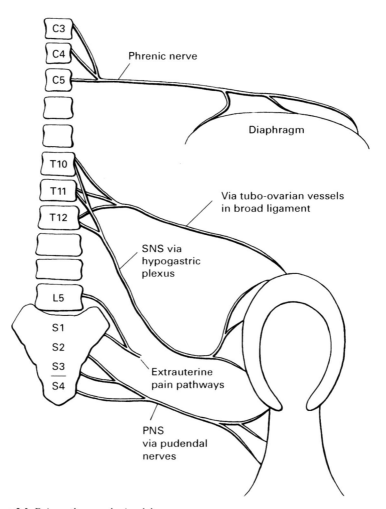

Figure 8.1 Pain pathways during labour.

Second stage
- pain due to vaginal and perineal stretching and tearing
- pain transmitted via pudendal nerves to S_2–S_4.

Extrauterine pelvic structures supplied by L_5/S_1. Particularly stimulated by the fetal head in the occipitoposterior position to cause backache.

LSCS stimulates sensory nerves to T_{10} in addition to phrenic. Aim to block from T_8 to S_5.

Aortocaval compression may occur from 20 weeks onwards. In the presence of acute blood loss, cardiovascular compensation may be seriously impaired if the block is extensive. Delivery of the baby relieves the compression.

Epidural test dose

Recommended to avoid complications of inadvertent intravenous injection of bupivacaine. Usually use a dose insufficient to cause total spinal anaesthesia if injected into the intrathecal space.

Catecholamines

Addition of adrenaline (>15 µg) or isoprenaline to the test dose may cause tachycardia within 1 min following intravenous injection. However, this sign may be unreliable because pregnancy may alter physiological changes to catecholamines and the pain of contraction may also cause sudden tachycardia. Catecholamines have also been shown to reduce placental blood flow in animal studies. Therefore, their use is controversial. If used, give between contractions and avoid in hypertensive or pre-eclamptic patients.

Opioids

The addition of 100 µg fentanyl to a test dose has been reported as a reliable indicator of intravascular injection by causing sedation and altered perception.

Air

Air (1 mL) injected intravenously and detected by parasternal Doppler has been proposed as an effective marker of inadvertent intravenous injection. There appear to be no adverse maternal or fetal effects from this small dose of air.

Regional anaesthesia

Platelet count <100 000, abnormal clotting or prolonged bleeding time is a relative contraindication to regional anaesthesia.

Epidurals are best established early and generally unsuitable for emergency procedures. Provide less effective anaesthesia than subarachnoid block and are more likely to require conversion to GA. Epidurals are the technique of choice for labour or LSCS in pre-eclamptic toxaemia (PET), where they provide better haemodynamic stability and improved uteroplacental flow, with avoidance of intubation risks from laryngeal oedema. L-bupivacaine 0.5% is as effective as bupivacaine 0.5% with less risk of CNS or CVS toxicity. Ropivacaine 0.75% is equipotent with bupivacaine 0.5%.

Spinals are the commonest form of anaesthesia for LSCS. Pencil point needles now reduce incidence of post-dural puncture headache requiring blood patch to <0.5%. Colloid fluid preload is more effective than crystalloid in preventing hypotension, but greater risk of anaphylaxis. Avoidance of aortocaval compression and use of vasopressor (e.g. phenylephrine 50–100 µg) significantly reduces hypotension. 2.25 mL 0.5% heavy bupivacaine achieves an adequate block to T4 at term, but larger volumes may be required earlier in pregnancy because of less venous congestion reducing the volume of the epidural space. Addition of opioids (fentanyl/morphine/diamorphine) reduces the incidence of intraoperative visceral pain with little risk of respiratory depression.

Combined spinal-epidural anaesthesia (CSE) may provide better anaesthesia than epidural alone. In a needle-through-needle technique, the spinal needle is advanced <15 mm beyond tip of Tuohy. Alternatively, puncture the subarachnoid space with spinal needle and replace the stylette immediately, then site epidural catheter via Tuohy needle at difference space. Give epidural test dose and then follow with subarachnoid injection. A smaller intrathecal dose (e.g. 1.0 mL 0.5% bupivacaine) followed by epidural increments improves haemodynamic stability; 0.25 mg intrathecal diamorphine ≡ 5 mg epidural diamorphine. There is some concern regarding breaching of the dura increasing infection risk and the complexity of the technique.

Epidural volume extension (EVE) A low subarachnoid block can be extended in a cephalad direction by an epidural injection of 10 mL of normal saline given within 5 min of the initial subarachnoid block. Probably related to compression of the subarachnoid space by the epidural saline, resulting in cephalad spread of local anaesthetic within the subarachnoid space. EVE allows CSE to be performed with small initial intrathecal doses of local anaesthetic and, as saline is used for the epidural 'top-ups', the total dose of local anaesthetic used is reduced.

Continuous spinal anaesthesia using an ultra fine bore catheter threaded through a spinal needle has been associated with cauda equine syndrome and is little used in the UK.

General anaesthesia

Technique of choice for emergency LSCS. Probably safer than an epidural if there is severe hypertension, uncorrected hypovolaemia, fetal distress, coagulopathy or risk of convulsions. GA morbidity most commonly due to anaphylaxis or airway crises. Short-acting antihypertensive drugs may be necessary to prevent intubation-induced hypertension, which causes CVA, pulmonary oedema and reduced placental blood flow. (Unlike thiopentone induction or lidocaine, remifentanil 1 μg.kg^{-1} prevents the haemodynamic changes at intubation). Beware of laryngeal oedema. Magnesium increases sensitivity to non-depolarizing neuromuscular blockers by inhibiting presynaptic calcium-facilitated neurotransmitter release.

Postoperative. Pre-eclampsia may not begin to resolve until 3–4 days post-delivery. Therefore, monitor BP and urine output carefully; 60% of patients who develop pulmonary oedema do so >48 h after delivery.

Failed intubation

Difficult intubation occurs in 1:300 (1:2000 in normal population). More common in Africans and Afro-Caribbeans.

It is the commonest cause of anaesthetic-related maternal deaths (it is not failure of intubation but subsequent failure of oxygenation that kills). Difficult intubation is due to left lateral tilt, increased weight, increased breast size, full dentition, laryngeal oedema, incorrect application of cricoid pressure, minimum dose of induction agent and attempted intubation before onset of neuromuscular blockade.

Perform no more than three attempts at intubation. Know the failed intubation drill which is being modified in many hospitals to use the laryngeal mask. Maintain cricoid pressure (if it does not prevent LMA insertion) which reduces aspiration risk and stops gastric distension if the patient is being bagged).

Aspiration

Incidence

In 1946, Mendelson described an asthma-like syndrome in 0.15% of deliveries using GA by mask due to aspiration of gastric contents. In more recent studies, the incidence of pulmonary aspiration syndrome is reported as 0.01%. More common with coughing during direct laryngoscopy and emergency surgery, even with cricoid pressure.

Symptoms

Of patients who aspirate, 63% are asymptomatic. Commonest symptoms are cough, bronchospasm, hypoxaemia and X-ray changes.

Gastric volumes

It is traditionally taught that >0.4 mL/kg aspirate of pH <2.5 is needed to cause symptoms, but these figures were based on a study from a single Rhesus monkey. Now thought to be a larger volume of at least 0.8 mL/kg.

Prophylaxis

A dose of 30 mL 0.3 M sodium citrate has replaced magnesium-based antacids, which did not mix with gastric contents and caused pneumonitis themselves if aspirated. Also give H_2 antagonist, e.g. ranitidine 150 mg p.o. (avoid cimetidine, which increases blood levels of bupivacaine), together with a gastric prokinetic, e.g. metoclopramide. Avoid prolonged fasting which is associated with increasing gastric volume and decreased pH. Anticholinergics only inhibit vagal stimulation and have little effect on gastric pH.

Anaesthetic manoeuvres reducing risk

Pre-oxygenation, rapid sequence induction with cricoid pressure (44 N), avoiding bagging following suxamethonium, avoiding attempts at intubation before patient is fully paralysed and extubating awake.

Postpartum

Assuming no opioids are present, rate of emptying, gastric pH and volume of stomach contents rapidly return to normal values within about 6–8 h. However, reflux (80% of women at term) may persist for up to 48 h. Therefore, anti-aspiration measures necessary for 48 h postpartum.

OAA/AAGBI GUIDELINES FOR OBSTETRIC ANAESTHESIA SERVICES

Association of Anaesthetists of Great Britain and Ireland and the Obstetric Anaesthetists Association 2005

1. A duty anaesthetist should be immediately available for the Delivery Suite 24 h/day.
2. There should be a nominated consultant in charge of obstetric anaesthesia.
3. There should be a clear line of communication from the duty anaesthetist to the supervising consultant at all times.
4. Women should have antenatal access to information about the availability and provision of all types of analgesia and anaesthesia.
5. There should be an agreed system whereby the anaesthetist is given sufficient advanced notice of all potential high-risk patients.
6. Where a 24-h epidural service is offered, the time from the anaesthetist being informed about an epidural until being able to attend the mother should not normally exceed 30 min, and must be within 1 hour except in exceptional circumstances.
7. Separate staffing and resources should be allocated to elective caesarean section lists to prevent delays due to emergency procedures and provision of regional analgesia in labour.
8. The assistant to the anaesthetist must have no other conflicting duties, must be trained to a recognized national standard and must work regularly in the obstetric unit.
9. The training undergone by staff in the maternity recovery unit and the facilities provided must be to the same standard as for general recovery facilities.
10. Appropriate facilities should be available for the antenatal and peripartum management of the sick obstetric patient.

Amniotic fluid embolus

Amniotic fluid may cause amniotic fluid embolus characterized by sudden cardiorespiratory collapse and coagulatory abnormalities. It is thought that the amniotic fluid itself is relatively non-toxic, even in volumes as large as 500 mL. Toxicity appears to be determined by the meconium content. In a pig model, 10 mL.kg^{-1} of meconium-free amniotic fluid caused few problems, whereas just 3 mL.kg^{-1} of meconium-contaminated amniotic fluid caused severe cardiorespiratory and coagulatory abnormalities.

Bibliography

American Society of Anesthesiologists: Practice guidelines for obstetrical anesthesia. A report by the American Society of Anesthesiologists, *Task Force on Obstetrical Anesthesia. Anesthesiology* 90:600–611, 1999.

Association of Anaesthetists of Great Britain and Ireland and the Obstetric Anaesthetists Association: Revised Guidelines 2005, OAA/AAGBI guidelines for obstetric anaesthesia services. Reproduced with the kind permission of the Association of anaesthetists of Great Britain and Ireland.

Bogod DG: The postpartum stomach – when is it safe? Editorial, *Anaesthesia* 49:1–2, 1994.

Comparative Obstetric Mobile Epidural Trial (COMET) Study Group UK: Effect of low-dose mobile vs traditional epidural techniques on mode of delivery: a randomized controlled trial, *Lancet* 358:19–23, 2001.

Duley L, Neilson JP: Magnesium sulphate and pre-eclampsia, *BMJ* 319:3–4, 1999.

Gomar C, Fernandez C: Epidural analgesia–anaesthesia in obstetrics, *Eur J Anaesth* 17:542–558, 2000.

Levy DM: Emergency caesarean section: best practice, *Anaesthesia* 61:786–791, 2006.

McDonnell NJ, Keating ML, Muchatuta NA, et al: Analgesia after caesarean delivery, *Anaesth Intensive Care* 37:539–551, 2009.

McGlennan A, Mustafa A: General anaesthesia for caesarean section, *Contin Edu Anaesth, Crit Care Pain* 9:148–151, 2009.

Ong K-B, Sashidharan R: Combined spinal–epidural techniques, *Contin Edu Anaesth, Crit Care Pain* 7:38–41, 2007.

Levy DM: Anaesthesia for caesarian section, *BJA CEPD Rev* 1:171–176, 2001.

Macarthur AJ: Gerard W. Ostheimer 'What's new in obstetric anesthesia' lecture, *Anesthesiology* 108:777–785, 2008.

McGrady E, Litchfield K: Epidural analgesia in labour, *Contin Edu Anaesth, Crit Care Pain* 4:14–17, 2004.

May A: Obstetric anaesthesia and analgesia, *Anaesthesia* 58:1186–1189, 2003.

Morris S: Management of difficult and failed intubation in obstetrics, *BJA CEPD Rev* 1:117–121, 2001.

Turner JA: Severe preeclampsia: anesthetic implications of the disease and its management, *Am J Ther* 16:284–288, 2009.

MATERNAL AND FETAL PHYSIOLOGY

Maternal physiology
Cardiovascular

- Cardiac output 30–40% above normal by 32 weeks. Aortocaval compression is sufficient to reduce cardiac output from 20 weeks
- ↑ heart rate of 15%, ↑ stroke volume of 30%. Fall in SVR results in unchanged BP
- Cardiac hypertrophy and dilation cause ECG changes of left axis deviation, ST depression and flattening/inversion of T wave in III

- Albumin is diluted, reducing plasma oncotic pressure and predisposing to pulmonary oedema at lower pressures
- ↑ progesterone due to pregnancy and reduced protein binding increases myocardial sensitivity to bupivacaine
- Aortocaval compression significant from mid-pregnancy.

Respiratory

- Reduction in lung volume by a 4 cm elevation of diaphragm compensated for by increased transverse and AP diameter of the chest due to hormonal effects that loosen ligaments
- Increased minute volume by 40%, ↑ tidal volume and 15% ↑ respiratory rate. Causes respiratory alkalosis and shifts O_2 dissociation curve to the left. Increase in P_{50} from 3.5 to 4.0 facilitates oxygen unloading across the placenta
- ↑ tidal volume with ↑ FRC results in faster pre-oxygenation in 2 min of tidal breathing (more effective than four vital capacity breaths) and quick gas induction, accelerated by reduced MAC
- Increased CC which may exceed FRC
- Increased O_2 consumption.

Gastrointestinal

- Uterine pressure increases intragastric pressure and distorts lower oesophageal sphincter, causing incompetence
- Delayed gastric emptying and increased acid production.

Blood

- Increased red cell mass by 20–30% and increased plasma volume by 40–50% at term, causing dilutional anaemia
- Hypercoagulable state with increased fibrinogen and factors VII, VIII, X, and XIII. Platelet, clotting and fibrinolytic systems all activated.

Renal

- Increase in GFR of 60% reduces plasma urea and creatinine by 40%.

Epidural

- Volume of epidural space is decreased due to distended venous plexus, reducing the volume of LA needed for epidurals by 30% and increasing the risk of epidural vein catheterization.

Metabolism

- Increased volume of distribution of intravenous agents prolongs their elimination half-lives. Elimination $t_{1/2}$ for thiopentone is doubled at term
- Serum cholinesterase levels fall by 25% during the first trimester and fall further by 33% during the first 7 postpartum days. The decreased levels

of enzymes are adequate for normal hydrolysis of suxamethonium during gestation, but may prolong duration of action in 10% of patients in the postpartum period.

Fetal physiology

- Fetus exists in a hypoxic environment. Oxygenation enhanced by left shift of O_2 dissociation curve with fetal $P_{50} = 2.6$ compared with maternal value of 4.0.
- Uterine vascular bed is maximally dilated at term but remains responsive to the effects of catecholamines. Ephedrine acts on $\beta > \alpha$ receptors and has less effect on placental flow than other vasopressors which act by α stimulation, e.g. methoxamine.
- Fetal acidosis results in more local anaesthetic taken up by the fetus with increased risk of toxicity.

Effect of anaesthesia and surgery on the fetus during LSCS

- Maternal catecholamine levels are lower with epidural/spinal than with GA.
- IPPV lowers cardiac output and reduces placental flow, especially with hypovolaemia. Minimize effects by reducing mean intrathoracic pressure.
- Hyperventilation shifts maternal O_2 dissociation curve to the left, reducing placental O_2 transfer and umbilical blood flow, and causes fetal acidosis. Slight maternal hypercapnia may benefit the fetus by improving oxygen delivery.
- Maternal P_aO_2 <13 kPa reduces fetal oxygenation and delays onset of spontaneous ventilation in the newborn. A maternal F_iO_2 >0.65 was shown to improve Apgar scores and reduce fetal acidosis at delivery, but the study did not control for aortocaval compression or F_iN_2O.
- Aortocaval compression occurs in 15% of women at term. When lying supine, the pregnant uterus at term almost completely obstructs the inferior vena cava. Reduced with lateral tilt, more effective to the left.
- Degree of fetal acidosis on delivery is related to the time from uterine incision to delivery. Induction–delivery time has little effect on acidosis if using left lateral tilt.

Effect of anaesthetic drugs on the fetus during LSCS

- Placental transfer of drugs is influenced by protein binding, high lipid solubility, low ionization and kPa.
- Fetus is not anaesthetized by i.v. induction agents because hepatic extraction and dilution of drugs with blood from the lower limbs and upper body reduce the concentration of drug delivered to the fetal CNS.

- Injection of induction agent at the onset of a contraction reduces the dose delivered to the fetus. Fetal plasma levels of induction agents follow the same pattern as in adults by 2–3 min.
- Thiopentone reduces placental blood flow and may reduce fetal O_2 delivery. Ketamine increases placental flow, but increased force of uterine contraction may worsen cord prolapse or abruptio placentae.
- N_2O may reach equilibrium in the fetus with a possible risk of diffusion hypoxia in the fetus upon delivery which should therefore have O_2. There is no evidence of methionine synthetase depression when N_2O is used for LSCS. Less than 1.0 MAC halothane, enflurane or isoflurane does not increase perioperative blood loss and is not detrimental to the fetus. Minimal fetal fluoride levels with enflurane.
- Neuromuscular blocking drugs are large highly ionized molecules with minimal placental transfer. However, fetal paralysis has been reported following extremely high doses of non-depolarizing drugs, e.g. when given in error. Suxamethonium administration to patients with homozygous plasma cholinesterase deficiency may result in fetal paralysis.
- Opioids rapidly cross the placenta to achieve fetal levels equal to those of the mother. Fentanyl 1 µg/kg at induction does not affect fetal Apgar score, neurobehavioural scores or acid–base status. Opioids may reduce the maternal stress response and lessen catecholamine-induced placental vasoconstriction.

Fetal and maternal effects of epidurals

- Improve coordination of uterine contraction by reducing noradrenaline levels
- Relief of pain reduces maternal hyperventilation
- Improve placental blood flow in pre-eclampsia and reduce fetal acidosis in the second stage of labour
- Fetal acidosis accelerates transfer of LA across placenta
- General anaesthesia is associated with lower Apgar scores at 1 min compared with regional techniques, but both techniques have similar scores by 5 min. Therefore, use a regional technique if possible when delivering a baby with fetal distress, but remember further fetal deterioration may occur while epidural is inserted.

Cardiotocograph

- Type I decelerations (early) – head compression causing vagal reflex
- Type II decelerations (late) – uteroplacental insufficiency
- Type III decelerations (variable) – umbilical cord compression.

INTRAOPERATIVE BLOOD CELL SALVAGE IN OBSTETRICS
National Institute for Clinical Excellence 2005 (www.nice.org.uk/ IPG144distributionlist)

Guidance

Intraoperative blood cell salvage is an efficacious technique for blood replacement and its use is well established in other areas of medicine, but there are theoretical safety concerns when it is used in obstetric practice.

Procedure

It has not been routinely adopted in obstetrics because of specific concerns about amniotic fluid embolism and about haemolytic disease in future pregnancies as a result of re-infusing amniotic fluid or fetal red blood cells.

Data collection is therefore important and clinicians should report all complications to the Medicines and Healthcare Products Regulatory Agency (www.mhra.gov.uk).

Pregnancy-induced hypertension

Incidence

- Pre-eclampsia – 5% all pregnancies
- Eclampsia – 0.05% all pregnancies.

Associations

Associated with positive family history, young primiparous, elderly, multiparous, diabetes, pre-existing hypertension, renal disease and collagen vascular disease. There is some evidence to suggest that there is an autosomal recessive predisposition to an immune response within the placenta.

Characterized by a *triad* of:

- *hypertension* – ↑ BP >30/15 mmHg; ↑ systolic above 160 mmHg, ↑ diastolic >15 mmHg
- *oedema*
- *proteinuria* – >0.3 mg/kg; severe >5 g/day.

Pathophysiology

Thought to be triggered by an autoimmune reaction against the placenta (Fig. 8.2).

Airway. Facial and laryngeal oedema may make intubation difficult. Consider awake fibreoptic intubation in elective patients undergoing GA.

Cardiovascular. In untreated patients, cardiac index (CI) is low/normal, SVR is normal/high and PCWP is low/normal due to contraction of intravascular volume by as much as 30–40% in severe cases. Fluid challenge may improve cardiovascular stability, increase CI and reduce SVR to more normal levels.

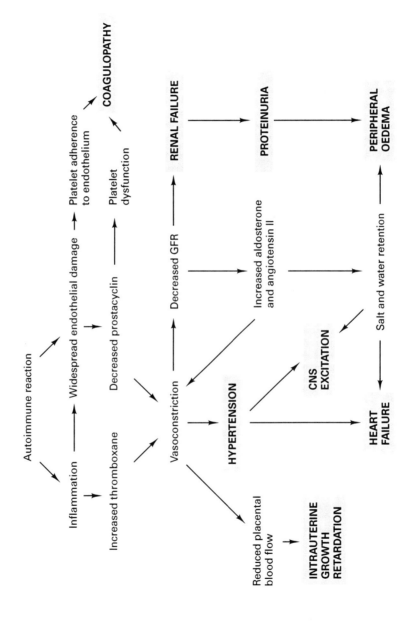

Figure 8.2 Pathophysiology of pre-eclampsia.

PCWP becomes normal/high, but CVP correlates poorly. Consider invasive monitoring if oliguria persists following 500 mL fluid challenge.

Treat hypertension with hydralazine 5–10 mg i.v. boluses or 5–40 mg/h infusion. Causes headache, tremor and vomiting, mimicking symptoms of eclampsia. Also consider labetalol up to 1 mg/kg (reports of fetal bradycardia if used in the presence of fetal distress) or sodium nitroprusside 0.3–8 μg/kg/min. Nifedipine may cause severe hypotension if used with magnesium.

Central nervous system. Cerebral vasospasm, microinfarcts, petechial haemorrhage and oedema cause CNS irritability, visual disturbance and headache. May be worsened by hypertension following pressor response to intubation. Fits are more common in teenage mothers and multiple pregnancies. CNS haemorrhage is a major cause of maternal deaths.

Treat CNS irritability with magnesium sulphate 4 g loading dose then 1–3 g/h which suppresses EEG excitatory activity, aiming for therapeutic blood level of 2–4 mmol/L. Titrate against deep tendon reflexes. Also vasodilates uterine vessels and attenuates uterine vascular response to catecholamines. May accumulate in renal failure. Excess (>4 mmol/L) causes respiratory paralysis, heart block and fetal weakness. Treat with calcium gluconate 1 g i.v.

Coagulation. Thrombocytopenia <100 000 is common. Normal platelet counts are associated with prolonged bleeding times in 10–25% of pre-eclamptics; 34% of patients with severe eclampsia have prolonged bleeding times. Low-grade DIC is common.

Recent Collaborative Low Dose Aspirin Study (CLASP) cast doubt on the efficacy of aspirin in reducing the incidence of pre-eclampsia.

Hepatic. Abnormal LFTs due to oedema and hepatic congestion. Associated with HELLP syndrome (**H**aemolysis, **E**levated **L**iver enzymes, **L**ow **P**latelets).

Renal. Decreased glomerular filtration, acute tubular necrosis and increased permeability to proteins causing proteinuria.

Bibliography

Gaiser RR: Old concepts applied to new problems: the fetus as a patient, *Curr Opin Anaesth* 11:251–253, 1998.

Heidemann BH, McClure JH: Changes in maternal physiology during pregnancy, *BJA CEPD Rev* 3:65–68, 2003.

NICE: *Intraoperative blood cell salvage in obstetrics. Interventional Procedures Guideline, 144*, London, 2005, National Institute for Health and Clinical Excellence.

9 Paediatrics

GENERAL PAEDIATRICS

Definitions

- *Neonate* – first 28 days of life or <44 weeks post-conception
- *Infant* – 1 month to 1 year
- *Child* – >1 year to adolescence
- *Low birth weight* – 2500 g at birth
- *Premature* – less than 37 weeks.

Physiological changes at birth

- Tactile stimulus triggers respiratory centre. Inflation of lungs reduces pulmonary vascular resistance.
- Increased flow to lungs increases left atrial pressure, closing the foramen ovale.
- Cessation of placental flow increases SVR. Combined with decreased PVR, flow through ductus arteriosus reverses. High P_aO_2 causes ductal smooth muscle to constrict, and closure occurs (reversible for several days).

Fetal circulation is shown in Figure 9.1.

Neonatal physiology
CVS

- Tendency to revert to fetal circulation for 2 weeks is triggered by acidosis and $\uparrow P_aCO_2$.
- Relatively little contractile tissue in heart (30%), so increased cardiac output achieved by increased heart rate rather than stroke volume. Ventricular thickness equal by 6 months.
- Cardiac index is 2–3 times that of an adult.
- Heart rate at term is 120/min. Rises to 160/min by 1 month and decreases to adult rates by 15 years.
- PNS more developed than SNS. Therefore there is a tendency to bradycardia. Response to adrenergic drugs is diminished.
- Ductus arteriosus reopens following fluid overload.

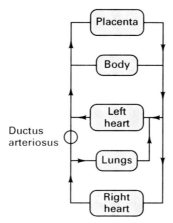

Figure 9.1 Fetal circulation.

Respiratory

- Obligatory nasal breathing until 5 months. Nasal passages account for 30–50% of airway resistance. May be unable to convert to mouth breathing if there is nasal obstruction.
- Large tongue obstructs the airway and makes laryngoscopy difficult. Epiglottis is longer, narrower and angled away from the axis of the trachea.
- Larynx is higher (C_3–C_4) and more anterior than in adults (C_4–C_5).
- Narrowest part of upper airway is cricoid cartilage. Even minimal oedema causes a large increase in airway resistance (Hagen–Poiseuille law).
- Short trachea at term: ≈4 cm.
- Tendency to apnoea if <50 weeks post-conceptual age, due to immature respiratory centre.
- Negative pressure of 40–80 cmH$_2$O is required for initial lung expansion.
- Surfactant produced from 32 weeks by type II alveolar pneumocytes.
- No bucket handle rib movement, therefore increased minute volume is achieved by increasing respiratory rate.
- Diaphragmatic > intercostal respiration. Fewer type I muscle fibres used in prolonged work so earlier diaphragm fatigue.
- Rapid respiratory rate of 32 breaths/min.
- FRC <CC due to decreased outward recoil of chest wall.
- Small FRC, high O$_2$ consumption; therefore rapid desaturation.
- Increased laryngeal irritability with susceptibility to laryngospasm.
- Increased susceptibility to respiratory infection.

GI

- Acute gastric dilatation is common, so consider a NG tube.
- Lower oesophageal sphincter incompetence predisposes to aspiration pneumonia.
- Immature hepatic function and reduced blood flow, increasing half-life of drugs excreted by hepatic metabolism. Phase I reactions attain adult levels within 1 week; phase II reactions within 3–4 months.

Renal

- Immature renal function with reduced GFR; therefore reduced ability to excrete drugs, dependent upon renal clearance.
- Reduced concentrating ability.
- 50% N_2 forms new tissue; therefore less renal N_2 load.

CNS

- Immature blood–brain barrier with increased permeability to lipid-soluble drugs.
- Motor nerve endings differentiate to form end plates at 26–28 weeks, but process still incomplete at term.
- Increased risk of intraventricular haemorrhage, particularly with abrupt fluctuations in cerebral blood flow and CVP, due to underdeveloped perivascular connective tissue.
- Increased proportion of low-affinity μ_2 opiate receptors (mediate respiratory depression).
- Increased sensitivity to volatiles due to increased progesterone, increased β-endorphins, immature blood–brain barrier and decreased protein binding.

Blood

- 70% HbF at term; P_{50} = 2.7 kPa (3.5–4.0 kPa in adult) with leftward shift of O_2 dissociation curve.
- Blood volume 80 mL.kg^{-1} at term.
- Physiological anaemia is greatest at 3–4 months, with Hb = 10 g.dL^{-1}.

Change of haematocrit with age is shown in Figure 9.2.

Temperature

- Increased surface area:body weight ratio. Therefore increased heat loss.
- Thermoneutral temperature at term = 33°C.
- Noradrenaline > adrenaline released with stress to trigger non-shivering thermogenesis in brown fat. Brown fat stores are limited. Shivering does not occur before 3 months.
- Immature thermoregulatory mechanisms, further inhibited by GA.
- Hypothermia causes acidosis, persistent fetal circulation, hypoxia, diaphragm fatigue, intraventricular haemorrhage and coagulopathy.

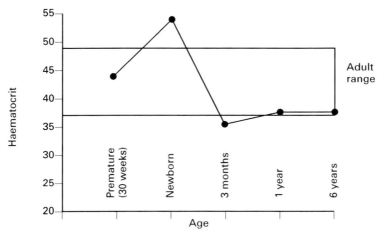

Figure 9.2 Changes in haematocrit with age.

Glucose

* Minimal glycogen reserves for gluconeogenesis.
* Poorly developed glucose homeostasis.
* High glucose requirements at term. Tendency to hypoglycaemia in small-for-dates babies, infants of diabetic mothers and sick neonates.

Pharmacokinetic and pharmacodynamic differences

* Decreased lean body mass.
* Increased total body water (increased central volume by 50%).
* Decreased total body fat. Therefore, increased V_D of water-soluble drugs, decreased V_D of fat-soluble drugs.
* Decreased protein binding.

General anaesthesia

NCEPOD RECOMMENDATIONS FOR PAEDIATRIC ANAESTHESIA

* Anaesthetist must have sufficient paediatric experience
* One anaesthetist in each hospital must be responsible for paediatric anaesthesia
* Most problems occur in children <3 years
* Neonates (<28 days) must be anaesthetized in specialist units.

Weight (kg)

- 1–8 years = (age + 4) × 2
- >9 years = age × 3

Preoperative fasting

Half-life of gastric fluid (saline) is 11 min, prolonged by fat and glucose. Recent studies show that prolonged fasting may actually decrease gastric pH and increase volume. Clear fluids administered 2–3 h preoperatively do not alter gastric residual volume and cause less distress. See Association of Paediatric Anaesthetists Guidelines 2007 (below) for preoperative fasting guidelines.

CONSENSUS GUIDELINE ON PERIOPERATIVE FLUID MANAGEMENT IN CHILDREN, V1.1

Association of Paediatric Anaesthetists of Great Britain and Ireland 2007

Executive summary

1. Children can safely be allowed clear fluids 2 h before surgery without increasing the risk of aspiration.
2. Food should normally be withheld for 6 h prior to surgery in children aged 6 months or older.
3. In children under 6 months of age it is probably safe to allow a breast milk feed up to 4 h before surgery.
4. Dehydration without signs of hypovolaemia should be corrected slowly.
5. Hypovolaemia should be corrected rapidly to maintain cardiac output and organ perfusion.
6. In the child, a fall in blood pressure is a late sign of hypovolaemia.
7. Maintenance fluid requirements should be calculated using the formula of Holliday and Segar

Body weight	Daily fluid requirement
0–10 kg	4 mL/kg per h
10–20 kg	40 mL/h + 2 mL/kg per h above 10 kg
>20 kg	60 mL/h + 1 mL/kg per h above 20 kg

8. A fluid management plan for any child should address three key issues:
   i. any fluid deficit which is present
   ii. maintenance fluid requirements
   iii. any losses due to surgery, e.g. blood loss, 3rd space losses.
9. During surgery, all of these requirements should be managed by giving isotonic fluid in all children over 1 month of age.
10. The majority of children over 1 month of age will maintain a normal blood sugar if given non-dextrose containing fluid during surgery.

11. Children at risk of hypoglycaemia if non-dextrose containing fluid is given are those on parenteral nutrition or a dextrose containing solution prior to theatre, children of low body weight (<3rd centile) or having surgery of more than 3 h duration and children having extensive regional anaesthesia. These children at risk should be given dextrose containing solutions or have their blood glucose monitored during surgery.
12. Blood loss during surgery should be replaced initially with crystalloid or colloid, and then with blood once the haematocrit has fallen to 25%. Children with cyanotic congenital heart disease and neonates may need a higher haematocrit to maintain oxygenation.
13. Fluid therapy should be monitored by daily electrolyte estimation, use of a fluid input/output chart and daily weighing if feasible.
14. Acute dilutional hyponatraemia is a medical emergency and should be managed in paediatric intensive care.

Preoperative assessment

Examine for congenital defects, cardiorespiratory pathology due to prematurity, hypoglycaemia and hypocalcaemia.

Premedication

Bradycardia secondary to cholinergic effects of drugs (halothane, suxamethonium) and upper airway stimulation is reduced with anticholinergic premedication.

Intubation

- Tracheal tube size (>1 year) = age/4 + 4 mm
- Tracheal tube length = age/2 + 12 cm.

Volatiles

MAC is lower in the neonate, but increases to a peak at 6 months before declining. Age-related change in MAC of sevoflurane is less pronounced. Gas induction is fast because alveolar ventilation is large compared with FRC, high cardiac output and lower blood:gas solubility of volatiles in neonates. Sevoflurane produces less laryngeal irritation than desflurane and is more suitable for gas induction. Baroreflex response is maintained with isoflurane and sevoflurane but not with halothane or desflurane.

Volatiles depress respiration, depress intercostal muscles and ventilation becomes diaphragmatic. Therefore, intubate if <5 kg or <44 weeks post-conceptual age. Volatiles reduce SVR, worsening a right-to-left shunt if persistent fetal circulation is present.

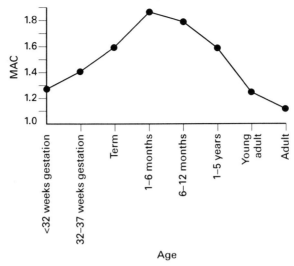

Figure 9.3 Variation in the MAC of isoflurane with age.

MAC of nitrous oxide is not related to age. N_2O may cause marked cardiovascular depression in neonates and diffusion into bowel may impair ventilation. Variation in MAC of isoflurane with age is shown in Figure 9.3.

Barbiturates

Reduced V_D of lipid-soluble drugs reduces redistribution of thiopentone thus prolonging recovery. Induction doses: 2–4 mg/kg in neonates; 7–8 mg/kg in infants; 5–6 mg/kg in older children.

Propofol

Pain on induction, more excitatory phenomenon and less postoperative nausea and vomiting than with thiopentone. Greater depression of laryngopharyngeal reflexes than with thiopentone so more suitable for use with laryngeal mask. Larger V_D, faster metabolism and clearance. Therefore, a larger induction dose of 2.5–3.5 mg/kg is required.

Only licensed as an induction agent in children >3 years because of case reports of a syndrome of lactic acidaemia, bradyarrhythmias, hypotension, lipaemia and oliguria.

Benzodiazepines

Diazepam has similar V_D to adult values but greatly prolonged $t_{1/2}$ (20–50 h in neonates; 8–14 h in children). Midazolam is more suitable in children, with a $t_{1/2}$ of 1.5 h.

Opioids

Increased sensitivity due to immature blood–brain barrier, reduced protein binding and decreased glucuronidation. Reduced clearance of all opioids. High doses reduce stress response and prevent pulmonary hypertension associated with airway instrumentation.

Muscle relaxants

Depolarizing. Decreased plasma cholinesterase but minimal effect on hydrolysis. Decreased sensitivity to suxamethonium due to increased V_D and immature neuromuscular junction. Therefore use a higher dose of 2 mg/kg.

Non-depolarizing. Atracurium has an increased V_D but increased clearance, so elimination half-life is unchanged and thus little change in overall pharmacokinetics. Sensitivity to, and action of, vecuronium is increased in children <1 year.

Ensure complete reversal before extubation with glycopyrrolate 0.01 mg/kg.

Local anaesthetics

Reduced protein binding and reduced metabolism increase risk of toxic side-effects.

Oxygen toxicity

Neonates <2 kg or <35 weeks are particularly susceptible to retinal damage by exposure to high P_aO_2. It is related to the level and duration of raised oxygen tension. Other risk factors are prematurity, twins, hypoxaemia, hyper/hypocarbia, sepsis and transfusion. S_aO_2 of 90–94% is considered optimal.

Fluid management

Insensible losses are greater due to:

- increased surface area:body ratio, increasing evaporation
- immature skin – loses more water
- increased alveolar ventilation – increases water lost via the lungs
- kidneys less able to concentrate urine.

Short operations <1 h in healthy children do not usually require fluids if preoperative fasting was not excessive. For longer procedures, an i.v. infusion is necessary. When calculating perioperative fluid requirements, add fluid lost during preoperative fasting to the operative regime. Maintain haematocrit >0.30.

Analgesia in neonates

Significant pain is not only unacceptable, but will produce a 'pain memory' with an exaggerated response to subsequent pain for as long as 6 months. Neonates and infants mount a graded hormonal stress response to surgery and adequate analgesia modifies the stress response and reduces morbidity and mortality. Multi-modal analgesia, using local anaesthetics, opioids, non-steroidal anti-inflammatory drugs (NSAIDs), and paracetamol is an effective approach for most infants. A local/regional analgesic technique should be used in *all* cases unless specifically contraindicated.

Opioids

Avoid painful i.m. injections. Subcutaneous delivery via cannula may be useful in some patients. Use of i.v. techniques is tempered by the risk of respiratory depression. Monitoring of respiratory frequency is an insensitive indicator of respiratory depression, and pulse oximetry in a high-dependency unit should be used when administering i.v. opioids. Patient-controlled analgesia has been used successfully in children as young as 5 years of age. Use of NSAIDs and regional/local blocks with their opioid-sparing effects is becoming much more widespread.

Table 9.1 Opioids: relative potency and dosing

Drug	Potency relative to morphine	Single dose	Continuous infusion
Morphine	1	$0.05-0.2\,mg.kg^{-1}$	$10-40\,\mu g.kg^{-1}.min^{-1}$
Alfentanil	10	$5-10\,\mu g.kg^{-1}$	$1-4\,\mu g.kg^{-1}.min^{-1}$
Fentanyl	50-100	$0.5-1\,\mu g.kg^{-1}$	$0.1-0.2\,\mu g.kg^{-1}.min^{-1}$
Remifentanil	50-100	$0.1-1\,\mu g.kg^{-1}$	$0.05-4\,\mu g.kg^{-1}.min^{-1}$

Non-steroidal anti-inflammatory drugs

These appear to provide analgesia in children as young as 3 years. Ketorolac, indometacin, diclofenac and ibuprofen have all been shown to reduce post-operative opioid requirements. The degree of gastric irritation, renal impairment and fluid retention is not known. Immature renal and hepatic function may impair excretion. Caution is required in those with asthma, severe eczema, multiple allergies and those with nasal polyps.

Regional techniques

Nerves are less myelinated, resulting in a faster onset of block and an adequate block at lower concentrations of LA. Reduced plasma protein results in higher blood levels of LA. All routes cause less hypotension than in adults because of an immature SNS and less developed capacitance vessels. Postoperative numbness over wide areas may cause confusion and restlessness (3% of patients).

Spinal cord ends at L_3; dura ends at S_4.

Spinal

- Consider atropine premedication $(20\,\mu g.kg^{-1})$
- 0.5% heavy bupivacaine at $L_{3/4}$ or $L_{4/5}$
  <4kg: $0.13\,mL.kg^{-1}$
  >4kg: $0.07\,mL.kg^{-1}$
  $+0.1\,mL$ needle deadspace.

Caudal

- 0.25% plain bupivacaine $\pm$ 0.05 mg.kg^{-1} morphine
  - block to lumbosacral region: $0.5\,mL.kg^{-1}$
  - block to thoracolumbar region: $1.0\,mL.kg^{-1}$
  - block to low thoracic region: $1.25\,mL.kg^{-1}$
- Urinary retention in up to 65% of patients and persistent motor block in up to 30%.

Epidural

- 0.5% bupivacaine at $0.5\,mL.kg^{-1} \pm 0.05\,mg.kg^{-1}$ morphine.

Table 9.2 Maximum dosages of bupivacaine, levobupivacaine and ropivacaine in neonates and children

	Single bolus injection	Continuous postoperative infusion
	Maximum dosage	Maximum infusion rate
Neonates	$2\,mg.kg^{-1}$	$0.2\,mg.kg^{-1}.h^{-1}$
Children	$2.5\,mg.kg^{-1}$	$0.4\,mg.kg^{-1}.h^{-1}$

GUIDELINES ON THE PREVENTION OF POSTOPERATIVE VOMITING (POV) IN CHILDREN

The Association of Paediatric Anaesthetists of Great Britain and Ireland, Spring 2007

Children at high risk of POV

- POV risk increases markedly at >3 years old and continues to rise throughout early childhood and into adolescence.
- Previous history of motion sickness is likely an independent risk factor of subsequent POV.
- Previous history of POV is an independent risk factor of subsequent POV in children.
- Post-pubertal girls have an increased incidence of POV.

Surgical procedures associated with high risk of POV

- Strabismus surgery
- Tonsillectomy ± adenoidectomy
- Surgical procedures >30 min duration.

What anaesthetic factors affect POV in children?

- Volatile anaesthesia is associated with increased POV risk, particularly in children with other risk factors.
- Opioids are associated with increased POV risk, particularly if longer-acting agents are used postoperatively.
- Mandating oral fluids may be associated with increased POV risk. Intraoperative i.v. fluids may reduce POV risk.
- N_2O is not associated with a high risk of POV.
- Anticholinesterases may be associated with an increased POV risk.

Recommendations for prevention of POV in children

- Children at increased risk of POV should be given i.v. ondansetron 0.15 mg.kg^{-1} prophylactically.
- Children at high risk of POV should be given prophylactically i.v. ondansetron 0.05 mg.kg^{-1} and i.v. dexamethasone 0.15 mg.kg^{-1}.
- Adenotonsillectomy or strabismus surgery: consider i.v. anaesthesia and alternatives to opioid analgesia in children at high risk of POV.

Recommendations for the treatment of established POV in children

- Ondansetron i.v. 0.15 mg.kg^{-1} should be given to children who have not already been given ondansetron for prophylaxis of POV.
- For children who have already been given ondansetron, a second antiemetic from another class should be given, such as dexamethasone i.v. 0.15 mg.kg^{-1} injected slowly.

Prematurity (37 weeks)

Associated with:

- Aspiration pneumonia, respiratory distress syndrome
- Apnoea
- Hypoglycaemia, hypocalcaemia, hypomagnesaemia
- Congenital defects.

Ex-premature baby for surgery

Preoperative assessment should include respiratory system, venous access and frequency of any apnoeic attacks. Assess gestational and chronological age.

Pulmonary function is often abnormal, with a higher respiratory rate, lower compliance and impaired gas exchange which may persist for several years. Risk of life-threatening apnoea is present until 45 weeks post-conceptual age. Use apnoea alarm for at least 24 h postoperatively.

Risk of postoperative apnoea in 30–40% of babies due to immature respiratory control mechanisms, impaired respiratory function, airway obstruction, anaemia and the residual effects of anaesthetic gases (reduced chemoreceptor response to hypoxia, increased paradoxical chest wall movement, depressed intercostal muscle activity). Caffeine 10 mg/kg i.v. at induction may reduce the risk of apnoea. Regional anaesthesia reduces but does not remove the risk of postoperative respiratory depression and apnoea.

Infections and sudden death more common.

Tracheo-oesophageal fistula (Fig. 9.4)

Presentation

Incidence of 1:3000 live births. Presents as excess oral secretions causing frothing at mouth, regurgitation of first feed and later as recurrent pneumonia; 30% are born prematurely, and 25% with major CVS abnormalities.

Associated with VATER syndrome (**V**ertebral abnormalities, **A**nal atresia, **T**racheo-o**E**sophageal fistula, **R**adius abnormalities) and musculoskeletal and craniofacial malformation.

Diagnosis

- Inability to pass NG tube
- Barium swallow.

Preoperative

- Nurse head-up to reduce risk of aspiration
- Continuous suction of upper oesophageal pouch
- Physiotherapy and antibiotics if there is evidence of aspiration
- Intravenous fluids to correct dehydration and prevent hypoglycaemia
- If IPPV is planned, gastrostomy under LA may be necessary preoperatively.

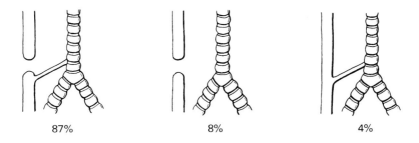

Figure 9.4 Anatomical variants of tracheo-oesophageal fistulae.

General anaesthesia

Right-sided thoracotomy. Left precordial stethoscope detects ETT displacement. Awake intubation or gas induction (sevoflurane) with spontaneous respiration avoids IPPV, which causes gastric distension and respiratory impairment. IPPV may also be ineffective in patients with a gastrostomy tube as gas escapes through the tube. Intravenous induction is safe if a fistula is not present because IPPV is effective. If a fistula is present, allow the baby to breathe spontaneously until the fistula is closed.

The opening of the fistula is usually located on the posterior distal wall of the trachea. Intubate the right main bronchus and withdraw the ETT until breath sounds are heard in both lungs so that the tip of the ETT then occludes the fistula.

Aim for early extubation postoperatively to minimize suture line stress. Postoperative respiratory complications (aspiration, pneumonia) are common.

Congenital diaphragmatic hernia

Incidence of 1:3000 live births. Associated with 50% mortality within 6 h. Caused by early gut return or delayed diaphragm closure.

Sites of herniation (Fig. 9.5)

* Posterolateral foramen of Bochdalek (left >> right) – 85%
* Anterior foramen of Morgagni – 10%
* Oesophageal hiatus – <5%.

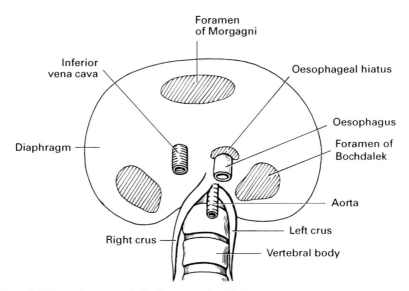

Figure 9.5 Sites of congenital diaphragmatic herniation.

Embryology of diaphragm

Comprises three structures:

- Septum transversum
- Pleuroperitoneal membrane
- Thoracic myotomes.

Sequelae

Ipsilateral alveolar and bronchial hypoplasia and decreased surfactant. Contralateral lung may also be affected. Usually presents as cyanosis, dyspnoea and cardiac dextroposition. Bowel sounds in thorax with reduced breath sounds.

A total of 23% are associated with cardiovascular abnormalities. Abnormalities of most other organ systems are also described; also trisomy 18 and 21.

Symptoms depend upon degree of hypoplasia:

- *Severe* – hypoplasia incompatible with life
- *Moderate* – respiratory distress, tachypnoea and cyanosis
- *Mild* – less severe symptoms, not always presenting immediately.

Pulmonary hypoplasia and pulmonary artery hypertension worsen any right-to-left shunt and cause respiratory acidosis, which predisposes to persistent fetal circulation. The degree of shunting may be reduced with bicarbonate infusion:

$$NaHCO_3 \text{ (mEq) required} = \text{body weight (kg)} \times \text{base deficit} \times 0.3$$

(Dilute in equal volume of 10% glucose prior to i.v. administration.)

General anaesthesia

- Emergency surgery is no longer recommended as mortality is reduced by preoperative resuscitation
- Monitoring: S_aO_2, ECG, invasive BP (one preductal, one post-ductal to assess shunt), urinary catheter
- Good venous access above IVC, which is compressed postoperatively by gut
- NG tube to decompress stomach
- Avoid IPPV which inflates the stomach and worsens respiratory distress. Therefore, awake intubation. Ventilate by hand to detect sudden changes in compliance, e.g. pneumothorax. Barotrauma, will further damage the hypoplastic lung and must be avoided.
- Avoid N_2O, which distends bowel. SNS stimulation worsens pulmonary vasoconstriction and is reduced by opioids, e.g. fentanyl
- Pulmonary vasodilators (tolazoline (α-antagonist), PGE_1, nitroprusside, nitroglycerine) improve oxygenation and acidosis, reducing airway pressure and risk of barotrauma
- Some success with ECMO, but mortality from anticoagulation causing bleeding

- Necessity for postoperative ventilation depends upon severity of abnormalities
- Successful *in utero* surgical correction reported.

ECMO has been used both as a rescue therapy in those with severe hypoxia after surgical repair and in the preoperative stabilization of infants before surgery. A recent UK study showed that infants who had received ECMO for CDH had a significant mortality in the first year of life, with long-term physical and neurodevelopmental morbidity in the majority of survivors.

Hypertrophic pyloric stenosis

Incidence 1:5000 live births. Occurs in males more than females. Due to hypertrophy of muscularis layer of pylorus. Associated anomalies in 6–20% cases include oesophageal atresia and congenital cardiac abnormalities. Usually presents in weeks 2–6 with non-bilious projectile vomiting.

Results in:

- dehydration
- metabolic disturbance
- aspiration risk.

Characterized by hypochloraemic hypokalaemic metabolic alkalosis with acidic urine. Due to bicarbonate initially excreted with K^+ and Na^+. Once K^+ becomes depleted, the kidneys excrete H^+ in an attempt to save Na^+, worsening the alkalosis. Increased urinary H^+ acidifies the urine. Prerenal renal failure and metabolic acidosis occur in severe cases.

Resuscitate preoperatively with normal saline 0.9% to correct acid–base balance and dehydration:

Deficit (mmol)×body wt (kg)×0.6 = mmol Na^+ needed to correct deficit

Aspirate stomach with large-bore NG tube preoperatively.

Gaseous induction risks vomiting and aspiration. Therefore, use awake intubation or rapid sequence induction. Balanced anaesthesia during surgery. Extubate awake.

Upper airway obstruction

Resulting large negative inspiratory intrathoracic pressure may cause pulmonary oedema. If bronchoscopy is required, intubate first to establish airway then exchange ETT for a ventilating bronchoscope. If child desaturates, remove bronchoscope back into trachea and re-oxygenate.

Epiglottitis

Usually 1–7 years. Of rapid onset and progression. Upper airway obstruction (inspiratory stridor, tachypnoea, intercostal recession) and difficulty swallowing with drooling. Systemically unwell.

Usually caused by *Haemophilus influenzae* type B. Chloramphenicol now superseded by third-generation cephalosporin, e.g. cefuroxime.

Keep the child and parents calm. No preoperative X-ray. Establish i.v. access only if the child is calm. Perform a gas induction in the sitting position with halothane in 100% O_2. Then establish i.v. and give atropine $20\mu g.kg^{-1}$ before laryngoscopy. Use oral ETT one size smaller than usual. If unable to pass, try intubating bronchoscope or cricothyroidotomy. Change to nasal ETT if easy intubation. Steroids are controversial. Intubate for 24–48 h. Examine larynx before extubation.

Laryngotracheobronchitis (Croup)

Occurs at 6 months–6 years. Slow onset with inspiratory stridor and intercostal recession. Mild pyrexia. Usually viral.

Treat with cool humidified air and O_2; nebulized adrenaline as appropriate (may initially improve, then worsen obstruction). If there is still no improvement, it is probably due to inspissated secretions (6% of cases). If so, treat as for epiglottitis.

Foreign body aspiration

Often a history of coughing, choking or cyanosis while eating. Most foreign bodies are not radiopaque. Hyperinflation and atelectasis on CXR. Specific problems are:

- Potential loss of airway
- Risk of full stomach
- V / Q mismatch prolonging gas induction.

Give atropine premedication. Avoid opioids. Gaseous induction as for epiglottitis. *Gentle* bagging if necessary to avoid driving foreign body distally. Insert Storz ventilating bronchoscope once airway is secured.

Peanut oil causes intense inflammation with rapid airway obstruction if not removed early. Consider the possibility of airway obstruction due to foreign body in oesophagus compressing trachea.

Bibliography

Al-Rawi O, Booker PD: Oesophageal atresia and tracheo-oesophageal fistula, *Contin Edu Anaesth, Crit Care Pain* 7:15–19, 2007.

American Society of Anesthesiologists' Task Force on Preoperative Fasting: Practice guidelines for preoperative fasting and the use of pharmacologic agents to reduce the risk of pulmonary aspiration: application to healthy patients undergoing elective procedures, *Anesthesiology* 90:896–905, 1999.

Association of Paediatric Anaesthetists of Great Britain and Ireland: *APA consensus guideline on perioperative fluid management in children*, v1.1 London, 2007, APAGBI. www.apagbi.org.uk.

Association of Paediatric Anaesthetists of Great Britain and Ireland: *Guidelines on the prevention of post-operative vomiting in children*, London, 2007, APAGBI. www.apagbi.org.uk.

Bingham B: Paediatric anaesthesia: past, present and future, *Anaesthesia* 58:1194–1196, 2003.

Fell D, Chelliah S: Infantile pyloric stenosis, *BJA CEPD Rev* 1:85–88, 2001.

Gormley SM, Crean PM: Basic principles of anaesthesia for neonates and infants, *BJA CEPD Rev* 1:130–134, 2001.

Holliday MA, Segar WE: The maintenance need for water in parenteral fluid therapy, *Pediatrics* 19:823–832, 1957.

King H, Booker PD: Congenital diaphragmatic hernia in the neonate, *Contin Edu Anaesth, Crit Care Pain* 5:171–174, 2005.

Lönnqvist PA, Morton NS: Postoperative analgesia in infants and children, *Br J Anaesth* 95:59–68, 2005.

Marsh DF, Hodkinson B: Remifentanil in paediatric anaesthetic practice, *Anaesthesia* 64: 301–308, 2009.

Rowney DA, Doyle E: Epidural and subarachnoid block in children, *Anaesthesia* 53:980–1001, 1998.

PAEDIATRIC CARDIOLOGY

Anaesthesia for congenital cardiovascular disease

Approximately 8000 infants born in the UK each year have some form of congenital heart disease, of which one-third will require cardiac surgery.

- *Cyanotic lesions* – Fallot's tetralogy, transposition of great vessels, tricuspid atresia, Eisenmenger's syndrome.
- *Acyanotic lesions* – ASD, VSD, PDA, aortic coarctation.

Assessment

History

- Ability to play with peers usually suggests adequate cardiac reserve
- Cyanosis, squatting, syncope, exercise/feeding intolerance, tachypnoea and failure to thrive all suggest varying degrees of cardiac failure.

Examination

- Previous scars
- Respiratory rate and pattern (nasal flaring, recession, grunting)
- Peripheral pulses, e.g. coarctation
- Pulse pressure, e.g. aortic regurgitation, PDA
- Enlarged liver/spleen
- Respiratory system for signs of LVF.

Investigation

- ECHO, cardiac catheterization
- Haematocrit is the best indicator of severity of right-to-left shunt (increased haematocrit causes renal, pulmonary and CNS thrombosis, especially with dehydration)
- Clotting – coagulopathies are common.

General anaesthesia

General aims

- Maintain adequate perfusion of systemic and pulmonary circulation
- If pulmonary hypertension is present, aim to reduce pulmonary artery pressures
- In the presence of an obstructive lesion, maintain filling pressures, HR and coronary perfusion pressure
- Careful purging of air bubbles from all lines to avoid systemic embolization.

Premedication

- None for babies <6 months or if there is minimal anxiety
- Morphine 0.1 mg/kg is well tolerated
- Glycopyrrolate as an antisialogogue.

Monitoring

- ECG, precordial/oesophageal stethoscope, NIBP, ± arterial line, CVP, temperature, pulse oximeter, capnograph and urinary catheter
- Consider pre- and post-ductal pulse oximeters to detect degree of right-to-left shunt.

Induction

- Intravenous is best for cardiovascular disease
- Gaseous induction risks desaturation, especially with severe disease. Slow if right-to-left shunt. If there is no venous access with severe disease, use 100% O_2, i.m. ketamine and i.m. suxamethonium.

Maintenance

High-dose fentanyl, 100% O_2, pancuronium technique provides good cardio-vascular stability and decreases the stress response. (Pancuronium offsets the vagotonic effects of fentanyl.)

Degree of shunting in PDA, ASD and VSD depends upon the pressure difference between the systemic and pulmonary circulations:

- Increase PVR by decreasing F_iO_2, use of PEEP and high P_aCO_2
- Decrease PVR by increasing F_iO_2, no PEEP, alkalosis, decreasing P_aCO_2 and nitric oxide
- Increase SVR by vasoconstrictors and flexing hips
- Decrease SVR by inhalational agents and vasodilators.

IPPV can reverse left-to-right shunt and therefore cause air bubbles to enter the arterial circulation.

Ventricular septal defect (Fig. 9.6)

Commonest congenital heart lesion (2/1000 births); 50% close spontaneously within 1 year. Often associated with more complex lesions. Results in gradually increasing left-to-right shunt as RV pressure falls below LV pressure after birth. High pulmonary blood flow causes heart failure and pulmonary oedema. Treat with digoxin and diuretics or pulmonary artery banding to reduce pulmonary blood flow if severe.

Patent ductus arteriosus

Similar pathophysiology to VSD. Pulmonary function is compromised because of pulmonary oedema, and reduced systemic flow may impair renal function. Give indometacin, avoid fluid overload and consider digoxin.

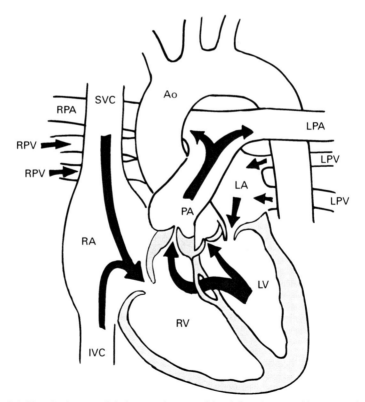

Figure 9.6 Ventricular septal defect – pulmonary blood flow increased by systemic vasoconstriction or pulmonary vasodilation.

Transposition of the great vessels (Fig. 9.7)

Aorta arises from RV and pulmonary artery arises from LV. Unless there is a shunt present (ASD, VSD, PDA), there is no communication between the two circuits and closure of the ductus arteriosus results in death. Balloon septostomy creates an atrial septal defect as a temporary measure. Definitive surgery involves switching PA and aorta or creating shunts to establish single circulation (Blalock shunt followed by Rastelli procedure).

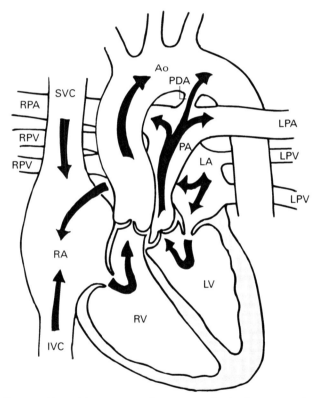

Figure 9.7 Transposition of the great vessels – communication between pulmonary and systemic circulations provided by the ASD and PDA.

Tetralogy of Fallot (Fig. 9.8)

- Overriding aorta
- Right ventricular hypertrophy
- VSD with right-to-left shunt
- Pulmonary stenosis.

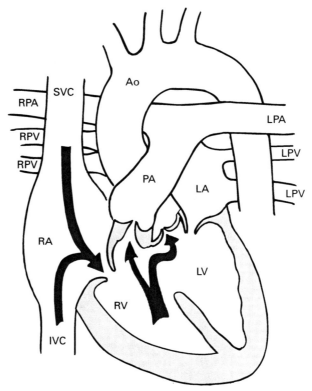

Figure 9.8 Tetralogy of Fallot – blood flow showing right-to-left shunt through the VSD.

Both ventricles are at the same (systemic) pressure. Increasing systemic vascular resistance (SVR) reduces right-to-left shunt and increases pulmonary blood flow. Acidosis and hypoxia cause infundibular spasm and worsen shunt. Squatting increases SVR and reduces return of acidotic venous blood from the IVC. Hyperviscosity from raised haematocrit is common. Avoid dehydration, which may cause hypotension and thrombotic complications. Cyanotic spells may be reversed with propanolol 0.025–0.1 mg/kg i.v.

Pulmonary hypertension

Common problem associated with VSD, total anomalous pulmonary venous drainage, truncus arteriosus, atrioventricular septal defect and hypoplastic left heart. Defined as PAP >50% of the systemic pressure. Usually associated with excess pulmonary blood flow and poor arborization of the pulmonary vasculature.

Minimize all stimuli which cause a rise in PAP, e.g. physical contact, suctioning, physiotherapy, hypoxaemia, hypercapnia and metabolic acidosis. Ensure baby is well sedated and paralyse if ventilatory pressures are high. Hyperventilate to achieve a moderate respiratory alkalosis (P_aCO_2 = 3.5 kPa, pH 7.50) and aim for P_aO_2 of 15–25 kPa. The only specific pulmonary vasodilator is nitric oxide (NO) at 2–10 ppm. Other vasodilators (prostacyclins, phenoxybenzamine, milrinone, sildenafil) cause pulmonary > systemic vasodilation.

Bibliography

Greenley WJ, Kern FH: Anesthesia for pediatric cardiac surgery. In: Miller RD, editor: *Anesthesia*, Edinburgh, 1994, Churchill Livingstone, pp 1811–1850.

Javorski JJ, Burrows FA: Pediatric cardiac anesthesia, *Curr Opin Anaesth* 8:62–67, 1995.

Long TJ: Pediatric cardiology and cardiac surgery update, *Curr Opin Anaesth* 10:221–226, 1997.

10 Pain

PAIN ASSESSMENT

Observation of the patient
Behavioural

- Time to sit/stand
- General activity
- Time to get in/out of bed.

Analgesic requirements

- Time to first dose of analgesia
- Total dose of analgesia over a given period
- Number of demands from PCA pump.

Measurement of the patient
Physiology

- Autonomic: BP, heart rate, respiratory rate
- Stress response: cortisol, ACTH, adrenaline
- Neuropharmacological: endorphins, skin temperature
- Neurological: nerve conduction, PET scan of CNS blood flow, skin conduction.

Measurement by the patient
Self-reporting

- Verbal, numerical tests
- Visual analogue scale
- McGill Pain Questionnaire: rows of words, each with a specific score. Add up scores from each section (sensory, emotive, evaluative)
- Minnesota Pain Inventory Score (for chronic pain)
- Pain diary.

Assessment of children

- COMFORT Pain scale: scores alertness, calmness/agitation, respiratory distress, crying, physical movement, muscle tone, facial tension, arterial pressure and heart rate.
- Face-Legs-Activity-Cry-Consolability. Assesses five categories of pain behaviour: facial expression; leg movement; activity; cry; and consolability.
- Visual scales:
  - Oucher Scale (picture scale)
  - Faces Pain Rating Scale
  - Colour matching charts
- Voice spectral analysis (research tool only).

Bibliography

Breivik H, Borchgrevink PC, Allen SM, et al: Assessment of pain, *Br J Anaesth* 101:17–24, 2008.

Cardno N, Kapur D: Measuring pain, *BJA CEPD Rev* 2:7–10, 2002.

PHYSIOLOGY AND TREATMENT OF PAIN

Definition of Pain International Association for the Study of Pain:
"An unpleasant sensory or emotional experience associated with actual or potential tissue damage."

Pathophysiology

Acute pain is only the initiation phase of an extensive, persistent nociceptive and behavioural cascade triggered by tissue injury. Failure to suppress acute pain may lead to amplification of tissue responses and development of chronic pain. Mechanical, thermal or chemical damage causes nociceptive neurones to increase their firing rate. Local inflammatory cascades sensitize these neurones and may recruit dormant ones. Sensitized neurones increase their basal discharge rate, have a lowered stimulus threshold and an exaggerated response to a stimulus.

- *Nociceptive pain* – activation of somatic or visceral sensory nerve fibres by noxious stimuli
- *Neuropathic pain* – due to abnormalities or damage to nerve fibres, e.g. mononeuropathies, polyneuropathies, deafferentation or reflex sympathetic dystrophy. May also involve central mechanisms

(sensitization of spinal cord neurons ('wind-up') and loss of central inhibitory mechanisms increase nociceptive transmission), e.g. phantom limb pain, trigeminal neuralgia, post-herpetic neuralgia, post-stroke pain

- *Inflammatory pain* – hypersensitivity state in which normally innocuous stimuli produce pain. Due to changes in the sensitivity of nociceptive neurons.

Pain pathways

C and Aδ fibres convey nociceptive information from visceral and somatic sites to the dorsal horn of the spinal cord. Ascending fibres then relay nociceptive information to thalamic, limbic and cortical structures. Descending noradrenergic pathways release noradrenaline to cause analgesia directly and to stimulate acetylcholine release to produce analgesia.

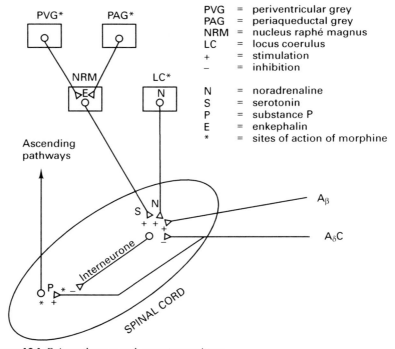

PVG	=	periventricular grey
PAG	=	periaqueductal grey
NRM	=	nucleus raphé magnus
LC	=	locus coerulus
+	=	stimulation
–	=	inhibition
N	=	noradrenaline
S	=	serotonin
P	=	substance P
E	=	enkephalin
*	=	sites of action of morphine

Figure 10.1 Pain pathways and neurotransmitters.

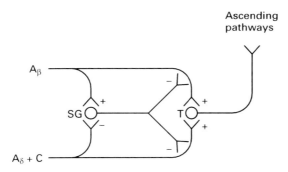

SG = substantia gelatinosa

T = intermediate transmission cell

Figure 10.2 Gate control theory of pain.

Gate control theory of pain

Proposes that pain pathways ($A\delta$ + C) are blocked by the stimulation of touch fibres ($A\beta$), which inhibit transmission to ascending pathways via an interneurone in the substantia gelatinosa (Fig. 10.2).

Effects of pain

- Patient discomfort and distress
- Hyperventilation, causing respiratory alkalosis (reduces placental flow)
- Increases O_2 demand, causing metabolic acidosis
- Thoracic pain impairs lung expansion and reduces compliance
- Increases neuroendocrine stress response
- Reduces immunological function
- Delays postoperative mobilization
- Increases DVT risk
- Prolongs hospital stay.

Pain in neonates

Neonates are thought to have reduced sensitivity due to incomplete myelination, high levels of endogenous endorphins and underdeveloped pain pathways. However, several studies now show that analgesia is important in neonates:

- Neonates undergoing PDA ligation anaesthetized with fentanyl in addition to N_2O/O_2/pancuronium show less stress response and less postoperative bradycardia, apnoea and poor perfusion.

- Neonatal heel lancing produces weeks of local sensitivity.
- Infant circumcision without analgesia is associated with altered behavioural responses to pain months later.

ANAESTHETISTS AND NON-ACUTE PAIN MANAGEMENT
Association of Anaesthetists 1993

Pain management is poorly taught, at both undergraduate and postgraduate levels, as a result of which it is poorly funded and not available to many patients who may benefit from its provision. Pain treatment and management should be available to all patients who require it.

Techniques in pain treatment
Pre-emptive analgesia

Concept introduced by Crile in 1913. Delivering pre-emptive analgesia was thought to reduce postoperative problems such as phantom limb pain, but subsequent studies have not confirmed this.

Combination analgesia

Combinations of opioids, NSAIDs and nerve blocks result in improved pain relief and fewer adverse side-effects. Most effective to use a combination strategy using multimodal drugs of increasing potency (Fig. 10.3).

Interruption at specific sites

Reduced peripheral stimulus (e.g. NSAIDs), interrupted peripheral pain transmission (e.g. local anaesthetic), interrupted central pain transmission (e.g. anterolateral cordotomy), stimulation of inhibitory pathways (e.g. acupuncture, opioids), or alteration of emotional or behavioural response.

Specific drugs
NSAIDs

NSAIDs are analgesic, anti-inflammatory and antipyretic. Act to inhibit cyclo-oxygenase in the spinal cord and periphery to decrease prostanoid synthesis and diminish post-injury hyperalgesia at these sites. NSAIDs reversibly inhibit cyclo-oxygenase to reduce prostaglandin and thromboxane synthesis (Fig. 10.4). Type 1 cyclo-oxygenase (COX-1) is present in gastric mucosa to produce protective prostaglandins and modulates renal function and platelet adhesiveness. Type 2 cyclo-oxygenase (COX-2) is responsible for inflammatory prostaglandins. Drugs which inhibit only COX-2 (rofecoxib, parecoxib)

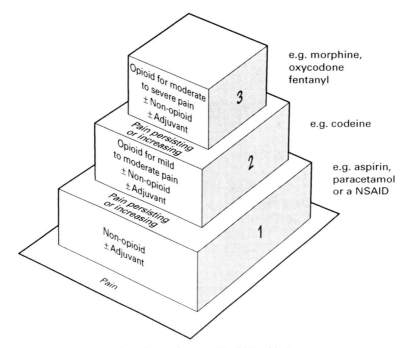

e.g. morphine,
oxycodone
fentanyl

e.g. codeine

e.g. aspirin,
paracetamol
or a NSAID

Figure 10.3 Pain ladder of escalating therapy (World Health Organisation).

cause fewer gastric, renal and haemorrhagic side-effects. NSAIDs also inhibit neutrophil activation by inflammatory mediators and act centrally on the thermoregulatory centre. There is minimal protein binding with subsequent large volume of distribution.

Not generally as effective as opioids for acute pain, but reduce opioid requirements by 30–50%. May be useful in day-case surgery to avoid opioids.

Side-effects

- GI bleeding, fluid retention, asthma
- Renal failure (PGI_2 enhances Na^+, Cl^- and water excretion; PGE_2 vasodilates to maintain GFR)
- Inhibit platelet function
- Blood dyscrasias
- Bowel enteropathy
- Pancreatitis
- Erythema multiforme
- Reye's syndrome

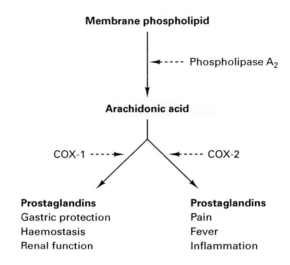

Figure 10.4 Cyclo-oxygenase (COX) pathways.

- Anaphylaxis, urticaria
- Aseptic meningitis
- Delayed spontaneous labour.

There is no evidence that i.m. or rectal preparations reduce risk of side-effects. Advice from the Committee on Safety of Medicines recommends using the lowest possible doses to reduce the risk of GI complications.

GUIDELINES FOR THE USE OF NON-STEROIDAL ANTI-INFLAMMATORY DRUGS IN THE PERIOPERATIVE PERIOD
Royal College of Anaesthetists 1998

Usage
NSAIDs are not sufficiently effective as the sole agent after major surgery in most patients, but are often effective after minor or moderate surgery. NSAIDs are the drug of choice after many day-case procedures.

NSAIDs often decrease opioid requirements and enhance the quality of opioid-based analgesia.

Gastrointestinal effects

GI bleeding or ulceration should be a prominent differential diagnosis in all patients receiving NSAIDs. NSAIDs should not be given to patients with a history of GI ulceration or bleeding.

Haematological effects

NSAIDs increase bleeding time and may increase blood loss. The clinical significance of a tendency to increased bleeding is unclear. It should not inhibit the use of NSAIDs in most cases if there are no specific contraindications. However, NSAIDs should not be given prior to surgery if there is an increased risk of intraoperative bleeding.

Renal effects

NSAIDs are contraindicated in renally compromised patients. Renal function should be monitored regularly in all patients taking NSAIDs after major surgery. Any increase in urea, creatinine or potassium or decreased urine output is an indication for discontinuing NSAIDs.

Other contraindications

NSAIDs are contraindicated in patients with hypovolaemia, pre-eclamptic toxaemia or uncontrolled hypertension. NSAIDs are contraindicated in aspirin-sensitive asthmatics and should be used with caution in other asthmatics. NSAIDs should be used with caution in the elderly, in patients with diabetes or vascular disease and after cardiac, hepatobiliary, renal or major vascular surgery.

Epidural anaesthesia

It is impossible to give meaningful recommendations on the safe use of NSAIDs with epidural anaesthesia.

Drug interactions

Patients taking NSAIDs should be monitored closely if they are also taking antihypertensive medication, ciclosporin (renal function) or lithium (lithium levels). NSAIDs used in the perioperative period have little clinical effect on warfarin, but INR should be checked after the start or withdrawal of treatment. Low-molecular-weight heparin may be affected by NSAIDs.

Opioids

- Narcotic – from Greek *narco*, meaning deaden/numb
- Morphine – from Greek *Morpheus*, god of dreams, son of the god of sleep.

Pharmacology. Protein binding is a major determinant of drug distribution. Albumin binds acidic drugs (e.g. morphine); α_1 acid glycoprotein (AAG) binds basic drugs (e.g. fentanyl, alfentanil, sufentanil). Neonatal albumin and AAG levels reach adult levels by 1 year.

Opioid receptors are found in high concentrations in the limbic system and spinal cord:

- μ (mu) – analgesia (μ_1), respiratory depression (μ_2), constipation
- δ (delta) – analgesia, respiratory depression, euphoria
- κ (kappa) – spinal analgesia, miosis, sedation, dysphoria, diuresis.

These opioid receptors have recently been reclassified by the International Union of Pharmacology (IUPHAR) as OP_1 (δ), OP_2 (κ) and OP_3 (μ).

Actions

- Cardiovascular: ↓ SNS drive, direct effect on vagal nucleus to ↓ HR, direct effect on SA node
- Respiratory: ↓ rate, dyscoordination, respiratory depression mediated by μ receptors. CO_2 response curve shifted to right. Depression of cough reflex
- Analgesia
- Anxiolysis (shift towards δ rhythm on EEG)
- Euphoria/dysphoria
- Histamine release via opioid receptors on mast cells. Blocked by naloxone
- GI: smooth muscle spasm, ↓ lower oesophageal sphincter tone, nausea and vomiting
- Miosis via opioid receptors on Edinger–Westphal nucleus
- Hormonal effects via D_2 receptors in hypothalamus: ↑ ADH, ↑ GH, ↑ prolactin; ↓ ACTH, ↓ FSH, ↓ LH
- Muscle rigidity via (?) opioid receptors in substantia nigra.

Routes of administration. Up to eightfold variation in minimum analgesic blood levels between patients. Therefore, no one regimen is suitable for all patients.

Oral. Delayed postoperative gastric emptying results in delayed absorption followed by large bolus absorbed when motility returns. May be of more use in the late postoperative period once bowel motility returns.

Nausea and vomiting prevent oral intake. Poor bioavailability because of first pass.

Sublingual. Systemic absorption avoids first pass. Dry mouth reduces absorption.

PR. Systemic absorption avoids first pass. Not affected by GI motility or nausea and vomiting. Slow absorption delays onset.

Transdermal. Rate of absorption $\propto$ lipid solubility. Reduced absorption with vasoconstriction.

Inhalational. Used for relieving symptoms of dyspnoea and postoperative pain. Some lost on expiration, widely variable absorption, nasal pruritis and cough limit its clinical application.

Intra-articular. Action via intra-articular opioid receptors.

Intranasal. Rapid onset of lipid-soluble drugs. Systemic absorption avoids first pass. Useful route for postoperative pain in children.

Subcutaneous. Useful for pain relief in children since small cannulae can be inserted with minimal distress. Use with continuous infusion or intermittent bolus.

Intramuscular. Pain of injection, erratic uptake if poor tissue perfusion, wide fluctuations in blood levels and thus degree of analgesia and side-effects. Often administered too infrequently if 'prn'.

Intermittent intravenous injections. Avoids pain of injection but has similar problems to i.m. route. Needs 1:1 nursing care to monitor respiratory depression.

Continuous intravenous infusion. May need initial i.v. bolus dose since steady state takes five half-lives to establish. More stable blood levels, but risk of insidious onset of respiratory depression and obstructive apnoea greater than that with PCA.

Patient controlled analgesia (Fig. 10.5).

Route of choice. Less overall opioid requirements than other routes. Patient acts as feedback to prevent overdose. Patients do not have to wait after onset of pain to receive analgesia, and immediate administration gives patients a greater sense of control. Requires loading dose and correct settings of lockout time (5–10 min), dose per bolus (morphine 0.01–0.025 mg/kg) and maximum dose/hour. Suitable for most children over 5 years. Background dose increases risk of respiratory depression and does not affect total dose. Fentanyl PCA reduces pruritis compared with morphine and may also be more appropriate in renal failure. Less incidence of respiratory depression

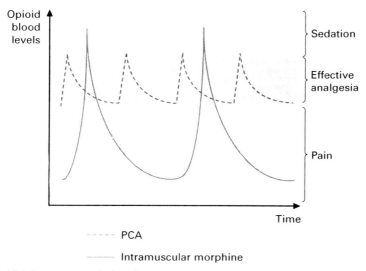

Figure 10.5 Patient controlled analgesia with intramucular morphine.

(0.1–0.8.%) when compared with i.m. opioid boluses (0.2–0.9%) or i.v. opioid infusion (1.7%). Patient concerns regarding addiction and overdose may limit effective use.

Intrathecal/extradural. Most effective when combined with local anaesthetics. Side-effects are common, especially pruritis. Respiratory depression up to 24 h.

FENTANYL PATCHES: SERIOUS AND FATAL OVERDOSE FROM DOSING ERRORS, ACCIDENTAL EXPOSURE, AND INAPPROPRIATE USE
MHRA Guidance 2007

- Healthcare professionals, particularly those who prescribe fentanyl patches, must fully inform patients and caregivers about directions for safe use:
  - Follow the prescribed dose
  - Follow the correct frequency of patch application
  - Ensure that old patches are removed before applying a new one
  - Patches must not be cut
  - Avoid touching the adhesive side of patches and wash hands after application
  - Follow instructions for safe storage and disposal of used or un-needed patches.
- Increased body temperature, exposure of patches to external heat sources, and concomitant use of CYP3A4 inhibitors may lead to potentially dangerous rises in serum fentanyl levels. Concomitant use of other CNS depressants might also potentiate adverse effects from fentanyl
- Healthcare professionals, particularly those who prescribe fentanyl patches, should ensure that patients and caregivers are aware of the signs and symptoms of fentanyl overdose, i.e. trouble breathing or shallow breathing; tiredness; extreme sleepiness or sedation; inability to think, walk, or talk normally; and feeling faint, dizzy, or confused. Patients and caregivers should be advised to seek medical attention immediately if overdose is suspected. Patients who experience serious adverse events should have the patches removed immediately and should be monitored for up to 24 h after patch removal.

α_2-Agonists (e.g. clonidine)

α_2-adrenergic receptors are located at peripheral (primary afferent terminals), spinal (neurones in the superficial laminae of the spinal cord) and brainstem sites (brainstem nuclei) where they are involved in nociceptive modulation. α_2

adrenoceptors are devoid of respiratory depressant and addictive effects, but sedation and hypotension are limiting their clinical use as an effective analgesic agent.

α_2-agonists have the following characteristics:

- Haemodynamic stabilizing properties decrease arrhythmias caused by halothane and reduce labetalol requirements in hypotensive anaesthesia
- Sedative and anxiolytic (via activation of postsynaptic α_2-adrenoceptors in the locus coeruleus of the brainstem)
- Analgesic – inhibit substance P release at dorsal root ganglia, enhance and prolong duration of epidural
- Reduced sympathetic tone (via activation of postsynaptic α_2-adrenoceptors in the nucleus tractus solitarius and locus coeruleus of the brainstem) and reduced cortisol release
- Decreased volatile and i.v. induction agent doses, decreased intraocular pressure and attenuated rise in IOP with intubation, decreased shivering.

NMDA receptor antagonists

NMDA receptors on the postsynaptic membrane of dorsal horn neurones are activated by glutamate to stimulate ascending pathways. Activation of NMDA receptors results in induction and maintenance of central sensitization during pain states. NMDA antagonists (especially those acting on the NR2β receptor subunit) may be useful in the treatment of chronic pain.

Ketamine blocks the open calcium channel of the NMDA receptor. Psychotomimetic side-effects, salivation and cardiac stimulation limit its use.

Gabapentin

Introduced for epilepsy in 1990s. High binding affinity for the $\alpha_2\delta$ subunit of the presynaptic voltage-gated calcium channels, binding to which inhibits calcium influx and subsequent release of excitatory neurotransmitters in the pain pathways. At least as effective as morphine for postoperative analgesia and may also prevent opioid tolerance. May cause dizziness and somnolence.

Capsaicin receptor antagonists

Capsaicin is a vanilloid found in chilli peppers. Capsaicin activates the transient receptor potential ligand-gated ion channel family (TRPV1), as does heat, acidosis, cannabinoids and NADA (N-arachidonoyl-dopamine). Prolonged application of an agonist, e.g. capsaicin leads to release of central transmitters (glutamate and substance P) from nociceptive afferents and loss of function of the afferents due to exhaustion of neurotransmitters. This is the basis of the use of capsaicin cream where it has been shown to be of benefit in osteoarthritis, diabetic neuropathy, psoriasis and post-herpetic neuralgia.

The TRPV1 receptor may be upregulated in some disease states e.g. osteoarthritis, post-herpetic neuralgia, cancer-induced bone pain. TPRV1 antagonists may be an important new class of analgesic agents.

Transcutaneous electrical nerve stimulation (TENS)

May act through the gate control theory of pain and by release of endorphins. Usually applied at 70Hz. May take several days of use to achieve maximal effect. Most effective with neurogenic pain, such as phantom limb pain, postherpetic neuralgia or nerve damage. Little evidence of efficacy in severe pain, e.g. childbirth.

Chronic pain

Defined as pain which persists past the time when healing is expected to be complete, usually more than 6 months.

Definition of pain terms

- *Allodynia* – pain due to a stimulus which does not normally cause pain
- *Dysaesthesia* – an unpleasant abnormal sensation, whether spontaneous or evoked
- *Hyperpathia* – a painful syndrome, characterized by increased reaction to a stimulus, as well as increased threshold
- *Hyperalgesia* – an increased response to a stimulus which is normally painful

Neuropathic pain is defined as: pain initiated or caused by a primary lesion or dysfunction in the nervous system. Covers a wide spectrum of clinical conditions:

- Trauma: spinal cord injury, phantom limb pain, reflex sympathetic dystrophy
- Ischaemic injury: painful diabetic neuropathy
- Infection/inflammation: post-herpetic neuralgia, reflex sympathetic dystrophy
- Cancer: invasion/compression of neuronal structures
- Drugs: vinca alkaloids
- Compression: sciatica, trigeminal neuralgia
- Unknown: trigeminal neuralgia, multiple sclerosis.

Reflex sympathetic dystrophy

Reflex sympathetic dystrophy (RSD) is now classified by the International Association for the Study of Pain as complex regional pain syndrome (CRPS) type I, and when associated with nerve injury (i.e. causalgia) it is known as CRPS type II.

CRPS type I (RSD). A syndrome that usually follows an initiating noxious event, with spontaneous pain or allodynia/hyperalgesia occurring in a regional distribution and not limited to the territory of a single peripheral nerve. Results in continuous pain in a portion of an extremity (not involving nerve damage), associated with sympathetic hyperactivity.

Characterized by:

1. *Pain.* Initial pain and burning become more diffuse and aching. Hyperalgesia and allodynia may be present.
2. *Autonomic dysfunction.* Abnormal skin blood flow causes both warm red skin and cold, cyanotic changes. Oedema occurs in 50% due to postcapillary vasoconstriction. Following nerve damage, C-polymodal nociceptors in the dorsal horn of the spinal cord develop increased sensitivity to sympathetic stimulation. Stimulation of these causes excess firing, which then causes increased pain and discharge of sympathetic neurones to the traumatized tissue. The increased sympathetic tone sensitizes peripheral chemoreceptors to such an extent that they fire without a stimulus, causing chronic sympathetically mediated pain. (This concept of central sensitization of the CNS may also be involved with mechanisms of pre-emptive analgesia.)
3. *Trophic changes.* Muscle wasting, thin shiny skin, coarse hair and thickened nails are late manifestations.
4. *Motor impairment.* Weakness and tremor (not necessary for diagnosis). Traditionally divided into three stages, but may not progress beyond the second:
   - *Acute stage* – days to months after injury. Pain and oedema. Warm, dry red skin. Treatment most effective at this stage: physiotherapy, NSAIDs, antidepressants and sympathetic nerve block.
   - *Dystrophic stage* – 3–6 months after onset of symptoms. Burning pain may spread to involve whole limb. Muscle wasting, pale cyanotic skin associated with increased sympathetic activity. Decreased hair and nail growth, muscle wasting and disuse osteoporosis.
   - *Atrophic stage* – 6–12 months after onset of symptoms. Pain may diminish. Cool limb, contractures and severe osteoporosis. Physiotherapy is the most effective treatment at this stage.

CRPS type II (causalgia – Greek: *kausis* = burning; *algos* = pain). Similar to RSD but associated with traumatic nerve injury. Onset may be delayed for several months. Commonest nerves are median, sciatic, tibial and ulnar.

Postherpetic neuralgia

Pain in the area of acute herpes zoster for at least 1 month after the initial infection. Incidence increases with age; female > male. Pain intensity during acute herpes zoster predicts severity of post-herpetic neuralgia. Predilection for thoracic dermatomes and ophthalmic division of trigeminal nerve. Sharp, burning pain. Due to damage of large myelinated fibres which removes inhibition to nociceptive input. Central neurones also expand receptor fields to produce allodynia and hyperpathia.

Early aggressive treatment reduces incidence of pain. Use antidepressants, anticonvulsants, neuroleptics, TENS, sympathetic blocks and topical local anaesthetics. Capsaicin cream enhances release and prevents reaccumulation of substance P from central and peripheral nerve terminals and may be of benefit.

Trigeminal neuralgia

Usually a primary neuralgia, but 3% of cases are due to MS, tumours, vascular malformation or dental lesions. Paroxysmal lancing pain, triggered by tactile stimulation, lasting a few seconds. Increasing severity and frequency of attacks as disease progresses. Anticonvulsants such as carbamazepine block sodium channels to reduce neuronal firing. Phenytoin, sodium valproate and clonazepam may also be effective. Vascular decompression and radiofrequency ablation may benefit some patients.

Postoperative pain

In a UK study (Kuhn et al 1990), 93% of patients described their postoperative pain as moderate (53%) or very painful (40%). Attempts have therefore been made to improve pain services.

PAIN AFTER SURGERY
Royal College of Surgeons of England and College of Anaesthetists 1990

Recommendations
- Extension of acute pain services needed
- Improve education of doctors, nurses and patients
- Designate a person in charge of acute pain services and set up pain team
- Monitor pain, including pain charts
- Encourage use of PCA
- Further research needed into pain management.

ANAESTHESIA UNDER EXAMINATION – THE EFFICIENCY AND EFFECTIVENESS OF ANAESTHESIA AND PAIN RELIEF SERVICES IN ENGLAND AND WALES
Audit Commission 1997

Findings
- Many patients still suffer postoperative pain and some hospitals are better at controlling it than others.
- Some hospitals do not have guidelines regarding postoperative pain management and those that do often do not follow them.
- The availability of PCA pumps varies between hospitals. The majority of patients are more satisfied with PCA than with conventional administration of analgesics. There are, however, significant numbers of patients using PCA experiencing poor analgesia or nausea and vomiting.

- The use of epidural analgesia for major abdominal and thoracic surgery is increasing, but its use is limited by inadequate numbers of nurses trained in its management.
- Patients' analgesia is often changed too quickly from strong opioids to minor analgesics, allowing breakthrough of pain.

Recommendations

- Develop specific targets to reduce the number of patients in severe pain after an operation.
- Identify one doctor with specialist knowledge of pain relief techniques to promote good practice.
- Carry out regular audit of pain relief targets.
- Develop evidence-based guidelines on effective analgesic therapies.
- The acute pain team should provide written information and guidelines, coordinate and educate staff, and provide leadership and a focus for improved team working.
- Develop a programme of continuing education in pain management for trainee doctors and nurses.

Bibliography

www.aagbi.org/publications/guidelines/docs/epidanalg04.pdf. Reproduced with the kind permission of the Association of anaesthetists of Great Britain and Ireland.

Bridges D, Thompson S, Rice A: Mechanisms of neuropathic pain, *Br J Anaesth* 87:12–26, 2001.

Carr DB, Goudas LC: Acute pain, *Lancet* 353:2051–2058, 1999.

Cervero F, Laird JMA: Visceral pain, *Lancet* 353:2145–2148, 1999.

Collett BJ: Chronic opioid therapy for non-cancer pain, *Br J Anaesth* 87:133–143, 2001.

Dickenson AH: Gate control theory of pain stands the test of time, *Br J Anaesth* 88:755–756, 2002.

Freynhagen R, Bennett MI: Diagnosis and management of neuropathic pain, *BMJ* 339:391–395, 2009.

Gajraj NM: Cyclooxygenase-2 inhibitors, *Anesth Analg* 96:1720–1738, 2003.

Grass JA: Patient-controlled analgesia, *Anesth Analg* 101:S44–S61, 2005.

Harden R: Complex regional pain syndrome, *Br J Anaesth* 87:99–106, 2001.

Kharasch E: Perioperative COX-2 inhibitors: knowledge and challenges, *Anesth Analg* 98:1–3, 2004.

Kidd BL, Urban LA: Mechanisms of inflammatory pain, *Br J Anaesth* 87:3–11, 2001.

Kong VKF, Irwin MG: Gabapentin: a multimodal perioperative drug? *Br J Anaesth* 99:775–786, 2007.

Kuhn S, Cooke S, Collins M, et al: Perceptions on pain relief after surgery, *BMJ* 300:1687–1690, 1990.

Lambert DG: Capsaicin receptor antagonists: a promising new addition to the pain clinic, *Br J Anaesth* 102:156–167, 2009.

Lynch L, Simpson KH: Transcutaneous electrical nerve stimulation and acute pain, *BJA CEPD Rev* 2:49–52, 2002.

Macintyre PE: Safety and efficacy of patient-controlled analgesia, *Br J Anaesth* 87:36–46, 2001.

Macrae WA: Chronic post-surgical pain: 10 years on, *Br J Anaesth* 101:77–86, 2008.

Maze M, Kamibayashi T: Clinical uses of α_2 adrenergic agonists, *Anesthesiology* 92:934–936, 2001.

McQuay HJ, Poon KH, Derry S, et al: Acute pain: combination treatments and how we measure their efficacy, *Br J Anaesth* 101:69–76, 2008.

Nikolajsen L, Jensen TS: Phantom limb pain, *Br J Anaesth* 87:107–116, 2001.

Nurmikko TJ, Eldridge PR: Trigeminal neuralgia – pathophysiology, diagnosis and current treatment, *Br J Anaesth* 87:117–132w, 2001.

Petrenko AB, Yamakura T, Baba H, et al: The role of N-methyl-D-aspartate (NMDA) receptors in pain: a review, *Anesth Analg* 97:1108–1116, 2003.

Royal College of Anaesthetists: Guidelines for the use of non-steroidal anti-inflammatory drugs in the perioperative period, London, 1998, Royal College of Anaesthetists.

Royal College of Surgeons of England and Royal College of Anaesthetists: Commission on the Provision of Surgical Services, Report of the Working Party on Pain after Surgery London, 1990, HMSO.

Stone M, Wheatley B: Patient-controlled analgesia, *BJA CEPD Rev* 2:79–82, 2002.

Walker SM: Pain in children: recent advances and ongoing challenges, *Br J Anaesth* 101:101–110, 2008.

White PF: The role of non-opioid analgesic techniques in the management of pain after ambulatory surgery, *Anesth Analg* 94:577–585, 2002. World Health Organisation Pain Relief Ladder (http://www.who.int/cancer/palliative/painladder/en).

EPIDURAL AND SPINAL ANAESTHESIA

Anatomy

Spinal dura is continuous with the meningeal layer of the dura mater of the brain. Vertebral canal periosteum is continuous with the outer layer of the cerebral dura.

Boundaries of the epidural space are:

- superior: foramen magnum
- inferior: sacrococcygeal membrane
- lateral: intervertebral foramina and pedicles
- anterior: posterior longitudinal ligament.

Epidural space contains dural sac, spinal nerve roots, spinal arteries, venous plexus, fat and lymphatics. It is widest in the mid-lumbar region (5–6 mm) and narrows cranially to 1.5–2 mm in the lower cervical spine. Veins are valveless; therefore fluid/air injected into vein passes to intracerebral vessels. Veins drain via azygous vein to IVC. Vena caval obstruction, e.g. pregnancy, distends veins. Intervertebral foramina smaller and calcified in the elderly; therefore smaller volumes of LA required.

Negative pressures in epidural space may be due to coning of the dura at the tip of the epidural needle, pressure transmitted from the thorax, drag of gut viscera on paravertebral spaces or differential growth of the subarachnoid space more than the spinal cord.

When supine, highest point on curve of spine is at L_3; lowest point is at T_6.

Indications for regional anaesthesia

Patient assessment

Allows assessment of mental state during surgery, e.g. TURP, carotid endarterectomy, diabetes. Avoids risks of aspiration and management of difficult airway.

Cardiac disease

Avoids haemodynamic response to intubation and hypotensive effects of induction and maintenance agents. Can therefore give greater haemodynamic stability than GA for patients with ischaemic heart disease or failure if managed carefully. May reduce early postoperative mortality compared with GA in high-risk patients. Not shown to reduce reinfarction rate compared with GA, but when used for general and vascular surgery, may reduce postoperative cardiac failure (Yeager et al 1987).

Decreased SVR increases cardiac output providing venous return is maintained. Reduced diastolic may reduce coronary artery perfusion pressure. Blockade of cardioaccelerator fibres (T_1–T_4) may cause bradycardia and impaired cardiovascular response to hypovolaemia.

Pregnant patients with severe cardiac disease, e.g. aortic stenosis, Fallot's, Eisenmenger's and pulmonary hypertension, require good analgesia during labour to prevent potentially dangerous hypertension and tachycardia. However, serious complications can occur following large decreases in systemic vascular resistance and cardiac output.

Respiratory disease

Epidurals produce longer analgesia and better respiratory function (FEV_1 and PEFR) than i.v. morphine. May reduce postoperative respiratory complications by avoiding effects of systemic opioids.

Gastrointestinal

For GI surgery, an epidural results in good operating conditions, reduces blood loss and gives good postoperative analgesia. However, any hypotension may reduce mesenteric blood flow, and sympathetic blockade may result in a relative increase in parasympathetic activity, causing anastomotic disruption.

Obesity

Regional anaesthesia avoids managing a difficult airway with risk of aspiration. Postoperative analgesia using epidural opioids provides earlier ambulation, fewer respiratory complications and earlier discharge compared with i.m. opioids.

Pregnancy

Avoids difficult airway, risk of aspiration and fetal depression with GA. Good postoperative analgesia avoids use of systemic opioids, which contaminate breast milk and impair maternal nursing (drowsiness, nausea and vomiting).

Malignant hyperthermia

Local anaesthetics do not trigger malignant hyperthermia. Use of epidural avoids triggering agents used for GA.

Muscle disease

Epidurals allow avoidance of muscle relaxants in myasthenia gravis, muscular dystrophy and myotonic dystrophy.

Other advantages of regional anaesthesia

* Decreases neuroendocrine stress response and postoperative negative nitrogen balance with less hyperglycaemia because of reduced catecholamine release
* Decreases blood loss
* Decreases incidence of DVT and avoids morbidity of general anaesthetic
* May have a role in pre-emptive analgesia
* Reduces incidence of phantom limb pain if established >3 days prior to limb amputation.

Yeager et al (1987) investigated 53 high-risk patients. One group had epidural with LA combined with light GA, while a second group had GA with high-dose fentanyl. Postoperative analgesia was given with i.m./i.v. opioids ± epidural. Those with epidural had significantly reduced postoperative complications, cardiovascular failure, infection and hospital costs.

Contraindications

Cardiac disease

Fixed output states, e.g. aortic or mitral stenosis, are poorly tolerated if the patient is hypovolaemic or becomes hypotensive.

Respiratory disease

Respiratory failure is worsened as more intercostal muscles are paralysed.

Neurological

Epidural or intrathecal injections can cause transient increases in intracranial pressure. Avoid if there is any unstable neurological deficit, e.g. multiple sclerosis. Carefully document any stable deficits preoperatively. Back pain and previous back surgery are generally not contraindications.

Gastrointestinal

Unopposed parasympathetic activity results in bowel contraction, and in the presence of a perforation, bowel contents are expelled into the peritoneal cavity.

Septicaemia and local infection

Both contraindicate epidural and spinal anaesthesia.

Coagulopathy

Epidural/spinal contraindicated if platelets <100000 or bleeding time prolonged.

Aspirin

Low-dose aspirin (75 mg o.d.) prolongs bleeding time only slightly, so it is not necessary to perform a bleeding time. There is no evidence that aspirin at normal doses causes complications with epidurals. Normal bleeding time = 2–9 min.

Heparin

Insertion of a regional block or removal of an epidural catheter should be avoided if prophylactic doses of unfractionated heparin (5000 U b.d.) have been administered within 4 h or low molecular weight heparin within 12 h. There is no evidence of complications at this dose of unfractionated heparin, although 10–20% of patients will have abnormal PT/PTT. Low-molecular-weight heparin does not produce any anticoagulant effects, so it may be safer.

In one study, 30000 patients in whom heparin was given following epidural catheter insertion showed no adverse sequelae (Rao et al 1981). A study from India showed no complications of epidural catheter insertion in 1200 fully anticoagulated patients!

Effects of regional blockade

Local sites of action

Epidural

- Anterior and posterior spinal roots via root cuffs
- Spinal roots in paravertebral space
- Spinal cord.

Spinal

- Lateral, anterior and posterior columns
- Dorsal roots, dorsal root ganglia.

Regional effects

Loss of neuronal transmission occurs in the following order: B → C and Aδ → Aδ → Aβ → Aα, i.e. autonomic → temperature and pain → proprioception → touch and pressure → motor.

Aα = motor, fast sensory

Aβ = touch, vibration, pressure

Aδ = pain, temperature (laminae I and V)

Aγ = muscle spindles

B = autonomic preganglionic fibres

C = autonomic postganglionic fibres, pain (laminae II (substantia gelatinosa)).

Systemic effects

Cardiovascular and CNS side-effects, usually following inadvertent intravenous injection.

Epidural

Methods of detecting the epidural space

- Loss of resistance to needle
- Loss of resistance to air/saline (described by Dogliotti 1933)
- Drip indicator (by Baraka 1972) – sudden flow as epidural space entered
- Hanging drop technique (by Gutierrez 1932) – withdrawal of hanging drop of fluid
- Odom's indicator (1936) – air bubble movement in clear tube attached to needle
- Macintosh balloon (1950) – small rubber balloon attached to needle reduces in size as space entered
- Macintosh spring-loaded trocar (1953)
- Spring-loaded syringe (by Iklé 1949)
- Amplification of the sound of air entering the epidural space (by Sagarnaga 1971).

Midline approach results in the needle entering the epidural space where epidural veins are the least dense.

Adrenaline decreases systemic absorption and reduces the risk of toxicity. It also increases the spread, duration and intensity of the block and perhaps protects against cardiac toxicity. Adrenaline may worsen arterial hypotension through β effects on resistance vessels and increasing the intensity of the sympathetic block.

Early symptoms and signs of intravascular or intrathecal injection are missed if the patient is asleep. Therefore, insert the epidural prior to any GA.

Factors affecting block

Age. Occlusion of intervertebral foraminae in patients >60 years results in more variable, and usually smaller, doses required.

Height. Increased dose, but poor correlation with height.

Weight. Lower blocks in obese patients if performed erect, but not if performed while supine.

Direction of bevel. Spinal blocks using isobaric bupivacaine with a cranially directed bevel may result in a higher sensory block with shorter duration than when the bevel is directed caudally. Not found in all studies.

Rate of injection. No effect.

Total amount (mg) of drug. Determines level of sensory block, rate of onset and duration of block.

Concentration of drug. Determines level of motor block.

Pharmacological modification. Bicarbonate reduces the latency and increases the duration of the block by increasing extracellular pH and thus percentage of free base.

Carbonation reduces the latency and increases the duration of block by decreasing intraneuronal pH:

$$pKa - pH = \log \frac{\text{ionized drug}}{\text{unionized drug}}$$

Pharmacokinetics and dynamics

Uptake of drugs into CSF

- Via dura
- Via arachnoid granulations and radicular arteries
- Diffusion into epidural fat
- Nerve trunks in paravertebral space.

Increased epidural blood flow in pregnancy increases the rate of epidural absorption. Increased lipid solubility also causes increased fat absorption, preventing an overall increase in CSF delivery.

Uptake of epidural morphine is sufficient to cause analgesia through a systemic route of action.

Spread of epidural LA. Spreads in a cephalad and caudad direction from the site of injection. In the thoracic region, the spread is symmetrical, in the lumbar area it is mostly cephalad, and in the caudal area it is mostly cephalad.

Epidural dosage for a healthy adult

- 10–12 mL to block to T_{10}
- 20–25 mL to block to T_4.

Increase these doses by 0.1 mL/segment for each 2 inches over 5 feet in height. Decrease these doses by 30% in the third trimester (venous distension reduces volume of the epidural space, progesterone increases nerve sensitivity to LA), 50% if advanced arteriosclerosis, and 30–50% for thoracic epidurals.

Advantages of continuous epidural infusions

- Safer if migration of catheter into subarachnoid space
- Less motor block than with top-ups
- Better analgesia – avoids peaks and troughs
- Better cardiovascular stability
- Lower total dose of local anaesthetic required
- Avoids top-ups
- Fewer side-effects, e.g. less nausea, vomiting and pruritis with opioids.

Ropivacaine

Hyperbaric ('heavy') ropivacaine has demonstrated better recovery profile when compared with 'heavy' bupivacaine. A more rapid regression of sensory and motor block, earlier mobilization and shorter time to first micturition were all demonstrated using doses more commonly employed for spinal anaesthesia.

ULTRASOUND-GUIDED CATHETERIZATION OF THE EPIDURAL SPACE
National Institute for Clinical Excellence 2008

Guidance

Ultrasound guidance may be used in two different ways to facilitate catheterization of the epidural space.

One method is to use real-time ultrasound imaging to observe passage of the needle towards and into the epidural space.

The second method (prepuncture ultrasound) is to use ultrasound as a guide to the conventional technique.

Evidence on ultrasound-guided catheterization of the epidural space is limited in amount, but suggests that it is safe and may be helpful in achieving correct placement. The procedure may be used provided that normal arrangements are in place for clinical governance, consent and audit. Normal consent should include informing patients about the possibility of rare but serious complications of catheterization of the epidural space.

GOOD PRACTICE IN THE MANAGEMENT OF CONTINUOUS EPIDURAL ANALGESIA IN THE HOSPITAL SETTING
Royal College of Anaesthetists 2004

The potential complications of continuous epidural analgesia include:

- Hypotension
- Motor block
- Urinary retention
- Pruritis
- Pressure sores
- Respiratory depression
- Post dural puncture headache
- Epidural haematoma or abscess
- Neurological damage
- Inadequate analgesia.

Recommendations

Patient selection and consent

Patient selection for continuous epidural analgesia should be based on a careful risk/benefit analysis and specific consent should be obtained.

Personnel and staffing levels

There should be designated personnel and clear protocols to support the use of continuous epidural analgesia. One way of doing this is with a multidisciplinary Acute Pain Service. In the absence of an Acute Pain Service there should be a named consultant anaesthetist responsible for the supervision of acute pain management in the hospital. Doctors in training must possess defined competencies before performing epidural injections without the direct supervision of a consultant. There must be nurses with special training and skills in the supervision of epidural infusions available on the ward, throughout the 24-h period.

Wards and nursing areas

Continuous epidural analgesia should only be used in wards or units where the technique is employed frequently enough to ensure expertise and safety. Patients receiving continuous epidural analgesia must be nursed in a setting that allows close supervision. There must be 24-h access to anaesthetic advice, to staff competent to recognize and manage complications and 24-h availability of a resuscitation team.

Technique for catheter insertion

Epidural catheter insertion must be performed using an aseptic technique. The tip of the epidural catheter should be positioned at an appropriate spinal level. The dressing should allow inspection of the insertion site. Advice should be obtained from a bacteriologist about the need for antibiotic prophylaxis.

Equipment for continuous epidural analgesia

Equipment should be standardized throughout the institution and staff must be trained in its use. Pumps should be configured specifically for continuous epidural analgesia with pre-set limits for maximum infusion rate and bolus size. Epidural infusion lines should be clearly identified. The epidural system between the pump and the patient must be considered as closed and should not be breached. An anti-bacterial filter must always be used in the infusion line, at the junction of epidural catheter and infusion line. Resuscitation equipment must be readily available.

Drugs for continuous epidural analgesia

There should be a strict limitation on the number of drugs and the concentrations of these drugs used for epidural infusions. The drugs and concentrations should be described clearly in hospital protocols or guidelines. Solutions for continuous epidural analgesia should use the lowest possible effective concentration of local anaesthetic in order to preserve motor function as much as possible. This will aid detection of neurological complications that might otherwise be masked by epidural blockade. If infusions of higher concentrations are required, there should be periodic reduction of the infusion rate to allow assessment of motor block. Epidural solutions must be stored separately from those intended for any other use.

Monitoring of patients

There must be close monitoring and written observations of the patient, appropriate to the clinical circumstances, throughout the period of continuous epidural analgesia. Pain scores and sedation scores will help to identify inadequate or excessive epidural drug administration. Monitoring of sensory and motor block is essential so that potentially serious complications can be detected early. An increasing degree of motor weakness implies excessive epidural drug administration, dural penetration of the catheter, or the development of either an epidural haematoma or abscess. These are potentially serious and a senior anaesthetist must be informed immediately.

Documentation, guidelines and protocols

Contemporaneous records must be kept of events throughout the period that the continuous epidural is in use. This includes: obtaining consent, insertion of the catheter, prescription of the infusion, monitoring, additional doses and notes about any complications or adverse events.Comprehensive protocols and guidelines should cover all aspects of the management of continuous epidural infusions.

Audit

There should be audit of the efficacy of the epidural service, including audit of serious complications and adverse events.

Education

There should be formal induction course and regular updates for doctors and nurses who will be responsible for supervising patients receiving continuous epidural analgesia.

Spinal block

The degree of sympathetic block is greater and the onset of hypotension faster with spinal compared with epidural blockade.

Sympathetic block tends to be 2–3 segments above the level of sensory block, unlike epidurals where sensory and sympathetic blocks are usually at the same level.

Epidural and spinal opioids

Introduced by Yaksh and Rudy in 1976.

Neuraxial opioids decrease LA requirements, thereby reducing motor blockade and improving pain relief. Compared with parenteral administration, opioids increase the duration of block and may decrease serious morbidity and mortality in high-risk surgical patients, probably through improving postoperative pulmonary function. Epidural opioids also speed the onset of block.

Lipophilicity determines onset, speed and duration of analgesia. Increasing lipophilicity results in greater systemic action of opioids. Epidural fentanyl (intermediate solubility) is reported to be no more effective than parenteral administration.

Lipid solubility

The relative lipid solubility of certain drugs is as follows: morphine < pethidine < alfentanil < diamorphine < fentanyl < buprenorphine. There is an inverse relationship between lipid solubility and potency.

Low lipophilicity of morphine results in drug migrating rostrally in the CSF to cause delayed respiratory depression. Lipid-soluble drugs penetrate the dorsal horn faster with quicker onset of action. Early respiratory depression occurs via systemic absorption from vertebral veins and via azygous veins to superior vena cava. Systemic administration of NSAIDs may decrease opioid requirements and enhance analgesia.

Complications of spinal/epidural anaesthesia

Serious complications of central neuraxial block are rare. Incidence of death or paraplegia is reported as approximately 1:100 000.

Safety

Mechanisms of toxicity include vasoconstriction, vascular injury and alteration in blood flow to the spinal cord; also injection of incorrect solution, bacterial contamination and chronic inflammation from catheters.

2-Chloroprocaine and hypertonic saline both cause spinal cord damage. Cleaning acid descaler (not phenol as originally thought) contamination of intrathecal LA (described by Wooley and Roe in 1954).

Cardiac arrest

More common with spinal (0.06%) than with epidural (0.01%) anaesthesia. In some cases, associated with intraoperative sedation (fentanyl, thiopentone, diazepam). Cardiac arrest is often preceded by cyanosis, suggesting hypoventilation, hypotension and bradycardia.

Hypotension

Due to loss of tone in resistance and capacitance vessels, causing decreased venous return, vasodilatation and decreased cardiac output.

Block below sympathetic outflow tract (T_1-L_2) has no effect on BP. Hypotension is worse if cardioaccelerator fibres (T_2-T_4) are blocked, which removes the ability to compensate for other circulatory changes. Crystalloid preload has a variable effect on preventing hypotension following spinal anaesthesia. Fluids alone have been shown to be unable to maintain BP in 50% of patients, and ephedrine in 17%, but metaraminol maintained BP in all patients following spinal anaesthesia. If there is any delay in performing the regional block, much of the fluid preload is redistributed to the extracellular compartment, reducing any benefit of preloading. Fluids should therefore only be given after establishment of the block as the block evolves. Vagal overactivity may cause severe hypotension in some patients.

Hypotension following a regional block during pregnancy may be treated safely with small doses of ephedrine (3–6 mg) or phenylephrine (80–100 μg). The use of pure α-agonists at higher doses may be associated with reduced placental flow, despite an increased MAP. Hypotension following a combined spinal/extradural technique is less marked by rapid establishment of a low spinal block followed by careful extradural extension into higher segments. Ephedrine causes nausea more frequently when given as a bolus (36%), compared with an infusion (5%).

Respiratory system

Respiratory impairment will occur if the block is too high. Impairment of force of cough and bronchoconstriction. Brainstem depression of respiratory centre due to direct effect of LA.

Total spinal blockade

Characterized by rapid onset of hypotension, respiratory arrest and loss of consciousness. May not be revealed by test dose. Requires immediate intubation, i.v. fluids and vasopressors.

Backache

Significant increase in long-term backache if epidural given during labour (18.2% vs 10.2%), for instrumental delivery or emergency LSCS (19.2%). No increased risk if epidural used for elective LSCS.

Day-case spinals are associated with 37% headache and 55% backache; therefore avoid use for day cases. Quinke > Sprogt > Whitacre at 1 day but no difference by 1 week.

Headache

Postdural puncture headache is caused by loss of CSF through dural tear with loss of CSF cushion and traction on pain-sensitive intracranial structures. Occurs in 70–90% cases following accidental dural puncture with a Tuohy needle. Described by Bier in 1989 who suffered a severe postdural headache after an experiment on himself resulted in a dural tap. Traction above the tentorium is transmitted via the trigeminal nerve to the frontal region; traction below the tentorium is transmitted by the vagus to the occiput and neck. Incidence is not affected by posture following spinal. Incidence following spinal is reduced (0–2%) with small-gauge pencil point needles. Conversely, they are associated with an increase risk of neurological deficit because of contact with either the spinal cord or the nerve roots of the cauda equina. A new 26G spinal needle with a cutting point and a double bevel is associated with a higher fewer neurological symptoms than a 25G Whitacre needle epidural catheters introduced into the CSF following dural tap reduce incidence of headache, perhaps by a fibroblast reaction sealing the tear.

Dura usually seals spontaneously within 1 week, but in persisting cases may cause intracerebral haemorrhage, subdural haemorrhage and cranial nerve palsies. Bed rest and hydration may improve symptoms. Epidural saline infusion, i.v. caffeine and abdominal binders are also reported to reduce symptoms.

Treatment

General measures
Bed rest ineffective. Caffeine 500 mg p.o./i.v. b.d. may be of benefit in some patients.

Epidural blood patch
Perform an autologous blood patch at 1–3 days if symptoms do not resolve. Largest study from USA (American Society for Obstetric Anesthesia and Perinatology) showed 182 of 185 women completely and permanently cured of symptoms using an average of 10 mL of blood injected 4 days after the dural tear. Symptoms are often relieved immediately. MRI scanning shows that the clot has an initial mass effect, with anterior displacement and compression of the dura and nerve roots over a mean of 4.6 vertebral segments, mostly cephalad. Clot resolution occurs by 7 h to leave a thick mature clot over the dorsal dura. A small amount of blood may enter the CSF (which accelerates its clotting). Spread of blood back into subcutaneous fat may cause backache following blood patch. No residual adhesions are formed in the epidural space.

Neural damage

More common if associated with paraesthesia during puncture or local anaesthetic injection.

Direct trauma to the spinal cord may result if the needle is inserted above L_1. Causes severe lancinating pain in the dermatomes below the level of insertion.

Transverse myelitis is also documented.

Spinal haematoma

Rare but significant morbidity (irreversible neurological injury and paraplegia). Estimated as 1:150000 for epidural block and 1:220000 for spinal block. Risk factors include coagulopathies (antiplatelet or oral anticoagulant drugs, chronic alcohol abuse, chronic renal failure), anatomical abnormalities (7%), technical difficulties (25%), bloody tap (25%), multiple punctures (20%) and insertion of an epidural catheter (50%).

A recent USA series of 43 cases had a mean age of 74 years and 75% were female. Cases occurred up to 12 days after low-molecular-weight heparin (LMWH) was started, with diagnosis being made a median of 24h after onset of symptoms. Usually presenting as lower limb weakness or numbness and *not* severe radicular back pain as is traditionally taught. Requires immediate surgical decompression to avoid permanent neurological damage.

More case reports of spinal haematoma with LMWH than with unfractionated heparin. May be due to fibrinolytic activity of LMWH and greater inhibition of platelet binding to fibrinogen and endothelium. Combination of LMWH and NSAID may further increase risk.

Other complications

Spinal abscess. Onset of fever and back pain over 1–3 days. CSF leucocytosis. Main risk factors are immune deficiency, spinal column disruption, and sepsis/bacteraemia. Requires early surgical drainage and high dose parenteral antibiotics.

Horner's syndrome. Sympathetic blockade presumed due to tracking of LA.

Shivering. Reduced by warming i.v. solutions and adding fentanyl to the LA.

Urinary retention. Attributed to loss of bladder sensation but still occurs if sensation intact.

Gastrointestinal. Nausea and vomiting due to a central effect of LA. Dopaminergic stimulation by opioids. Loss of sympathetic inhibition results in small bowel contraction and expression of gut contents through a bowel perforation.

Foreign body. Breakage of catheter. Shearing of catheter if withdrawn back through the needle.

Prolonged labour. Most studies show an increased risk of instrumental delivery of LSCS.

MAJOR COMPLICATIONS OF CENTRAL NEURAXIAL BLOCKS (CNB)
Royal College of Anaesthetists 2009

The census phase produced a denominator of a little over 700000 CNB. Of these, 46% were spinals and 41% epidurals, and 45% were performed for obstetric indications and 44% perioperative.

Summary

- A total of 84 major complications were reported in the year of data collection, with 52 meeting all of the audit inclusion criteria. With the data interpreted 'pessimistically', there were 30 permanent injuries, and 'optimistically' 14.
- The incidence of permanent injury due to CNB (expressed per 100 000 cases) was 'pessimistically' 4.2 (95% confidence interval 2.9–6.1) and 'optimistically' 2.0 (1.1–3.3). These are equivalent to 1 in 24 000 and 1 in 54 000, respectively.
- 'Pessimistically' there were 13 deaths or paraplegias, 'optimistically' 5. The incidence of paraplegia or death was 'pessimistically' 1.8 per 100 000 (1.0–3.1) or 1 in 50 000 and 'optimistically' 0.7 (0–1.6) or 1 in 140 000.
- In the 30 patients with permanent harm (judged 'pessimistically'), 60% occurred after epidural block, 23% after spinal anaesthesia and 13% after CSE. More than 80% of these patients had a CNB placed for perioperative analgesia.
- Two-thirds of injuries judged initially as severe, resolved fully.

Interpretation of results

- Two-thirds of patients with complications reported to the project made a full recovery. However, patients with vertebral canal haematoma and spinal cord ischaemia had a poor prognosis, with most patients being left with significant disability after these complications.
- Most complications leading to harm occurred following CNB performed in the perioperative setting. The incidence of complications in children, and after CNB for chronic pain or obstetric indications seems to be extremely low.
- The majority of complications after perioperative CNB occurred after epidurals. Perioperative epidurals represent approximately 1 in 7 of all CNB, but accounted for more than half of complications leading to harm. The data do not clarify whether this is because perioperative epidurals are intrinsically unsafe or because these patients have particularly high risk.
- Considering the relatively small number of combined spinal epidurals performed (<6% of all CNB), the number of associated reports of harm (>13%) is concerning.
- Several reported cases illustrate that failure to identify and understand the relevance of inappropriately weak legs (including unilateral weakness) after CNB or during continuous postoperative CNB can lead to avoidable harm.
- Organizational deficiencies contributed to delays in diagnosis and intervention in several cases and led to avoidable harm. Delays included failure to monitor, poor understanding of abnormal findings (by nurses and doctors), poor interdepartmental referral processes, scanning equipment which was routinely unavailable out of hours or broken, and lack of availability of beds in tertiary referral centres for patients requiring specialized emergency surgery.
- A care bundle for CNB might usefully be developed.

Side-effects of central opioids

Respiratory depression

There is an 0.09% incidence with extradural morphine, and 0.36% following spinal morphine. Can occur up to 24 h, especially with water-soluble opioids.

Worse in the presence of other respiratory depressants, patient supine, rapid injection (intrathecal), elderly, respiratory disease and increased intra-abdominal pressure.

Pruritis

- Intrathecal – 46%
- Epidural – 8.5%.

Especially common with morphine. Less common if bupivacaine is mixed with opioid.

Can be reduced with naloxone (5–10 µg/kg per h), propofol (10 mg), droperidol (2.5 mg) or ondansetron (8 mg).

Nausea and vomiting

Much more common with intrathecal opioids than with epidural opioids. Occurs in 20% of patients given epidural morphine.

Scopolamine patch decreases incidence in labour.

Bibliography

Ballantyne JC: Does epidural analgesia improve surgical outcome? *Br J Anaesth* 92:4–6, 2004.

Cook TM, Counsell D, Wildsmith JAW; on behalf of the Royal College of Anaesthetists Third National Audit Project: Major complications of central neuraxial block: report on the Third National Audit Project of the Royal College of Anaesthetists, *Br J Anaesth* 102:179–190, 2009.

Grewal S, Hocking G, Wildsmith JAW: Epidural abscesses, *Br J Anaesth* 96:292–302, 2006.

Guay J: The epidural test dose: a review, *Anesth Analg* 102:921–929, 2006.

Liu SS, McDonald SB: Current issues in spinal anesthesia, *Anaesthesiology* 94:888–906, 2001.

NICE: Ultrasound-guided catheterisation of the epidural space. Interventional procedure guidance, vol 249, London, 2008, National Institute for Health and Clinical Excellence. www.nice.org.uk/nicemedia/pdf/IPG249Guidance.pdf.

Rao TL, El-Etr AA: Anticoagulation following placement of epidural and subarachnoid catheters: an evaluation of neurologic sequelae, *Anesthesiology* 55:618–620, 1981.

Rathmell JP, Lair TR, Nauman B: The role of intrathecal drugs in the treatment of acute pain, *Anesth Analg* 101:S30–S43, 2005.

Royal College of Anaesthetists: 3rd National Audit Project. Major complications of central neuraxial blocks, London, 2009, Royal College of Anaesthetists. www.rcoa.ac.uk/docs/NAP3_Exec-summary.pdf.

Royal College of Anaesthetists, et al: Good practice in the management of continuous epidural analgesia in the hospital setting, London, 2004, Royal College of Anaesthetists. www.aagbi.org/publications/guidelines/docs/epidanalg04.pdf.

Sharpe P: Accidental dural puncture in obstetrics, *BJA CEPD Rev* 1:81–84, 2001.

Stone M, Wheatley B: Patient-controlled analgesia, *BJA CEPD Rev* 2:79–82, 2002.

Walker SM, Goudas LC, Cousins MJ, et al: Combination spinal analgesic chemotherapy: a systematic review, *Anesth Analg* 95:674–715, 2002.

Wheatley RG, Schug SA, Watson D: Safety and efficacy of postoperative epidural analgesia, *Br J Anaesth* 87:47–61, 2001.

Whiteside JB, Wildsmith JAW: Spinal anaesthesia: an update, *Contin Educ Anaesth, Crit Care Pain* 5:37–40, 2005.

Yeager MP, Glass DD, Neff RK, et al: Epidural anesthesia and analgesia in high-risk surgical patients, *Anesthesiology* 66:729–736, 1987.

11 Pharmacology

ANAESTHETIC GASES

Oxygen

Discovered by Joseph Priestley in 1777. Manufactured by:

- fractional distillation of liquid air
- passing air over an artificial zeolite, which entraps N_2, leaving a gas containing greater than 90% O_2.

Critical temperature: 119°C
Critical pressure: 50 bar
Boiling point: −182.5°C
Vacuum insulated evaporator (VIE) stores O_2 at −180°C at a pressure of ≈10 bar. One litre of liquid oxygen evaporates to give 842 L O_2 at standard temperature and pressure (STP). Contents of a VIE are measured by weighing scales on which the VIE sits.

GUIDELINE FOR EMERGENCY OXYGEN USE IN ADULT PATIENTS
British Thoracic Society 2008

Aims to ensure oxygen is prescribed according to a target saturation range and for those who administer oxygen therapy to monitor the patient and keep within the target saturation range.

Aim to achieve normal or near-normal oxygen saturation for all acutely ill patients apart from those at risk of hypercapnic respiratory failure or those receiving terminal palliative care.

Assessing patients

For critically ill patients, high concentration oxygen should be administered immediately.

Pulse oximetry must be available in all locations where emergency oxygen is used. Oxygen saturation should be checked by pulse oximetry in all breathless and acutely ill patients (supplemented by blood gases when necessary).

Oxygen prescription

The recommended target saturation range for acutely ill patients not at risk of hypercapnic respiratory failure is 94–98%.

For most patients with known chronic obstructive pulmonary disease (COPD) or other known risk factors for hypercapnic respiratory failure (e.g. morbid obesity, chest wall deformities or neuromuscular disorders), a target saturation range of 88–92% is suggested, pending the availability of blood gas results.

For patients with prior hypercapnic failure (requiring non-invasive ventilation or intermittent positive pressure ventilation), treatment should be commenced using a 24% Venturi mask at 2–4 L.min^{-1} in hospital settings with an initial target saturation of 88–92% pending urgent blood gas results.

Because oxygenation is reduced in the supine position, fully conscious hypoxaemic patients should ideally be allowed to maintain the most upright posture possible.

Nitrous oxide

Sweet-smelling, non-irritant colourless gas. First prepared by Joseph Priestley in 1772. First used as an anaesthetic agent in 1845 by Horace Wells. Now manufactured by heating ammonium nitrate with products washed through water and caustic soda to remove NO and NO_2:

$$NH_4NO_3 \xrightarrow{240°C} 2H_2O + N_2O$$

Critical temperature: 36.5°C
Critical pressure: 71.7 bar
Boiling point: −89°C
Blood:gas solubility: 0.42
MAC: 105%
Filling ratio: temperate, 0.75; tropics, 0.67

Exists in cylinder as a liquid so pressure in cylinder does not reflect contents. Measure contents by weight.

Entonox

- 500 L cylinders – store at >10°C for 2 h or, alternatively, place in water at 37°C for 5 min and invert three times before use
- 2000 and 5000 L cylinders – store at 10–45°C for 24 h in horizontal position. Do not store <0°C for >10 min after delivery.

Only Entonox cylinders contain a dip tube. If Entonox laminates, lower level of fluid contains ≈80% N_2O and 20% O_2, which is delivered to the patient via a dip tube. The mixture gradually becomes richer in O_2. If gas was withdrawn from the top of the cylinder, it would initially contain 20% N_2O and

80% O_2, but as this mixture was withdrawn, the remaining liquid would become very low in O_2 and a hypoxic mixture would eventually be delivered to the patient.

Analgesia is due to release of endogenous opioids and direct effect at opioid receptors.

Side-effects

- Diffusion hypoxia
- Diffusion into air-filled cavities (35 times more soluble in blood than N_2)
- Diffusion out of gas-filled pockets at end of surgery, e.g. retinal detachment
- SNS stimulant, but if SNS already stimulated, e.g. LVF, N_2O causes hypotension, particularly in the presence of opioids
- Reduced bowel motility
- Limits F_iO_2
- Increases intracranial pressure
- Nausea and vomiting. Meta-analyses show that omission of N_2O reduces the incidence of PONV by 30%
- Irreversibly inactivates cob(I)alamin, the active form of vitamin B_{12}, essential for methionine-synthase activity in the brain. Recurrent exposure to nitrous oxide has been documented to cause vitamin B_{12} deficiency (subacute combined degeneration of the cord, megaloblastic anaemia, spastic paraparesis, encephalopathy). Cobalamin-deficient patients are particularly susceptible (deficient B_{12} consumption, B_{12} malabsorption)
- High-dose (>70%) nitrous oxide is teratogenic in rats. There is concern over effects in humans
- Increased spontaneous abortion rate in female staff exposed to waste gas. Dental assistants exposed to >5 h/week of unscavenged N_2O take longer to become pregnant than those exposed to lesser amounts
- Greenhouse gas accounts for <1% of all N_2O omissions, but $t_{1/2}$ of 30 years.

NITROUS OXIDE: NEUROLOGICAL AND HAEMATOLOGICAL TOXIC EFFECTS, ESPECIALLY WITH PROLONGED USE
MHRA Guidance 2008

Neurological and haematological toxic effects can occur with prolonged use of nitrous oxide. For this reason, nitrous oxide should not be given continuously for >24 h, or more frequently than every 4 days, without close clinical supervision and haematological monitoring.
- Neurological toxic effects can occur without preceding overt haematological changes.
- Assessment of vitamin B_{12} levels should be considered before nitrous oxide anaesthesia in people with risk factors for deficiency of this vitamin. Specialist haematological advice should be sought as appropriate.

Xenon

Proposed as a replacement for nitrous oxide. The only inert gas with anaesthetic properties at ambient pressure, having a MAC of 71% and the lowest blood/gas partition coefficient of any anaesthetic gas, making induction and recovery very rapid. Minimal haemodynamic effects. Possibly some degree of neuroprotection. Prepared from air where it is present in a concentration of 0.000 009%, making it very expensive.

Carbon dioxide

Colourless, pungent gas. From a:

- by-product of beer fermentation
- waste gas from burning fuel
- by-product of H_2 manufacture.

Critical temperature: $-31°C$
Critical pressure: $73.8 \, bar$
Filling ratio: temperate, 0.75; tropics, 0.67.

Bibliography

Banks A, Hardman JG: Nitrous oxide, *Contin Educ Anaesth, Crit Care Pain* 5:145–148, 2005.

Harris PD, Barnes R: The uses of helium and xenon in current clinical practice, *Anaesthesia* 63:284–293, 2008.

Ma D, Wilhelm S, Maze M, et al: Neuroprotective and neurotoxic properties of the 'inert' gas, xenon, *Br J Anaesth* 89:739–746, 2002.

Maze M, Fujinaga M: Recent advances in understanding the actions and toxicity of nitrous oxide, *Anaesthesia* 55:311–314, 2000.

O'Driscoll BR, Howard LS, Davison AG on behalf of the: British Thoracic Society: British Thoracic Society guideline for emergency oxygen use in adult patients, *Thorax* 63(Suppl VI):vi1–vi68, 2008.

Sanders RD, Franks NP, Maze M: Xenon: no stranger to anaesthesia, *Br J Anaesth* 91:709–717, 2003.

Sanders RD, Weimann J, Maze M: Biologic effects of nitrous oxide: a mechanistic and toxicologic review, *Anesthesiology* 109:707–722, 2009.

Taneja R, Vaughan RS: Oxygen, *BJA CEPD Rev* 1:104–107, 2001.

DRUG INTERACTIONS

- *Pharmacokinetics* determine the relationship between dose administered and concentration delivered to site of action, i.e. effect of body on drug.
- *Pharmacodynamics* determine the relationship between concentration of drug at site of action and intensity of effect produced, i.e. effect of drug on body.

Monoamine oxidase inhibitors (MAOIS)

MAO-A is found in CNS, and MAO-B in liver, lungs and kidneys. Most new MAOIs are selective for type A and are reversible within 48 h.
   Actions:

- Decrease sympathetic tone with decreased ability to respond to stress
- Postural hypotension
- Decrease plasma cholinesterase and thereby prolong action of suxamethonium
- Synergistic with insulin to cause hypoglycaemia
- No serious interaction with common agents except pethidine. Reaction with pethidine (via norpethidine) causes pyrexia, hypertension, CNS excitation and coma. Unlikely to occur with other opioids
- Indirect sympathomimetics are contraindicated because they cause excess noradrenaline release.

Antiplatelet agents

Non-steroidal anti-inflammatory drugs, aspirin and clopidogrel are being pre-scribed with increasing frequency and are all implicated in increased surgical blood loss. Ideally, these drugs should be stopped before surgery to allow platelet function to return to normal.

- **NSAIDs** reversibly inhibit cyclo-oxygenase. Their antiplatelet effects are half-life dependent (usually hours).
- **Aspirin** causes irreversible cyclo-oxygenase inhibition, the effect lasting for the life span of the platelet ($\approx$10 days).
- **Clopidogrel** is a pro-drug whose action is to irreversibly inhibit the P2Y ADP receptor on platelet membranes to prevent the cross-linking of platelets by fibrin. The active metabolite circulates for approximately 18 h and permanently inhibits any platelets present during this time (whether endogenous or transfused). Delaying surgery for 24 h after the last dose of clopidogrel will improve the response to platelet transfusion.

There is growing evidence that haemorrhagic risk is increased when aspirin and clopidogrel are taken concomitantly. These drugs need to be stopped for 7 days to be confident of adequate platelet function. However, due consider-ation must be given to the risks associated with stopping these drugs in surgi-cal patients, particularly those with drug eluting coronary artery stents.

Tricyclics

- Inhibit reuptake of noradrenaline at nerve terminals, potentiating action of adrenaline, noradrenaline and other catecholamines
- Anticholinergic side-effects potentiate anticholinergic effect of other drugs, e.g. atropine, glycopyrrolate

- Quinidine-like membrane-stabilizing effects with prolonged PR interval, widened QRS complex and risk of VF.

Therefore tricyclics result in an increased risk of arrhythmias and hypotension.

Selective serotonin reuptake inhibitors (fluoxetine (Prozac), sertraline, paroxetine)

Second-generation antidepressants replacing tricyclics. Selectively inhibit pre-synaptic 5HT reuptake, causing an increase in serotonin at the synaptic cleft.

- Common side-effects include nausea, diarrhoea, headache, insomnia and syndrome of inappropriate ADH secretion (particularly in the elderly).
- Overdose is usually associated with few symptoms unless combined with MAOIs or tricyclics when a serotonin syndrome may occur, characterized by coma, hyperreflexia, autonomic instability (fever, diarrhoea, tachycardia, labile BP), DIC, myoglobinaemia, renal failure and death.
- P_{450} inhibition causes interaction with haloperidol, tricyclics, theophylline, phenytoin, carbamazepine and warfarin.

Anaesthetic implications

Exclude hyponatraemia and clotting abnormalities preoperatively. Inhibition of midazolam metabolism prolongs its action. Seratomimetic drugs (pethidine, pentazocine, dextromethorphan) may cause a serotonin syndrome. May antagonize the μ-opioid receptor to cause reduced effects of opioids.

Anticonvulsants

- Barbiturates and phenytoin induce P_{450} hepatic enzymes with increased dose requirements of anaesthetic drugs
- Also cause resistance to non-depolarizers (except atracurium) possibly via effect on ACh receptors
- No significant reaction of benzodiazepines with anaesthetic drugs.

Angiotensin-converting enzyme (ACE) inhibitors

May improve perioperative CVS stability but are associated with peri- and postoperative hypotension. Consider stopping drug 24 h before surgery.

Potassium channel activators

Nicorandil is a potassium-channel activator with a nitrate component. It activates an ATP-sensitive K^+ channel to cause K^+ efflux and subsequent cellular hyperpolarization. This reduces contractility and results in both arterial and venous vasodilation. It is effective in the treatment of angina. May exacerbate hypotension induced by GA.

Table 11.1 Drugs affecting hepatic enzymes

Hepatic enzyme induction	Hepatic enzyme inhibition
Alcohol	Cimetidine
Barbiturates	Erythromycin
Phenytoin	Ciprofloxacin
Carbamazepine	
Sodium valproate	

H$_2$ antagonists

Ranitidine. Causes sinus bradycardia and AV block, especially following i.v. administration.

Cimetidine. Inhibits hepatic cytochrome P$_{450}$, increasing levels and thus toxicity of lidocaine, nifedipine and propanolol (Table 11.1). Potentiation of action of warfarin and theophyllines. Cimetidine competes with creatinine for renal excretion.

Droperidol

Butyrophenone; used for neuroleptic anaesthesia and as an antiemetic. Causes:

- mental detachment
- catatonia
- dopaminergic antagonism (acts at chemoreceptor trigger zone)
- α-adrenergic antagonism, causing hypotension. Exacerbates hypotensive effects of anaesthetic agents
- amfetamine antagonism
- gamma-aminobutyric acid (GABA) antagonism.

Large doses cause extrapyramidal movements. Gives some protection against catecholamine-induced arrhythmias. Reduces oxygen uptake. Has minimal effects on CVS, respiratory or liver function.

Leucotriene antagonists (montelukast, zafirlukast)

Leucotriene receptor antagonists block receptors in bronchial smooth muscle and are therefore of use in treating asthma:

- Zafirlukast – inhibits cytochrome P$_{450}$ enzyme
- Montelukast – metabolized by cytochrome P$_{450}$ enzyme.

Bibliography

Fee JPH, McCaughey W: Preoperative preparation, premedication and concurrent drug therapy. In Nimmo WS, Rowbotham DJ, Smith G, editors: *Anaesthesia*, ed 2, Oxford, 1994, Blackwell Scientific, pp 677–703.

Kam PCA, Chang GWM: Selective serotonin reuptake inhibitors, *Anaesthesia* 52:982–988, 1997.

Licker M, Morel DR: Inhibitors of the renin angiotensin system: implications for the anaesthesiologist, *Curr Opin Anaesth* 11:321–326, 1998.

Vuyk J: Drug interactions in anaesthesia, *Curr Opin Anaesth* 10:267–270, 1997.

ECSTASY

Ecstasy (3,4-methylenedioxymethamfetamine, MDMA) is an amfetamine derivate with similar properties to sister drugs 'Eve' (3,4-methylenedioxyethamfetamine) and 'Ice' (3,4-methylenedioxyamfetamine). First produced in 1914 as an appetite suppressant but not used again until the 1970s when it was reintroduced for psychotherapy to give energy and euphoria.

Acute effects include empathy, heightened alertness, acute psychosis trismus and tachycardia. Positive effects tend to decrease with regular use, while negative effects increase. Hangover lasts 4–5 days and is associated with depression and impaired memory.

MDMA causes the release of 5HT, one of the neurotransmitters implicated in control of mood. In primates, it causes irreversible loss of serotonergic nerve fibres. 5HT is a neurotransmitter triggering the thermoregulatory centre in the hypothalamus to increase body temperature.

Main problems in the management of these patients are:

- Acute side-effects related to hyperpyrexia causing a syndrome similar to malignant hyperthermia with rhabdomyolysis, DIC and multiple organ failure. Mortality relates to the extent and duration of hyperthermia. Rapid cooling and use of dantrolene if core temperature >40°C have been recommended.

- Drinking of large amounts of water at 'raves' to prevent dehydration causes dilutional hyponatraemia and cerebral oedema. This may also be associated with the syndrome of inappropriate production of antidiuretic hormone.

- Acute liver failure may occur due to either a reaction to MDMA itself or a reaction to a contaminant.

Bibliography

Hall AP, Henry JA: Acute toxic effects of 'Ecstasy' (MDMA) and related compounds: overview of pathophysiology and clinical management, *Br J Anaesth* 96:678–685, 2006.

LEVOSIMENDAN

Levosimendan is an intravenous calcium sensitizer approved for the treatment of acute decompensated heart failure. It acts as a positive inotrope and vasodilator through calcium sensitization, avoiding the increase in free intracellular calcium caused by β-agonists which increases myocardial oxygen demand. Inotropic effects result from binding of levosimendan to cardiac troponin C to facilitate actin-myosin cross-bridge formation and also inhibition of phosphodiesterase-3. Vasodilation occurs as a result of the opening of K-ATP channels.

Some (LIDO, REVIVE I, REVIVE II, CASINO), but not all (SURVIVE) studies have shown improvement in symptoms and outcome when compared to conventional β-agonist therapy. Use currently limited by cost.

Bibliography

Mercer S, Rhodes A: Levosimendan. In Cashman J, Grounds M, editors: *Recent Advances in Anaesthesia and Intensive Care*, vol 24, Cambridge, 2007, Cambridge University Press, pp 131–142.

Salmenperä M, Eriksson H: Levosimendan in perioperative and critical care patients, *Curr Opin Anesth* 22:496–501, 2009.

INTRAVENOUS INDUCTION AGENTS

Thiopentone

Prepared as 6% anhydrous sodium carbonate in nitrogen to prevent thiopentone forming acid with the CO_2 present in air. pH of 2.5% solution = 10.8.

Highly lipid-soluble and rapidly distributed into the tissues. Pharmacokinetics are those of a three compartment model. Undergoes first-order kinetics.

80% protein bound; $t_{1/2}$ = 12h. Induction dose 4–5 mg.kg^{-1}. Oxidized by liver to inactive metabolites with renal excretion. Serious allergic reactions are rare but severe.

Physiological effects

- ↓ Myocardial contractility and peripheral vasodilation
- ↑ Bronchial muscle tone and laryngeal spasm
- ↓ ICP, ↓ CNS flow, ↓ CNS metabolism
- ↓ IOP
- ↓ SNS > PNS.

Accidental intra-arterial thiopentone injection

- Immediate pain and blanching
- Arterial obstruction due to vascular spasm and obstruction by thiopentone crystals.

Treatment

- Leave needle in place
- Irrigate with saline. Commence anticoagulation with heparin and then warfarin for 2 weeks
- Give 10 mL of 1% procaine to buffer thiopentone and act as LA
- Consider papaverine 40 mg, phenoxybenzamine 0.5 mg or urokinase
- Sympathetic block, e.g. brachial plexus block
- Keep limb warm, elevate and continue with the GA to dilate vessels.

Propofol (di-isopropylphenol)

Emulsified in soya bean oil and egg phosphatide (formerly Cremphor EL).
$t_{1/2}$ = 4 h. Induction dose 2–3 mg.kg^{-1}. Highly lipid-soluble.
Metabolized by liver and extrahepatic sites (?lung). Hepatic excretion.
Delay in loss of eyelash reflex. Short duration of action makes drug suitable for day-case anaesthesia and ITU sedation.

Physiological effects

- Hypotension due to vasodilation more than myocardial depression
- Tachycardia. Resets baroreceptors to allow ↓ BP
- Bronchial muscle tone unchanged. Less laryngospasm than other induction agents.

METABOLIC INFUSION SYNDROME RELATED TO PROPOFOL

Metabolic decompensation has been reported following long-term high-dose infusion in adults (>5 mg.kg^{-1}.h^{-1} for >2 days). Similar reports also received of similar reactions in children sedated on intensive care units. Characterised by

Sudden onset of marked bradycardia, progressing to complete heart block.

- Lipaemic plasma
- Hepatomegaly
- Cardiac failure
- Metabolic acidosis
- Rhabdomyolysis
- Myoglobinuria

Propofol is contraindicated for sedation in intensive care units for ventilated children ≤16 years. Propofol is also not recommended for sedation during surgical and diagnostic procedures in children as safety and efficacy have not been demonstrated. It remains licensed for induction and maintenance of GA in children ≥1 month of age.

Methohexitone

Prepared in 6% anhydrous sodium carbonate. pH of 1% solution = 11.1.

$t_{\frac{1}{2}}$ = 4 h. Induction dose 1–1.5 mg.kg^{-1}. Metabolized to 4-OH methohexitone (inactive). Causes involuntary muscle movement (including hiccough). Pain on injection.

Less cardiovascular depression than with thiopentone. Epileptiform EEG, therefore good for electroconvulsive therapy. Rapid recovery, therefore good for day-case surgery.

Etomidate

Carboxylated imidazole; pH 3.3. Dissolved in propylene glycol.

$t_{1/2}$ = 1.2h; 75% protein bound. Induction dose 0.3 mg.kg^{-1}.

Inhibits 17α- and 11β-hydroxylase, impairing adrenal function. Increases mortality when used for ICU sedation, but prospective study showed no difference when compared with ketamine for induction. Broken down by esterase hydrolysis in plasma and liver. Renal excretion.

Most haemodynamically stable of all i.v. induction agents. Causes postoperative nausea and vomiting. Venous thrombosis. Worst agent for pain on injection. Dose-related myoclonus.

Ketamine

Phencyclidine derivative; pH 4.0.

$t_{1/2}$ = 2.5h; 12% protein bound. Racemic mixture; S (+) form is now available which is 3–5 times more potent than R form. Although both enantiomers have similar side-effect profile for a given dose, the increased efficacy of S (+) ketamine allows smaller dose with reduced side-effects.

Physiological effects

- ↑ CNS metabolic rate
- ↑ BP, ↑ HR, ↑ CO (possibly secondary to ↑ Ca^{2+} flux modulated by cAMP)
- Salivation. Bronchial smooth muscle dilation
- Dissociative analgesia possibly via NMDA receptors.

Liver breakdown by demethylation and hydroxylation to form norketamine (active). Metabolism slowed in the presence of halothane and benzodiazepines. Renal excretion. Contraindicated with ischaemic heart disease, hypertension and in psychiatric patients. Historically contraindicated in patients with increased ICP, but reports of neuroprotective and neuroregenerative effects combined with cardiovascular stability and maintained CPP suggest it may have a role in head injury.

Midazolam

Addition of a fused imidazole ring to the benzodiazepine structure. Prepared as a solution at pH 3.5 with an open ring structure making the drug water-soluble. After injection, the change in pH closes the ring to form a highly lipophilic compound.

$t_{\frac{1}{2}}$ = 2.5 h; 94% protein bound. Hydroxylated by the liver to active metabolites. Renal excretion.

Hypnotic, anxiolytic, amnesic and anticonvulsant. Induction dose of 0.15–0.3 mg.kg^{-1}. Relatively slow induction. Hypotension due to vasodilation and negative inotropic effect. Causes apnoea on induction in 10–20% of patients. Minimal effect on ICP.

Reversed with the benzodiazepine antagonist, flumazenil.

Bibliography

Craven R: Ketamine, *Anaesthesia* 6(Suppl 1):48–53, 2007.

Jabre P, Combes X, Lapostolle F, et al: Etomidate versus ketamine for rapid sequence intubation in acutely ill patients: a multicentre randomised controlled trial, *Lancet* 374:293–300, 2009.

Kam PCA, Cardon D: Propofol infusion syndrome, *Anaesthesia* 62:690–701, 2007.

Mather LE, Edwards SR: Chirality in anaesthesia – ropivacaine, ketamine and thiopentone, *Curr Opin Anaesth* 11:383–390, 1998.

Morris C, McAllister C: Etomidate for emergency anaesthesia; mad, bad and dangerous to know, *Anaesthesia* 60:737–740, 2005.

Pai A, Heining M: Ketamine, *Contin Educ Anaesth, Crit Care Pain* 7:59–63, 2007.

Sneyd JR: Recent advances in intravenous anaesthesia, *Br J Anaesth* 93:725–736, 2004.

LOCAL ANAESTHETICS

Pharmacology and physiology

Local anaesthetics are weak bases. The proportion of drug existing in an ionized form is dependent upon the pH of the solution. The non-ionized form diffuses into the axoplasm where it becomes charged and binds with sodium channels.

$$pH - pKa = \log \frac{\text{ionized } [BH^+]}{\text{unionized} [B]}$$

Frequency-dependent block

Open sodium channels are more susceptible to local anaesthetic binding than those in a closed state. Thus, the higher the frequency of stimulation, the more intense the block. Nerves that carry high-frequency impulses, e.g.

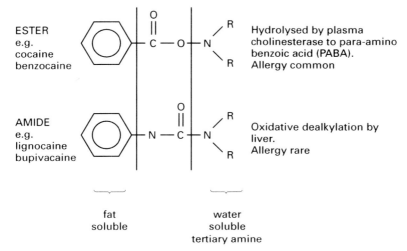

Figure 11.1 Structures of ester and amide local anaesthetics.

sensory nerves, are more susceptible to block than those carrying low-frequency impulses, e.g. motor nerves. This frequency-dependent block may explain why cardiac toxicity of local anaesthetics is more pronounced at faster heart rates.

Differential nerve block

Three successive nodes of Ranvier must be blocked by local anaesthetic to block nerve conduction. Thicker nerves have more widely spaced nodes and therefore take longer to be blocked. Thus small-diameter Aδ and C pain fibres are blocked earlier than large Aα motor fibres. If muscle relaxation in addition to analgesia is required (e.g. to reduce a dislocation), a higher dose of local anaesthetic is required.

pH effects

Local anaesthetics are usually prepared as the salt to provide solubility and stability. Most local anaesthetics dissolved in water have a pKa of ≈8. At a physiological pH of 7.4, more cation will be present than base. Addition of bicarbonate increases the proportion of drug present in the unionized form and increases the speed of onset. Local anaesthetics with low pKa have an increased speed of onset. Potency ∝ ↑ pKa.

Inflamed tissues have a low pH, so LA exists mostly in the ionized form and thus little drug reaches the sodium channels.

Vasoconstriction/dilation

All local anaesthetics cause vasoconstriction at very low doses, but vasodilate at higher doses. Cocaine causes vasoconstriction by inhibiting noradrenaline uptake.

Convulsions

Appear to be triggered by the limbic system to cause seizures electrographically resembling temporal lobe epilepsy: dysphoria, metallic taste in the mouth, circumoral numbness, slurred speech, dizziness, fine twitching of the small muscles of the face and hands, drowsiness, generalized convulsion. Highest blood levels seen after intercostal block, interpleural block and topical anaesthesia of upper airway. Lowest levels seen with spinal anaesthesia.

Cardiotoxicity

Unlike other local anaesthetics, bupivacaine toxicity usually manifests as myocardial depression rather than neurological symptoms. Highly protein bound to the sodium channel which is abundant in myocardial tissue. Limited animal and clinical studies suggest that Intralipid may be of benefit in cardiac arrest occurring due to local anaesthetic toxicity.

Specific drugs
Levobupivacaine

An amide anaesthetic, purified from its racemic mixture. Similar clinical profile to the racemic mixture, but with enhanced safety profile. CNS excitation and myocardial depression/arrhythmias occur at higher doses than the racemic mixture.

EMLA cream (eutectic mixture of local anaesthetic)

Eutectic means having a low melting point below that of either compound separately. Mixture of 2.5% lidocaine and 2.5% prilocaine. In addition to its use for venepuncture, has also been used for split-skin grafts, removal of anal warts and postherpetic neuralgia. Large doses can cause methaemoglobinaemia. Depresses local immune response when applied topically to open wounds.

Tetracaine gel

At 4%, tetracaine gel has a much more rapid onset than EMLA and is a vasodilator, but local histamine release may cause itching. It is rapidly absorbed from mucous membranes and should never be applied to inflamed, traumatized or highly vascular surfaces. Should not be left on for >45 min because of risk of methaemoglobinaemia.

Prilocaine

Prilocaine is metabolized to toluidine which reduces Hb to methaemoglobin. A dose >600 mg prilocaine risks methaemoglobinaemia (reduction of >1.5 mg/dL Hb). Treat with 1 mg/kg methylene blue i.v.

Ropivacaine

An amide anaesthetic structurally similar to bupivacaine, with similar potency and duration as bupivacaine but less cardiotoxicity (Fig. 11.2). This may be because it is manufactured in the S (–) form, whereas bupivacaine exists in the racemic (RS) form. The sensory block is similar to that provided by bupivacaine but the motor block is slower in onset, less intense and shorter in duration. It is an effective vasoconstrictor (bupivacaine vasodilates) and has no detrimental effect on placental blood flow. Cardiotoxicity and CNS symptoms occur at higher doses compared with bupivacaine.

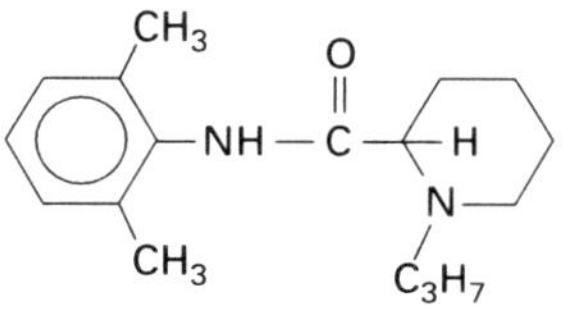

Ropivacaine

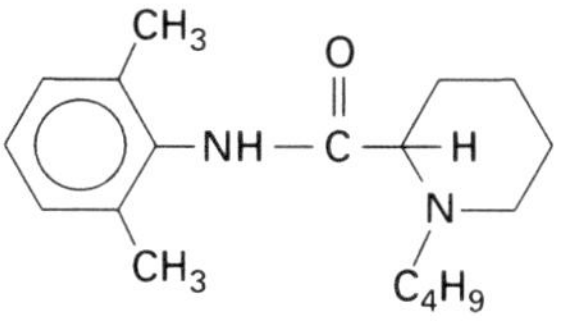

Bupivacaine

Figure 11.2 Ropivacaine and bupivacaine.

Maximum recommended doses

Table 11.2 Maximum recommended doses of some common local anaesthetics

	Plain	With adrenaline
Lidocaine	3 mg/kg	7 mg/kg
Bupivacaine	2 mg/kg	2 mg/kg
Prilocaine	5 mg/kg	8 mg/kg
Cocaine	2 mg/kg	
Tetracaine	1.5 mg/kg	

GUIDELINES FOR THE MANAGEMENT OF SEVERE LOCAL ANAESTHETIC TOXICITY
Association of Anaesthetists of Great Britain and Ireland 2007

Signs of severe toxicity:
- Sudden loss of consciousness, with or without tonic-clonic convulsions
- Cardiovascular collapse: sinus bradycardia, conduction blocks, asystole and ventricular tachyarrhythmias may all occur
- Local anaesthetic (LA) toxicity may occur some time after the initial injection.

Immediate management:
- Stop injecting the LA
- *Call for help*
- Maintain the airway and, if necessary, secure it with a tracheal tube
- Give 100% oxygen and ensure adequate lung ventilation (hyperventilation may help by increasing pH in the presence of metabolic acidosis)
- Confirm or establish intravenous access
- Control seizures: give a benzodiazepine, thiopentone or propofol in small incremental doses
- Assess cardiovascular status throughout.

Management of cardiac arrest associated with LA injection
- Start cardiopulmonary resuscitation (CPR) using standard protocols
- Manage arrhythmias using the same protocols, recognizing that they may be very refractory to treatment
- Prolonged resuscitation may be necessary; it may be appropriate to consider other options, e.g. cardiopulmonary bypass or treatment with lipid emulsion.

Treatment of cardiac arrest with lipid emulsion: (approximate doses for a 70-kg patient)
- Give an intravenous bolus injection of Intralipid 20% 1.5 mL.kg^{-1} over 1 min (give a bolus of 100 mL)
- Continue CPR
- Start an intravenous infusion of Intralipid 20% at 0.25 mL.kg^{-1}.min^{-1} (give at a rate of 400 mL over 20 min)
- Repeat the bolus injection twice at 5 min intervals if an adequate circulation has not been restored (give two further boluses of 100 mL at 5 min intervals)
- After another 5 min, increase the rate to 0.5 mL.kg^{-1}.min^{-1} if an adequate circulation has not been restored (give at a rate of 400 mL over 10 min)
- Continue infusion until a stable and adequate circulation has been restored.

Remember:

- Continue CPR throughout treatment with lipid emulsion.
- Recovery from LA-induced cardiac arrest may take >1 h.
- Propofol is not a suitable substitute for Intralipid.

Follow-up action:

- Report cases from the UK to the National Patient Safety Agency (via www.npsa.nhs.uk). Whether or not lipid emulsion is administered, please also report cases to the LipidRescue site: www.lipidrescue.org
- If possible, take blood samples into a plain tube and a heparinized tube before and after lipid emulsion administration and at 1 h intervals afterwards. Ask your laboratory to measure LA and triglyceride levels (these have not yet been reported in a human case of LA intoxication treated with lipid).

Bibliography

Association of Anaesthetists of Great Britain and Ireland: *Guidelines for the management of severe local anaesthetic toxicity*, 2007, Reproduced with the kind permission of the Association of anaesthetists of Great Britain and Ireland.

Heavener JE: Local anesthetics, *Curr Opin Anaesth* 20:336–342, 2007.

Leskiw U, Weinberg GL: Lipid resuscitation for local anesthetic toxicity: is it really lifesaving? *Curr Opin Anesth* 22:667–671, 2009.

McLeod GA, Burke D: Levobupivacaine, *Anaesthesia* 56:331–341, 2001.

Picard J, Harrop-Griffith W: Lipid emulsion to treat drug overdose: past, present and future, *Anaesthesia* 64:119–121, 2009.

Whiteside JB, Wildsmith JAW: Developments in local anaesthetic drugs, *Br J Anaesth* 87:27–35, 2001.

NEUROMUSCULAR BLOCKADE

Neuromuscular blocking drugs

Tubocurarine (dTC). Long-acting non-depolarizing quaternary ammonium compound. The first neuromuscular blocker was used clinically by Griffiths and Johnson in Montreal in 1942. Prepared from the plant *Chondrodendron tomentosum*; 50% protein bound. Hypotension secondary to histamine release and also SNS > PNS blockade, causing bradycardia. Minimal metabolism. Excreted in bile and urine.

Gallamine. Blocks vagus and acts as β_1-agonist to cause tachycardia and hypertension. Crosses placenta, so contraindicated in obstetrics. Renal excretion 85%; therefore avoid in renal failure.

Benzylisoquinoliniums

Doxacurium. Long-acting non-depolarizing drug with no cardiovascular side-effects; 25% recovery of twitch height in 2–3 h. Excreted by the kidney unchanged, with minor pathway via the liver. Therefore prolonged action in hepatic and renal failure.

Mivacurium. Short-acting non-depolarizing drug. Consists of three stereo-isomers, two with short elimination half-lives of 1.8–1.9 min, the third with an elimination half-life of 53 min but only one-tenth as potent. Hydrolysed by plasma cholinesterases to inactive metabolites. Duration of action prolonged by same factors that affect suxamethonium, e.g. atypical enzymes. Weak ability to release histamine.

Atracurium. Intermediate-acting non-depolarizing drug. Minimal cardiovascular effects. Amount of histamine release is proportional to the rate of injection. Spontaneous degradation by ester hydrolysis and Hofmann degradation. Breakdown product of laudanosine is known to cause cerebral irritation which may accumulate to significant levels when using prolonged infusions, e.g. ITU.

Cisatracurium. Purified form (1R-cis, 1R'-cis isomer) of one of the 10 stereoisomers of atracurium, accounting for about 15% of the racemic mixture. Intermediate-acting non-depolarizing drug. It is more potent and has a slightly longer duration of action than atracurium. It provides greater cardiovascular stability because it lacks histamine-releasing effects. Mostly broken down by Hofmann degradation to form laudanosine, with a small amount removed by the liver and kidney. Plasma esterases do not appear to hydrolyse cisatracurium directly. Hepatic or renal impairment have little pharmacokinetic effect.

Steroid derivatives

Pancuronium. Long-acting non-depolarizing drug; 80% protein bound. Deacetylated by liver to three inactive metabolites: 75% excreted in urine, 25% via bile. Indirect SNS effects (via release of noradrenaline from nerve endings) to cause ↑ CO, ↑ HR and ↑ BP. Potentiated by its additional vagal blockade. Minimal histamine release.

Vecuronium. Intermediate-acting non-depolarizing drug. No cardiovascular side-effects. Safe in liver failure. No histamine release. 60% eliminated in bile, half of which is broken down to the 3 OH-metabolite.

Pipecuronium. Long-acting non-depolarizing drug with no cardiovascular side-effects. Excreted by the kidney unchanged with minor pathway via the liver. Therefore prolonged in hepatic and renal failure. No histamine release.

Rocuronium. Intermediate-acting non-depolarizing drug. Neuromuscular blocking drugs of low potency are thought to have a faster onset of action because of the higher concentration gradient between plasma and postsynaptic nicotinic receptor (Bowman 1988). Similar kinetics to vecuronium but with faster biphasic onset (80% of block within 60 s followed by remainder over 2–3 min). Vagolytic action may cause 10–12% increase in HR. Does not cause histamine release. Not metabolized, and excreted unchanged in urine and bile. Prolonged action in liver failure but not in renal failure. Rocuronium 1.0 mg/kg can be used as an alternative to suxamethonium 1.0 mg/kg for rapid sequence induction provided there is no anticipated difficulty in intubation. The clinical duration of this dose of rocuronium is, however, 60 min. Classed as intermediate in its risk of causing anaphylaxis.

Table 11.3 Short-acting non-depolarizing neuromuscular blocking drugs

Drug	ED$_{95}$ (mg/kg)	Intubation (mg/kg)	Onset (s)	95% recovery (min)
Vecuronium	0.05	0.10–0.20	90–150	60–120
Atracurium	0.25	0.40–0.60	90–150	60–90
Cisatracurium	0.05	0.15	100–160	50–70
Rocuronium	0.30	0.60–1.00	60–90	60–120
Mivacurium	0.08	0.20–0.25	90–150	20–40

Table 11.4 Long-acting non-depolarizing neuromuscular blocking drugs

Drug	ED$_{95}$ (mg/kg)	Intubation (mg/kg)	$t_{1/2}$ β (min)
Pancuronium	0.06	0.10	≈100
Pipecuronium	0.05	0.10	≈100
Doxacurium	0.03	0.05	≈100

Priming

Priming accelerates onset of block by ≈30 s. Use dose of 20% ED$_{95}$, pre-oxygenate and keep priming interval <2 min. Also accelerate onset of block by using large (2–3 times ED$_{95}$) single doses of non-depolarizer, e.g. increasing dose of vecuronium from 0.1 to 0.4 mg/kg speeds onset from 3.5 to 1.5 min.

Suxamethonium

$$(CH_3)_3N^+ - CH_2 - O - \overset{\overset{\textstyle O}{\|}}{C} - CH_2$$
$$(CH_3)_3N^+ - CH_2 - O - \underset{\underset{\textstyle O}{\|}}{C} - CH_2$$

Stimulates all sympathetic and parasympathetic ganglia, cholinergic autonomic receptors, muscarinic receptors in the sinus node of the heart and nicotine receptors. In low doses, causes negative inotropic and chronotropic effects, attenuated by atropine.

Side-effects include:

- masseter muscle rigidity and malignant hyperthermia
- increased intraocular pressure
- increased intragastric pressure but increased lower oesophageal sphincter pressure
- increased intracerebral pressure
- myalgia and muscle damage
- anaphylactic reactions
- hyperkalaemia – raises plasma K^+ by 0.5–0.8 mmol, particularly in burns and renal failure
- bradycardia, particularly with second doses in neonates
- dual block.

Metabolized by plasma cholinesterase ($t_{1/2}$ = 2–4 min). Decreased plasma cholinesterase with congenital and acquired conditions.

Congenital. Several genes control the structure of plasma cholinesterase (Table 11.5). Normal homozygote genetic structure is $E1^U$, $E1^U$. Common abnormal variants are:

- atypical gene $E1^a$
- fluoride gene $E1^f$
- silent gene $E1^s$.

Commonest abnormality is the heterozygous state for the atypical gene ($E1^U$, $E1^a$) present in 4% of the Caucasian population. This results in prolongation of neuromuscular blockade for ≈30 min. Heterozygous forms of the other abnormal genes result in prolongation of neuromuscular blockade for >3 h.

In vitro, dibucaine prevents normal plasma cholinesterase breaking down benzoylcholine. Normal benzoylcholine breakdown produces a colour change, the percentage inhibition of which is related to the dibucaine number (DN). A dibucaine number >77 is present in normal homozygotes; lower numbers suggest impaired plasma cholinesterase activity. Use of fluoride instead of dibucaine allows detection of the abnormal fluoride gene, by measuring the fluoride number (FN).

Table 11.5 Common genotypes of plasma cholinesterase

	Incidence	DN	FN	Response to suxamethonium
$E1^U$, $E1^U$	96%	80	61	Normal
$E1^U$, $E1^a$	4%	62	50	Slightly prolonged
$E1^U$, $E1^f$	1:200	74	52	Slightly prolonged
$E1^a$, $E1^a$	1:2000	21	19	Prolonged
$E1^a$, $E1^f$	1:20000	53	33	Moderately prolonged

Acquired
- Liver disease, chronic renal failure, MI
- Pregnancy, oral contraceptive pill
- Haemodialysis, plasmapheresis, cardiopulmonary bypass
- Hypothyroidism
- Anaesthetic drugs metabolized by cholinesterase – etomidate, neostigmine, phenothiazines
- Propanolol
- Burns.

Decrease suxamethonium fasciculations with gallamine, benzodiazepines, lidocaine, calcium, magnesium or thiopentone.

Suxamethonium-induced hyperkalaemia due to:
- upregulation of extrajunctional ACh receptors, which leak K^+ in response to suxamethonium
- whole muscle cell membrane behaving as motor end-plate.

Autonomic effects of neuromuscular blockers

Autonomic ganglia

- Suxamethonium – stimulates
- dTC – blocks.

Cardiac muscarinic receptors

- Suxamethonium – stimulates
- Gallamine – strong block
- Pancuronium – moderate block
- Rocuronium – weak block
- Vecuronium – clinically insignificant block.

Onset of neuromuscular blockade

Relative sensitivity of muscles to neuromuscular blockade is as follows: muscles of upper airway > peripheral muscle and intercostal muscles > diaphragm. Therefore, optimal intubating conditions develop earlier than a similar depth of block in the hand. Sufficient relaxation for intubation is usually present well before complete loss of the TO4 in the adductor pollicis.

A normal tidal volume requires just 15% of maximum diaphragm strength, so adequate respiratory effort can still occur while limbs are still paralysed. Forearm/hand muscles are of comparable sensitivity to intercostals and may explain why ventilatory weakness is still present until the adductor pollicis muscle has recovered completely. Any weakness detectable in peripheral muscles is likely to be associated with difficulty in maintaining an airway.

Neonatal diaphragmatic paralysis occurs at the same time as peripheral muscle groups, making peripheral neuromuscular monitoring a good indicator of respiratory muscle reversal.

Reversal of neuromuscular blockade

Sustained head lift, tongue protrusion, hand grip, coughing and vital capacity of >10 mL/kg require patient cooperation and are only crude measures.

Inspiratory effort $> -25\,cmH_2O$ is required before spontaneous respiration becomes adequate (equates with 15 mL/kg vital capacity). Adequate gag/swallowing correlates with $> -40\,cmH_2O$. Five-second head lift equates to $-55\,cmH_2O$ inspiratory pressure.

In neonates and infants, hip flexion to >90° equates with a maximum inspiratory force of $-30\,cmH_2O$, which is adequate for spontaneous respiration.

Anticholinesterase agents

Main reversal agent is neostigmine, which inhibits acetylcholinesterase, preventing the breakdown of acetylcholine and resulting in re-establishment of neuromuscular transmission. Neostigmine causes muscarinic side-effect, necessitating the co-administration of anticholinergic drugs. Unable to reverse deep block and also associated with persistence of residual block.

Sugammadex

Sugammadex is a modified γ-cyclodextrin, a selective NMB binding agent, specifically developed to reverse aminosteroid NMBs (rocuronium/vecuronium). Block induced by rocuronium or vecuronium can be reversed from superficial or deep levels within 2–3 min using 4–8 mg.kg^{-1} or 16 mg.kg^{-1} sugammadex, respectively. The ability of sugammadex to reverse deep block with 3–5 min of administering 1.0–1.2 mg.kg^{-1} rocuronium makes use of rocuronium as an alternative to suxamethonium for rapid sequence induction a possibility. May bind to progestagen (oral contraceptive pill), fusidic acid and flucloxacillin to reduce their efficacy.

Neuromuscular blockade by other drugs

- Aminoglycosides – pre-junctional block
- Tetracyclines – post-junctional block
- Calcium-channel blockers – interfere with pre-junctional Ca^{2+} flux
- Magnesium – potentiates block
- Metoclopramide – prolongs action of suxamethonium by 50%.

Monitoring

Monitor to assess degree of relaxation, help adjust dosage, assess development of phase II block, provide early recognition of patients with abnormal cholinesterases, and to assess cause of apnoea.

Stimulate peripheral nerve and assess visually, by feeling the strength of contraction or mechanically (mechanomyography, electromyography). Ulnar nerve in forearm is motor only to adductor pollicis in hand, which is easily accessible. Facial nerve stimulation is a better indicator than ulnar nerve to predict when intubation is possible.

Patterns of nerve stimulation

All stimulation should be supramaximal. Achieved by increasing the intensity of the stimulus until twitch height increases no further.

- **Single twitch**. A 2 ms stimulus is applied every few seconds and subsequent contractions monitored. Insensitive since >75% of postsynaptic receptors must be blocked before there is any diminution in twitch height.
- **Train of four**. A 2 Hz stimulus is applied no more often than every 10 s. Compare first (T_1) and last twitch (T_4). TO4 ratio ($T_1:T_4$) indicates degree of neuromuscular blockade:
  - T_4 disappears at 75% depression of T_1 (1st, 2nd and 3rd twitches present)
  - T_3 disappears at 80% depression of T_1 (1st and 2nd twitches present)
  - T_2 disappears at 90% depression of T_1 (1st twitch only)
  - T_1 disappears at 100% depression of T_1 (no twitches).

A TO4 count of 0–1 is needed for adequate intubating conditions, but a count of three twitches provides adequate relaxation for most surgery. A TO4 ratio >0.70, or $T_1:T_0$ >0.75, corresponds to adequate clinical recovery, but normal pharyngeal function requires a ratio >0.90.

Neuromuscular reversal can be given when T_2 has reappeared, i.e. when T_1 is about 20% of its control height.

- **Tetanic stimulation**. Supramaximal stimulation of 50 Hz for 5 s. With non-depolarizing block, peak height is reduced and fades. Release of acetylcholine is reduced (possibly presynaptic effect) and postsynaptic receptors are blocked, limiting sustained contraction.
- **Post-tetanic count**. A 1 Hz stimulus is applied 5–10 s after tetanic stimulus. May result in response (post-tetanic potentiation), even if none is seen with original TO4. Due to increased synthesis and mobilization of acetylcholine following tetanus. Appearance of post-tetanic count precedes return of TO4 by 30–40 min.
- **Double-burst stimulation** (Engbaek et al 1989). Three 0.2 ms bursts of 50 Hz tetanus, each burst separated by 20 ms and repeated after 750 ms. Similar to TO4, but tactile evaluation is more sensitive because fade of the two resultant contractions is more marked.

Table 11.6 Depolarizing versus non-depolarizing block

Depolarizing block	Non-depolarizing block
Reduced twitch height	Reduced twitch height
No fade of TO4/tetanus	Fade of TO4/tetanus
No post-tetanic potentiation	Post-tetanic potentiation

Bibliography

Donati F, Bevan DR: Not all muscles are the same, Editorial, *Br J Anaesth* 68:235–236, 1992.

Fuchs-Buder T, Schreiber JU, Meistelman C: Monitoring neuromuscular block: an update, *Anaesthesia* 64(Suppl 1):82–89, 2009.

Kopman AF, Eikermann M: Antagonism of non-depolarising neuromuscular block: current practice, *Anaesthesia* 64(Suppl 1):22–30, 2009.

Kopman AF: Sugammadex: A revolutionary approach to neuromuscular antagonism, *Anesthesiology* 104:631–633, 2006.

Martyn JAJ, Fagerlund MJ, Eriksson LI: Basic principles of neuromuscular transmission, *Anaesthesia* 64(Suppl 1):1–9, 2009.

Martyn J, Durieux ME: Succinylcholine: new insights into mechanisms of action of an old drug, *Anesthesiology* 104:633–634, 2006.

McGrath CD, Hunter JM: Monitoring of neuromuscular block, *Contin Educ Anaesthesia, Crit Care Pain* 6:7–12, 2006.

Mirakhur RK: Sugammadex in clinical practice, *Anaesthesia* 64(Suppl 1):45–54, 2009.

Mirakhur RK, Harrop-Griffiths W: Management of neuromuscular block: time for a change? *Anaesthesia* 64(Suppl 1):iv–v, 2009.

OPIOIDS AND OTHER ANALGESICS

Fentanyl (anilino-piperidine)

Fentanyl was the first of the potent anilino-piperidine opioids, being 200 times as potent as morphine with a high therapeutic index. Its high lipid solubility causes accumulation of the drug in lipophilic tissues, particularly the lungs on first pass, with a resultant prolongation in elimination half-life (150–400 min); 84% is protein bound to albumin and α- and β-globulins; 80% undergoes N-dealkylation by liver metabolism to inactive norfentanyl, so it has prolonged duration of action with liver disease. Little change in drug kinetics in patients with renal disease.

Alfentanil (anilino-piperidine)

Alfentanil has 20% of the potency of fentanyl. Less lipid-soluble than fentanyl, with 90% bound to α_1-acid glycoprotein. It is shorter acting and 80% is biotransformed by liver metabolism, so has prolonged duration of action with liver disease. Little change in drug kinetics in patients with renal disease.

Sufentanil (anilino-piperidine)

Shorter acting than fentanyl, with an elimination half-life of 140–200 min. Some 80% is biotransformed by liver metabolism, so has prolonged duration of action with liver disease. Little change in drug kinetics in patients with renal disease except in uraemic patients.

Remifentanil (anilino-piperidine)

Remifentanil is an ultra-short-acting synthetic opioid with µ-specific opioid activity. Vials of remifentanil contain glycine which is an inhibitory neurotransmitter, making it unsuitable for subarachnoid and extradural injection; 70% bound to α_1-acid glycoprotein. It has cardiovascular and side-effect profiles similar to fentanyl. Not associated with histamine release. The ester linkage (shown by the dotted line) makes remifentanil susceptible to rapid hydrolysis by tissue and blood non-specific esterases (distinct from pseudocholinesterase) and it therefore has a rapid clearance (elimination $t_{\frac{1}{2}} = 5$ min) independent of renal and hepatic function. The major metabolite is a pure µ-opioid agonist excreted by the kidney, but with a potency 1/4600 of the parent compound. Placental transfer occurs rapidly, but metabolism and redistribution prevent adverse neonatal effects. Prolonged duration of action with liver disease. Little change in drug kinetics in patients with renal disease.

Allows more rapid recovery, but associated with increased postoperative analgesia requirements. Less nausea and vomiting than with other longer-acting opioids. As with other opioids, muscle rigidity at high dose may occur. When assessed by the effect on reduction in MAC, the relative potencies of sufentanil, fentanyl, remifentanil and alfentanil are 1:10:10:80.

Pethidine

Greater (>70%) protein binding (mostly α_1-acid glycoprotein) than morphine. Metabolized by N-demethylation to the active metabolite, norpethidine and inactive pethidinic acid and norpethidinic acid. Accumulation of norpethidine in renal impairment may prolong the action of pethidine and cause tremor, agitation and seizures. Despite significant pulmonary clearance, 80% is biotransformed by liver metabolism, so liver disease is associated with increased elimination half-life.

Said to be the opioid of choice for biliary colic because its atropine-like effect will counteract the opioid action on smooth muscle. Topical atropine, however, does not relax a contracted gall bladder and there no is evidence that pethidine is any better than equianalgesic doses of other opioids.

Morphine

Metabolized to morphine 3-glucuronide (M3G) and the active metabolite morphine 6-glucuronide (M6G). 10% of morphine conjugation occurs in extrahepatic and GI tissues; 80% biotransformed by liver metabolism, but kinetics of morphine remain unaltered until end-stage liver disease. Renal failure is associated with accumulation of M3G and M6G and prolonged action.

Diamorphine

3,6-diacetylmorphine (heroin). Hydrolysed in liver and blood to 6-monoacetyl morphine, a potent opioid.

Codeine

3-methoxymorphine. Approximately 10–20% of the potency of morphine. Methyl ether group reduces metabolism so increasing oral bioavailability. Undergoes extensive hepatic metabolism, mostly to inactive conjugated compounds but 10–20% metabolized to morphine.

Tramadol

A phenylpiperidine derivative with a structure similar to pethidine and elimination $t_{\frac{1}{2}}$ of 5–7 h. Same analgesic potency as pethidine. Analgesic effects through:

- moderate affinity at μ-receptors and weak activity at κ-receptors
- enhancing the function of the spinal descending inhibitory pathways and blocking spinal nociceptive pathways by inhibition of reuptake of both 5HT and norepinephrine at synapses
- presynaptic stimulation of 5HT release.

As it enhances monoaminergic transmission, it is contraindicated in patients taking MAOIs. Does not cause significant respiratory depression or histamine release. Exists as a chiral mixture with (+) form acting at μ-receptors and (–) form causing monoamine reuptake inhibition. Has 10–20% of the potency of morphine but causes less respiratory depression and less depression; 20% bound to plasma protein with an elimination $t_{\frac{1}{2}}$ of 5 h. Demethylation by the liver (P_{450}) accounts for 86% of the metabolism. The O-desmethyl-tramadol metabolite is active with a $t_{\frac{1}{2}}$ of 9 h. Most metabolites are excreted in the urine. Hepatic and renal impairment causes significant prolongation of action.

For moderate/severe pain, 3 mg/kg is an effective initial dose. Associated with common but mild side-effects of headache, nausea, vomiting and dizziness. Reduced side-effects with oral slow-release preparations.

Committee on Safety of Medicines (CSM) has received 27 reports of convulsions possibly associated with tramadol, although many of the patients were known epileptics. Some reports have shown interaction with coumarin anticoagulants to prolong the INR and there have also been reports of drug abuse.

Bibliography

Budd K, Langford R: Tramadol revisited, Br J Anaesth 82:493–496, 1999.
Komatsu R, Turan AM, Orhan-Sungur M, et al: Remifentanil for general anaesthesia: a systematic review, Anaesthesia 62:1266–1280, 2007.
Sear JW: Recent advances and developments in the clinical use of i.v. opioids during the preoperative period, Br J Anaesth 81:38–50, 1998.

VOLATILE AGENTS

Table 11.7 Physical properties of volatile agents

	Halothane	Enflurane	Isoflurane	Sevoflurane	Desflurane
Blood:gas solubility	2.3	1.9	1.4	0.6	0.42
MAC	0.75	1.68	1.15	2	7
Boiling point (°C)	50	56	48	58	24
Saturated vapour pressure (kPa)	32	24	32	21	88
% metabolism	20	2	0.2	2	0.02

Halothane

$$\begin{array}{ccc} & F & Br \\ & | & | \\ F - & C - & C - Cl \\ & | & | \\ & F & H \end{array}$$

Instability in light is improved by the addition of 0.01% thymol. Arrhythmogenicity associated with alkane structure. Maximum recommended safe dose of adrenaline is 0.1 mg/10 min. Least irritant of all the volatiles for gas induction.

Halothane hepatitis

The National Halothane Study (USA 1966) studied 750 000 anaesthetics. Spectrum of damage from minor derangement of LFTs to fulminant hepatic failure (FHF). There were seven cases of unexplained FHF (1:35 000 halothane exposures). Hepatitis was associated with more than one exposure to halothane, recent exposure to halothane, family history of halothane hepatotoxicity, obesity, female sex and drug allergies. Eosinophilia and autoantibodies were common.

There are two patterns of hepatitis:

- *mild* – usually subclinical with transient derangement in LFTs
- *fulminant hepatic failure* – defined by Neuberger & Williams (1988) as 'the appearance of liver damage within 28 days of halothane exposure in a person in whom other known causes of liver disease had been excluded'.

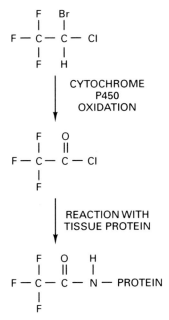

Figure 11.3 Proposed mechanism of formation of trifluoroacetyl halide antigen.

Some 75% of patients with halothane hepatitis have antibodies reacting to halothane-altered antigens. Route of metabolism of halothane depends upon O_2 tension in liver. At high O_2 tension, an oxidative route generates trifluoroacetyl halide (TFAH) (Fig. 11.3), which covalently binds to liver proteins, forming haptens. Halothane-directed antibodies detectable by ELISA test have been identified that are directed against TFAH antigens. Present in 70% of cases of halothane-induced FHF. The significance of the more minor reductive route at low O_2 tension is debated. It may be associated with direct liver damage with release of fluoride. National database of FHF patients set up at St Mary's Hospital, London (Prof. R.M. Jones), to whom these patients should be reported.

GUIDELINES FOR HALOTHANE EXPOSURE
Committee on Safety of Medicines 1997

Halothane is well known to be associated with hepatotoxicity, particularly if patients are re-exposed. This risk decreases as the time between halothane exposure increases, but a risk persists, regardless of the time since last exposure.

The Committee on Safety of Medicines (CSM) received reports of 15 cases of halothane-induced acute liver failure requiring liver transplants between 1985 and 1995. Ten patients had at least one previous halothane exposure of which four were in the preceding month, and six had previous adverse reactions to halothane.

The CSM recommend that halothane be avoided if there has been a previous exposure within 3 months, previous adverse reaction to halothane, family history of adverse reaction to halothane or pre-existing liver disease, unless there are overriding clinical needs.

Enflurane

Causes paroxysmal epileptiform EEG spike wave activity at >3%. Fluoride ions may approach toxic levels in prolonged or high-dose anaesthesia. May generate significant amounts of carbon monoxide in the presence of dry baralyme or soda lime.

Enflurane hepatitis

There are several reports of FHF. Patients tend to be older, have more rapid onset of symptoms and have postoperative pyrexia. Degree of hepatotoxicity is unsure.

Isoflurane

Isoflurane hepatitis

Limited number of reports of hepatotoxicity. Patients tend to be younger. May generate significant amounts of carbon monoxide in the presence of dry baralyme or soda lime.

Desflurane

Differs from isoflurane only by substitution of a fluorine for a chlorine atom. Change from partial chlorination causes ↓ potency, ↑ volatility, ↓ solubility, ↑ stability and ↑ SVP. The strength of the carbon–fluorine bond increases stability with 0.02% metabolism and stability in soda lime. Requires heated vaporizer because of high SVP.

Has similar CVS effects to isoflurane (↑ HR, ↓ SVR). Not arrhythmogenic, even with adrenaline. Coronary artery vasodilator (no evidence for coronary steal). Respiratory depression equivalent to isoflurane. Irritant to upper respiratory tract, therefore not suitable for gas induction. EEG effects similar to isoflurane with dose-related depression. No renal/hepatic toxicity reported.

May generate significant amounts of carbon monoxide in the presence of dry baralyme or soda lime (see Ch. 12).

Sevoflurane

Has similar CVS effects to isoflurane but less tachycardia and coronary vasodilation (no evidence for coronary steal). Less myocardial depression than halothane. Not arrhythmogenic, even with adrenaline. No more irritant than halothane to upper respiratory tract. Greater respiratory depression than halothane but faster elimination results in less postoperative respiratory depression. EEG effects similar to isoflurane, with dose-related depression. Decomposed by soda lime to compounds A and B (Fig. 11.4; and see Ch. 12); 2% metabolized. Levels of fluoride ions $>50\,\mu mol.L^{-1}$ (thought to be the threshold for nephrotoxicity) and post-anaesthetic albuminuria have been reported, but there is no evidence of significant post-anaesthetic renal impairment. However, consider avoiding in patients with renal failure (fresh gas flow rates $<1\,L.min^{-1}$ are not recommended). Also reported to cause small post-anaesthetic increase in serum ALT, suggesting mild transient hepatic injury.

Use of sevoflurane is associated with more rapid recovery than either propofol or isoflurane.

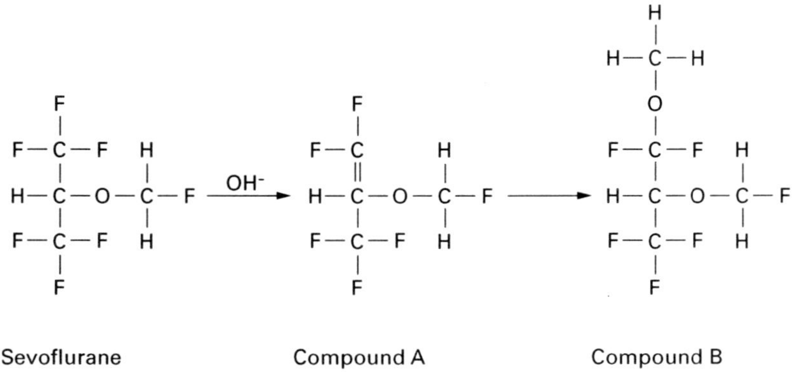

Sevoflurane   Compound A   Compound B

Figure 11.4 Decomposition of sevoflurane (by soda lime) to compounds A and B.

Bibliography

Bedford RF, Ives HE: The renal safety of sevoflurane, *Anesth Analg* 90:505–508, 2000.

Committee on Safety of Medicines: Guidelines for halothane exposure, *Curr Prob* 23:7, 1997.

Coppens MJ, Versichelen LF, Rolly G, et al: The mechanisms of carbon monoxide production by inhalational agents, *Anaesthesia* 61:462–468, 2006.

Elliot RH, Strunin L: Hepatotoxicity of volatile anaesthetics. Review, *Br J Anaesth* 70:339–348, 1993.

Jones R: The new inhalational agents: desflurane and sevoflurane. What is the clinical role of 3rd generation fluorinated anaesthetics and how do they compare with 2nd generation agents, *Acta Anaesth Scand* 39(Suppl):130–131, 1995.

Kharasch ED: Adverse drug reactions with halogenated anesthetics, *Clin Pharmacol Ther* 84:158–162, 2008.

Langbein T, Sonntag H, Trapp D, et al: Volatile anaesthetics and the atmosphere: atmospheric lifetimes and atmospheric effects of halothane, enflurane, isoflurane, desflurane and sevoflurane, *Br J Anaesth* 82:66–73, 1999.

Neuberger J, Williams R: Halothane hepatitis, *Dig Dis* 6:52–54, 1988.

Smith I, Nathanson M, White PF: Sevoflurane – a long-awaited volatile anaesthetic, *Br J Anaesth* 76:435–445, 1996.

Terrell RC: The invention and development of enflurane, isoflurane, sevoflurane, and desflurane, *Anesthesiology* 108:531–533, 2008.

Young CJ, Apfelbaum JL: A comparative review of the newer inhalational anaesthetics, *CNS Drugs* 10:287–310, 1998.

12 Equipment

ANAESTHETIC EQUIPMENT

Gases

Cylinders

Gas cylinders are manufactured from chromium molybdenum steel as a seamless tube.

Colours. Conform to International Standards Organization (Table 12.1).

Marks on cylinders. Test pressure, dates of test, chemical formula of gas and tare weight (i.e. weight when empty).

Gas pressures

- N_2O – 51.6 bar (liquid). No reduction in cylinder pressure until 75% empty
- CO_2 – 44 bar (liquid)
- Cyclopropane – 4 bar (liquid)
- O_2 – 137 bar
- Entonox – 137 bar.

Filling ratio = weight of gas in cylinder/weight of water cylinder would hold. For CO_2 and N_2O, filling ratio = 0.75 in temperate climates and 0.67 in tropics.

Table 12.1 Gas cylinder colours

	Body	Shoulder
Oxygen	Black	White
Nitrous oxide	French blue	French blue
Air	Grey	Black/white
Carbon dioxide	Grey	Grey
Helium	Brown	Brown
Cyclopropane	Orange	Orange
Entonox	French blue	French blue/white
Nitric oxide	Pink	Pink

Vacuum

Vacuum required to give 0.53 kPa pressure below atmospheric pressure, producing 40 L/min suction of air.

Anaesthetic machine safety features

- Copper reinforced gas hoses to prevent kinking, with specific colours for each gas. Non-interchangeable Schraeder valves at wall with different threads to connect to the anaesthetic machine
- One-way valves at yokes to prevent leaks
- Pin index system for cylinders
- Pressure-reducing valves (from 137 to 4 bar)
- Sintered bronze filters proximal to rotameters to prevent ingress of dust
- Oxygen flow knob on rotameter more proud than others with serrated surface
- Oxygen enters fresh gas flow from rotameter last
- Rotameters have a stop to prevent bobbin disappearing from site at high gas flows
- Gold/tin coating on surface of rotameter to prevent static electricity causing bobbin to stick
- Flow restrictors sited proximal to rotameters to protect them from sudden surges in pressure and distal to rotameters to protect them from back pressure
- Interlocking vaporizers
- Oxygen failure alarm
- Emergency O_2 flush without locking valve (>35 L/min)
- Air entrainment if oxygen delivery fails
- Blow-off valve at 43 kPa to protect back bar
- Blow-off valve in patient circuit at 5 kPa.

CHECKING ANAESTHETIC EQUIPMENT 3
Association of Anaesthetists of Great Britain and Ireland 2004

Full checklist is the responsibility of the anaesthetist and should be performed prior to each operating session.

1. Check that the anaesthetic machine is connected to the electricity supply (if appropriate) and switched on

Note: Some anaesthetic workstations may enter an integral self-test programme when switched on; those functions tested by such a programme need not be retested.

- Take note of any information or labelling on the anaesthetic machine referring to the current status of the machine. Particular attention should be paid to recent servicing. Servicing labels should be fixed in the service logbook.

2. Check that all monitoring devices, in particular the oxygen analyser, pulse oximeter and capnograph, are functioning and have appropriate alarm limits
   - Check that gas sampling lines are properly attached and free of obstructions.
   - Check that an appropriate frequency of recording non-invasive blood pressure is selected.
3. Check with a 'tug test' that each pipeline is correctly inserted into the appropriate gas supply terminal

Note: Carbon dioxide cylinders should not be present on the anaesthetic machine unless requested by the anaesthetist. A blanking plug should be fitted to any empty cylinder yoke.

   - Check that the anaesthetic machine is connected to a supply of oxygen and that an adequate supply of oxygen is available from a reserve oxygen cylinder.
   - Check that adequate supplies of other gases (nitrous oxide, air) are available and connected as appropriate.
   - Check that all pipeline pressure gauges in use on the anaesthetic machine indicate 400–500 kPa.
4. Check the operation of flowmeters (where fitted)
   - Check that each flow valve operates smoothly and that the bobbin moves freely throughout its range.
   - Check the anti-hypoxia device is working correctly.
   - Check the operation of the emergency oxygen bypass control.
5. Check the vaporizer(s)
   - Check that each vaporizer is adequately, but not over, filled.
   - Check that each vaporizer is correctly seated on the back bar and not tilted.
   - Check the vaporizer for leaks (with vaporizer on and off) by temporarily occluding the common gas outlet.
   - Turn the vaporizer(s) off when checks are completed.
   - Repeat the leak test immediately after changing any vaporizer.
6. Check the breathing system to be employed
   - Inspect the system for correct configuration. All connections should be secured by 'push and twist'.
   - Perform a pressure leak test on the breathing system by occluding the patient-end and compressing the reservoir bag. Bain-type co-axial systems should have the inner tube compressed for the leak test.

Vaporizers

Because desflurane has such a high saturated vapour pressure (88 kPa), standard vaporizers are unsuitable for its storage and delivery. Use of a conventional vaporizer would require very high fresh gas flows to achieve 1 MAC equivalent of desflurane. The low boiling point of desflurane (24°C) also makes a conventional vaporizer unsuitable. The Tech 6 desflurane vaporizer

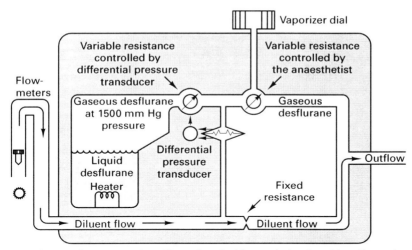

Figure 12.1 Desflurane vaporizer. (Reproduced with permission from New Generation Vaporizers, Pharmacia.)

(Fig. 12.1) uses a servo-controlled electronic system which heats the vaporizer chamber to a constant 39°C (higher than the boiling point) at a pressure of 1500 mmHg. The desflurane is delivered into the fresh gas flow (FGF) at equal pressures through a pressure-regulating valve which increases desflurane delivery as the FGF increases. Unlike conventional ventilators, use of the Tech 6 vaporizer at high altitude requires manual adjustment to increase desflurane concentrations.

Ventilators
Nuffield 200 series ventilator

This is a time-cycled pressure generator. It has variable expiratory and inspiratory timers and a variable inspiratory flow rate control (Fig. 12.2).

Paediatric Newton valve. Capable of delivering tidal volume between 10 and 300 mL at flow rates of 0.5–18 L/min. At small tidal volumes, pressure-controlled ventilation is preferable to volume-controlled ventilation because the final volume delivered is dependent upon circuit leaks, circuit compliance and fresh gas flow rates.

Bibliography

Andrews JJ, Johnston RV: The new Tech 6 desflurane vaporizer, *Anesth Analg* 76:1338–1341, 1993.

Association of Anaesthetists of Great Britain and Ireland: *Checking anaesthetic equipment*, vol 3, London, 2004, AAGBI.

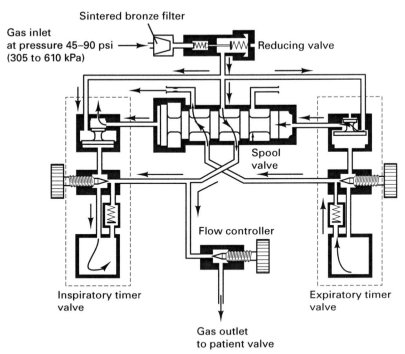

Figure 12.2 Nuffield Penlon 200 ventilator – inspiratory mode. (Reproduced with permission from Davey et al 1992.)

Cartwright DP, Freeman MF: Vaporisers, *Anaesthesia* 54:519–520, 1999.

Davey A, Moyle JT, Ward CS, editors: *Ward's anaesthetic equipment*, ed 3, London, 1992, WB Saunders.

Gardner MC, Adams AP: Anaesthetic vaporizers: design and function, *Curr Anaesth Crit Care* 7:315–321, 1996.

Howell RSC: Medical gases (1) Manufacture and uses. In Kaufman L, editor: *Anaesthesia review*, vol 7, Edinburgh, 1989, Churchill Livingstone, pp 87–104.

Howell RSC: Medical gases (2) Distribution. In Kaufman L, editor: *Anaesthesia review*, vol 8, Edinburgh, 1990, Churchill Livingstone, pp 195–210.

BREATHING CIRCUITS

Mapleson's classification of breathing systems

For all adult circuits, a 110 cm hose holds a volume of 550 mL. T-piece reservoir should equal the tidal volume (more reservoir volume causes increased resistance and re-breathing).

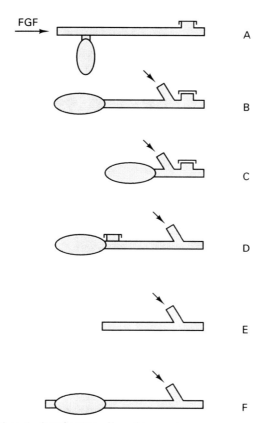

Figure 12.3 Mapleson's classification of breathing systems.

Table 12.2 Breathing circuit flow rates

Mapleson classification	Spontaneous ventilation	IPPV
A	70 mL/kg per min	2.5 × MV
B	2.5 × MV	2.5 × MV
C	2.5 × MV	2.5 × MV
D	2.5 × MV	70 mL/kg per min
E - Adult	2.5 × MV	2.5 × MV

Continued

Table 12.2 Breathing circuit flow rates—cont'd

Mapleson classification	Spontaneous ventilation	IPPV
E < 20 kg	3 (1000 + 100 mL/kg)	1000 + 100 mL/kg (minimum flow = 3 L)
or	3 (5 × frequency × kg)	5 × frequency × kg
Lack (coaxial A)	50 mL/kg per min	
Bain (coaxial D)		70 mL/kg per min

Paediatric circuits

Deadspace and resistance are most important during spontaneous respiration. Circuit resistance is higher with smaller circuits ($\propto 1/r^4$). Use of low flows with T-piece or Bain circuit results in carbon dioxide being re-breathed only at the latter part of inspiration, which may not affect alveolar ventilation. Re-breathed gas has the advantage of being warm and humidified.

CIRCLE SYSTEMS

Re-breathing was introduced by Snow in 1850. Circle systems were pioneered by Sword in 1926.

Anaesthetic circuits

- *Open circuit* – respiratory tract open to the atmosphere and no rebreathing, e.g. open drop mask for ether
- *Semi-open circuit* – anaesthetic gases carried by fresh gas but may be diluted with room air
- *Semi-closed circuit* – anaesthetic gases carried by fresh gas and no dilution with room air, e.g. Mapleson D
- *Closed circuit* – respiratory tract closed to the atmosphere on both inspiration and expiration.

Advantages of closed-circuit anaesthesia

- Conservation of heat
- Maintenance of humidity of inspired gases
- Additional monitoring of oxygen consumption, circuit leaks and tidal volume
- Oxygen reservoir if failure of supply
- Decreased pollution
- Less volatile agent used, with cost saving.

Disadvantages of closed-circuit anaesthesia

- Cost of circle system and soda lime
- Complexity of system
- Unsuitable for short operations when equilibration does not have time to occur
- Possible to deliver hypoxic mixtures of gases or mixtures with little volatile, leading to awareness
- Slow changes in depth of anaesthesia
- Accumulation of anaesthetic metabolites.

Carbon dioxide absorber

Soda lime contains:

- 94% $Ca(OH)_2$
- 5% NaOH
- 1% KOH
- trace of silicates (prevent powdering)
- 15% water (more efficient CO_2 absorption and less absorption of anaesthetic gases)
- pH indicator, e.g. Clayton Yellow turning from pink to white when exhausted.

Size 4–8 mesh (i.e. granules ¼ – ⅛ inch in diameter); 50% volume of canister is granules, 50% is air. Pack tightly to avoid channelling.

Reaction of soda lime

$$2NaOH + CO_2 \rightarrow Na_2CO_3 + H_2O + heat$$
$$Na_2CO_3 + Ca(OH)_2 \rightarrow CaCO_3 + 2NaOH$$

Temperature within canister may exceed 60°C. Canister should at least equal tidal volume. Therefore, minimum 500 g soda lime becomes exhausted after about 2 h; 100 g soda lime can theoretically absorb 25 L of CO_2, but this figure is reduced by channelling and uneven absorption. Large cylinders contain 2 kg soda lime which can be inverted once the upper chamber becomes exhausted. 'Regeneration' of soda lime on standing occurs due to migration of hydroxyl ions to the surface of granules.

Circle layout

There are 64 different possible combinations of layout. The most efficient has been found to be that shown in Figure 12.4.

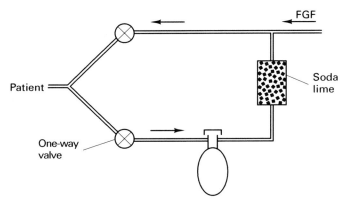

Figure 12.4 Layout for optimal circle system.

Equilibration of circle gases

The wash-in and wash-out curves for changes in vapour concentration within a closed circuit are exponential. Assuming net gas uptake is minimal:

$$\text{Time constant (Tc) for circle} = \frac{\text{volume of circle system}}{\text{FGF}}$$

- 1 Tc = 63% equilibration of FGF with circle gases
- 2 Tc = 86% equilibration of FGF with circle gases
- 3 Tc = 95% equilibration of FGF with circle gases.

For example, in a circuit of volume 4 L with FGF = 8 L/min, Tc = 0.5 min. Therefore, 95% of any change in the percentage of volatile selected will be reflected in the circuit within 1.5 min (Tc × 3). However, at low FGF, e.g. 1 L/min, Tc = 2 min and therefore 95% equilibration will not be achieved until 12 min. Hence, increase flow rather than volatile to deepen anaesthesia.

At low flow rates of O_2 and N_2O into a circle system, the uptake of N_2O exceeds that of O_2, and the $[O_2]$ in the circle exceeds that set by the rotameters. After 30 min equilibration, uptake of N_2O is less than that of O_2, and the $[N_2O]$ in the circle exceeds that set by the rotameters. After the start of an anaesthetic, 15 mL/kg N_2 will be released from tissues, lowering $[N_2O]$. This effect is lessened with denitrogenation prior to closing the circuit.

Thus it is difficult to predict exact concentrations of gases, so use of anaesthetic gas monitoring is mandatory to prevent hypoxic mixtures or mixtures that are deficient in volatile, resulting in awareness. Monitor *expired* gases, which are a better reflection of alveolar gas concentrations than inspired gases.

Principles of closed circuit volatile administration

$$Vo_2(mL / min) = kg^{0.75} \times 10$$

Direct administration of volatiles into the circuit was pioneered by Lowe.

Uptake of volatile $\propto 1/\sqrt{time}$, so the same dose of volatile is taken up between each square of time after induction, i.e. 1, 4, 9, 16, etc. min. Thus one dose is taken up by 1 min after induction, two doses by 4 min after induction, three doses by 9 min after induction, etc. This does not take into account the amount of volatile needed to prime the circuit or any uptake by soda lime or rubber in the circuit. Therefore, extra priming dose needs to be given within the first 9 min.

Aim for ED_{95} of volatile within circuit, i.e. ≈ 1.3 MAC. Thus, at any time after induction, volatile anaesthetic uptake is as follows:

$$Q_{AN} = (1.3 - \%N_2O / 100) \times MAC \times \lambda_{B/G} \times time^{-0.5}$$

where:
Q_{AN} = uptake of anaesthetic
$\lambda_{B/G}$ = blood/gas solubility of volatile.

Vaporizer outside circle (VOC)

At high FGFs, the volatile concentration inspired by the patient will approach that leaving the vaporizer (Fig. 12.5).

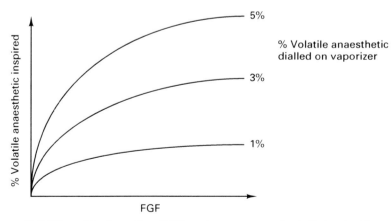

Figure 12.5 Effect of fresh gas flow (FGF) on the percentage of volatile inspired for vaporizers outside the circle.

Vaporizer inside circle (VIC)

At low FGFs, the volatile concentration inspired by the patient will be much higher than that leaving the vaporizer (Fig. 12.6).

Draw-over vaporizers for VIC must not have wicks, because water vapour from saturated gases condenses on them to cause inaccurate volatile delivery. Need draw-over vaporizer with low internal resistance if using spontaneous respiration, e.g. Goldman vaporizer. Plenum vaporizers have too high an internal resistance.

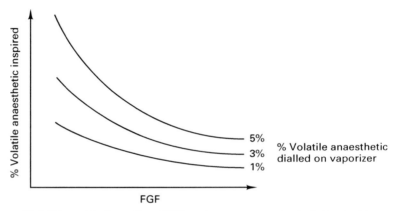

Figure 12.6 Effect of fresh gas flow (FGF) on the percentage of volatile inspired for vaporizers inside the circle.

Products of reactions with absorbents

Carboxyhaemoglobinaemia

In 1995, reports were received from the USA of patients developing significant carboxyhaemoglobinaemia during anaesthesia. This phenomenon was only observed while using halogenated volatile agents (enflurane, isoflurane, desflurane) in association with circle systems. Cases usually occurred on Monday mornings when oxygen had been left flowing through the circuit over the weekend.

Further investigation found that barium hydroxide (baralyme) in the canister was generating significant amounts of carbon monoxide, particularly at low water content as it dried out. Dry baralyme or soda lime (e.g. gas flowing through an anaesthesia circuit over a weekend period) results in excessive carbon monoxide formation due to reaction with KOH, which may reach fatal levels (35000 ppm CO documented with desflurane; safe limit is 35 ppm for 1h). In the UK, barium hydroxide is not available and soda lime (⅓ the amount of KOH compared with baralyme) only dries significantly (<2% water) in circuits where the FGF is placed upstream from the absorbent canister – an arrangement not found in circle systems in the UK. No cases of carboxyhaemoglobinaemia have been reported in the UK and it is thought unlikely that the problems seen in the USA will occur in the UK.

Compound A

Trichloroethylene is decomposed by soda lime to phosgene (toxic). Sevoflurane is decomposed by soda lime and baralyme to compounds A, B, C, D and methanol. Concentrations of compound A in circle systems produce renal injury in rats, but humans are less sensitive. Now believed that compound A has a considerable margin of safety in humans at the concentrations typically found during low-flow sevoflurane anaesthesia (around 15 ppm). Nevertheless, the Food and Drugs Administration (regulatory body for the USA) has set a 1 L. min^{-1} lower limit for gas flow during sevoflurane anaesthesia. No limit exists in the UK.

In 1999, a novel absorbent was introduced (Amsorb) which contains no strong alkali. Amsorb utilizes hygroscopic agents to ensure that the CaOH does not dry. Amsorb therefore produces no carbon monoxide or compound A.

Excessive heat

In November 2003, the Food and Drugs Administration issued a warning relating to 16 cases of overheating in breathing systems when sevoflurane was being used. The cause was a reaction between the volatile agent and dry KOH. The cases reported from the USA included melting of absorber canisters, smoke, and two explosions. No such incidents have ever been reported in the UK.

Bibliography

Baxter PJ, Garton K, Kharasch ED: Mechanistic aspects of carbon monoxide formation from volatile anesthetics, *Anesthesiology* 89:929–941, 1998.

Committee on Safety of Medicines: Circle systems and volatile agents, *Curr Prob* 23:7, 1997.

Jones MJ: Breathing systems and vaporizers. In Nimmo WS, Rowbotham DJ, Smith G, editors: *Anaesthesia*, ed 2, Oxford, 1994, Blackwell Scientific, pp 486–505.

Nunn G: Low-flow anaesthesia, *Contin Educ Anaesth, Crit Care Pain* 8:1–4, 2008.

Schober P, Loer SA: Closed system anaesthesia – historical aspects and recent developments, *Eur J Anaesthesiol* 23:914–920, 2006.

MONITORING

Inadequate monitoring or observation causes 8.2% of all anaesthetic fatalities; 90% of 'monitor-detectable' incidents would be picked up with the correct use of pulse oximetry or capnography.

RECOMMENDATIONS FOR STANDARDS OF MONITORING DURING ANAESTHESIA AND RECOVERY
Association of Anaesthetists of Great Britain and Ireland 2007 (4E)

The Association of Anaesthetists of Great Britain and Ireland regards it as essential that certain core standards of monitoring must be used whenever a patient is anaesthetized. These minimum standards should be uniform irrespective of duration, location or mode of anaesthesia.

- The anaesthetist must be present and care for the patient throughout the conduct of an anaesthetic.
- Monitoring devices must be attached before induction of anaesthesia and their use continued until the patient has recovered from the effects of anaesthesia.
- The same standards of monitoring apply when the anaesthetist is responsible for a local/regional anaesthetic or sedative technique for an operative procedure.
- A summary of information provided by monitoring devices should be recorded on the anaesthetic record. Electronic record-keeping systems are now recommended.
- The anaesthetist must ensure that all equipment has been checked before use. Alarm limits for all equipment must be set appropriately before use. Audible alarms must be enabled during anaesthesia.
- These recommendations state the monitoring devices which are essential and those which must be immediately available during anaesthesia. If it is necessary to continue anaesthesia without a device categorized as 'essential', the anaesthetist must clearly note the reasons for this in the anaesthetic record.
- Additional monitoring may be necessary as deemed appropriate by the anaesthetist.
- A brief interruption of monitoring is only acceptable if the recovery area is immediately adjacent to the operating theatre. Otherwise, monitoring should be continued during transfer to the same degree as any other intra- or inter-hospital transfer.
- Provision, maintenance, calibration and renewal of equipment is an institutional responsibility.

Inspired oxygen concentration
Fuel cell

In a fuel cell (Fig. 12.7), the current is proportional to the partial pressure of oxygen:

$$Pb + 2OH^- \rightarrow PbO + H_2O + 2e^-$$

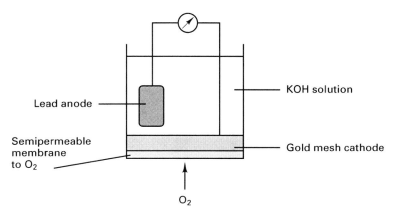

Figure 12.7 Fuel cell.

Clarke electrode

In a Clarke electrode (Fig. 12.8) the current is proportional to the partial pressure of oxygen. This type of electrode is usually used in blood gas machines.

$$2H_2O + O_2 + 4e^- \rightarrow 4OH^-$$

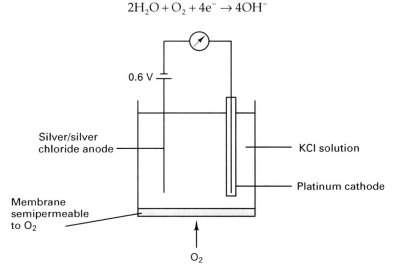

Figure 12.8 Clarke electrode.

Paramagnetic analysis

Based on the fact that oxygen is paramagnetic and attracted towards magnetic fields. Most other gases are diamagnetic and repelled from magnetic fields.

Dumb-bells analyser. Consists of nitrogen-filled dumb-bells with each ball resting within a magnetic field. Any oxygen in the sample gas is attracted into the magnetic field and displaces the nitrogen dumb-bells out of the magnetic field. As the dumb-bells swing, a mirror attached to them displaces a light beam onto photocells.

Datex analyser. The sample gas is separated from the reference gas by a thin diaphragm attached to a pressure transducer. An alternating current applied to the gases causes pressure oscillations across the diaphragm, which is displaced in proportion to the oxygen concentration in the sample gas.

Pulse oximeter

Mechanism

Light is transmitted through tissue at two alternating wavelengths:

- red at 660 nm
- near infrared at 940 nm (not visible).

Beer's law, used to calculate the absorption (Fig. 12.9), states:

$$I_t = I_o e^{-dce}$$

where:
I_t = intensity of reflected light
I_o = intensity of incident light
d = distance light is transmitted through liquid
c = concentration of solute
e = extinction coefficient of solute.

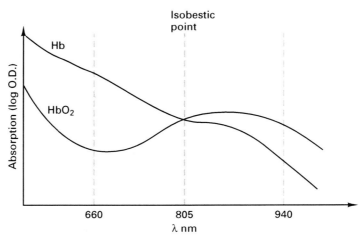

Figure 12.9 Absorption spectra of haemoglobin and oxyhaemoglobin.

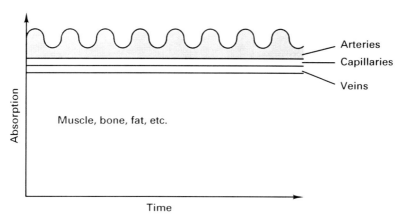

Figure 12.10 Composition of the absorption spectra. (Reproduced with permission from Davey et al 1992.)

The pulse oximeter measures the variation in absorption caused by the arterial pulse, cancelling out the effects of other tissues, venous blood and background light (Fig. 12.10). It is accurate to within 2%, but falls to ± 5% with saturations below 80%.

Factors affecting accuracy

- Smoking: overestimates the saturation by the percentage of HbCO present (≈3% in urban dwellers, 15% in heavy smokers)
- Methaemoglobin: saturation tends towards 85%
- Cardiac dyes: cause underestimation
- HbF and hyperbilirubinaemia have no effect on accuracy of readings
- Extraneous light, motion artefact and diathermy all interfere with absorption
- Atrial fibrillation and vasoconstriction result in a poor pulse volume, which causes errors in measurement.

Capnography

Uses spectrophotometry to measure absorption of CO_2 in sample chamber (Beer's law) and compares results with known CO_2 concentration in a reference chamber (Fig. 12.11).

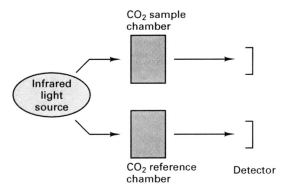

Figure 12.11 Infrared analyser for carbon dioxide.

Arrangement of sampling chamber

The sampling chamber can have one of two arrangements:

1. Attached close to endotracheal tube to measure absorption directly through fresh and expired gases. Avoids delays in sampling time but necessitates a heavy, bulky detector attached to the endotracheal tube.
2. Sampling tube attached close to endotracheal tube which continuously samples gases at 150 mL/min. Avoids bulky attachment but several seconds delay in measuring expired CO_2. If used with a circle system, sampled gas must be returned to the circuit to prevent emptying of the circle gases.

Factors affecting accuracy

- Length and size of sampling tubing and rate of sampling
- N_2O has similar absorption to CO_2 and therefore requires compensation in calculations
- High respiratory rate, e.g. children, can underestimate $P_{ET}CO_2$ if sampling rate is too slow
- PEEP and CPAP can cause overestimation of readings
- $P_{ET}CO_2$ is usually 0.3–0.6 kPa below P_aCO_2, but with severe COAD it may be >2 kPa.

Patterns of capnography displays

IPPV. During ventilation with a Bain circuit, $P_{ET}CO_2$ does not return to zero during inspiration because FGF is less than the minute volume. During inspiration, the trace is distorted by the mixing of expired and fresh gas.

Severe COAD causes a prolonged sloping expiratory phase because of the wide spread in V/Q values. Alveoli emptying last have the least ventilation, the lowest V/Q and thus the highest $P_{ET}CO_2$.

Pulmonary embolus causes a flat expiratory plateau that is lower than the true $P_{ET}CO_2$ because of dilution of expiratory gases with air from non-perfused alveoli.

Shunting, e.g. secretions blocking alveoli, causes a rise in $P_{ET}CO_2$, but the difference is only small since the AV difference is only ≈0.6 kPa.

Clinical uses

- Detection of oesophageal intubation
- Disconnection/apnoea alarm
- Estimation of P_aCO_2. $P_{ET}CO_2$ is 0.3–0.6 kPa less than P_aCO_2, with the least difference at large tidal volumes. $P_{ET}CO_2$ has been measured at higher values than P_aCO_2, possibly due to time-dependent mismatching of ventilation and perfusion occurring in normal lungs at large tidal volumes
- Monitoring IPPV and hyperventilation
- ↓ $P_{ET}CO_2$ with pulmonary embolus, ↓ cardiac output, hyperventilation, hypothermia or hypovolaemia
- ↑ $P_{ET}CO_2$ with hypoventilation, pyrexia or malignant hyperthermia
- Detection of re-breathing
- Monitors early return of spontaneous respiratory effort
- Detects soda lime exhaustion.

Volatile agent monitoring

Drager Narcotest halothane indicator

Uses a rubber band under tension attached to a pointer. Halothane is absorbed by rubber, causing change in elasticity and thus length of the rubber band. Only measures to 3%.

Infrared absorption spectroscopy

Asymmetric, polyatomic molecules absorb infrared radiation, e.g. CO_2, N_2O. H_2 and O_2 do not. Similar arrangement as the capnograph CO_2 detector. Volatile agents have overlapping absorption spectra (Fig. 12.12) and therefore the gas being measured must be specified.

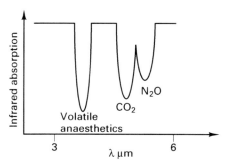

Figure 12.12 Infrared absorption spectrum.

Piezoelectric crystal

Quartz crystal coated in oil. Volatile agent absorbed into oil which changes the weight and thus the frequency of oscillation of the crystal.

Raman scattering

Argon laser beam is shone through the sample gas. It emerges at a different wavelength, the change being dependent upon the type of volatile agent.

Non-invasive blood pressure

Mercury manometer

Korotkoff sounds:

I   – first appearance of pulse
II – reduced intensity of pulsation
III – increased intensity of pulsation
IV – reduced intensity of pulsation
V   – loss of all sound ≡ diastole.

Finapres

Utilizes the technique of Penaz. Digital cuff is servo-controlled so that its pressure is equal to the blood pressure in that digit. The pressure waveform of the cuff is calibrated with the systolic, diastolic and mean blood pressures from a conventional cuff and displayed continuously on an oscilloscope. Less accurate with peripheral vasoconstriction and susceptible to movement artefact.

Arterial tonometry

Microtransducers compress a large artery, e.g. brachial, and continuously monitor the arterial blood pressure. Calibrated by standard BP cuff. Not yet available commercially.

Pulse wave detection velocity

Two photometric sensors at different sites, e.g. forehead and finger, compare rate of propagation of the arterial pulse, which is related to blood pressure. Viscoelasticity decreases with age and may affect accuracy in the elderly. Calibrated by standard BP cuff. Not yet available commercially.

Central venous pressure

IPPV increases intrathoracic pressure and overestimates mean CVP. Spontaneous respiration decreases intrathoracic pressure and underestimates mean CVP. Measure the peak pressure of the 'a' wave during the end-expiratory pause.

Right atrial pressure is a reasonable indicator of left atrial pressure with normal myocardial and pulmonary function.

Bibliography

Association of Anaesthetists of Great Britain and Ireland: Recommendations for standards of monitoring during anaesthesia and recovery: report of a Working Party, ed 4, London, 2007, AAGBI.

Lennmarken C, Vegfors M: Advances in pulse oximetry, *Curr Opin Anaesth* 11: 639–644, 1998.

Moyle JTB: Pulse oximetry. Principles and practice series, London, 1994, BMJ Publishing.

O'Flaherty D: Capnography. Principles and practice series, London, 1994, BMJ Publishing.

Runciman WB, Ludbrook GL: Monitoring. In Nimmo WS, Rowbotham DJ, Smith G, editors: *Anaesthesia*, ed 2, Oxford, 1994, Blackwell Scientific, pp 704–739.

PHYSICS

Gas laws

Henry's law. Amount of gas dissolved ∝ partial pressure of the gas.

Fick's law. Rate of diffusion across a membrane ∝ concentration gradient.

Graham's law. Rate of diffusion ∝ 1/molecular weight.

Charles' law. The volume of a gas changes in proportion to the change in temperature.

Boyle's law. The volume of a gas is inversely proportional to pressure.

Gay-Lussac's law. At constant volume, the absolute pressure of a given mass of gas varies directly with the absolute temperature.

Adiabatic change. A change in pressure, volume or temperature without changes in energy of gas (i.e. heat is lost or added).

Avogadro's hypothesis

Equal volumes of 'ideal' gases at the same temperature and pressure contain the same number of molecules. (Avogadro's number = 6.022×10^{23} molecules occupying 22.4 L at STP.)

Pressure

Dalton's law of partial pressures. The pressure exerted by a mixture of gases is equal to the sum of the pressures which each gas would exert on its own.

Vapour pressure. A vapour is saturated when it is in equilibrium with its own liquid, i.e. as many molecules leave the surface as rejoin it. When vapour pressure equals atmospheric pressure, the liquid boils.

Solubility

Ostwald solubility coefficient. The amount of gas that dissolves in unit volume of liquid under the stated temperature and pressure.
Bunsen solubility coefficient. The amount of gas that dissolves in unit volume of liquid at standard temperature (273 K) and pressure (101.3 kPa).

Temperature

Critical temperature. Temperature above which a gas cannot be liquefied.
Critical pressure. Pressure above which a gas at its critical temperature cannot be liquefied.
Pseudocritical temperature. Temperature at which a mixture of gases separate out into their separate components, e.g. N_2O and O_2 in Entonox at $-5.5°C$.
Specific heat capacity. Amount of heat required to increase the temperature of a substance by $1°C/kg$.

Gas flow

Hagen–Poiseuille equation. For laminar flow:

$$Q = \frac{P \times \pi \times r^4}{8 \times \eta \times L}$$

where P = pressure, r = tube radius, L = tube length, η = viscosity.

Liquid tends to flow smoothly in straight and uniform tubes. Abrupt changes in diameter or direction of flow cause turbulent flow, which is dependent upon density (ρ) rather than viscosity.

For turbulent flow:

$$Q \alpha \frac{\rho}{r^5}$$

When Reynold's number (R) exceeds 2000, flow becomes turbulent:

$$R = \frac{v \times \rho \times r}{\eta}$$

Bernoulli effect. Fall of pressure at a constriction in a tube. Increased gas/fluid velocity results in increased kinetic energy with a reduction in potential energy and thus a decrease in pressure.
Venturi devices use the Bernoulli effect for suction, e.g. Venturi oxygen mask.
Coanda effect. Streaming of gas at a division in tubing along only one of the divisions. Used as logic valve in some ventilators.

Poynting effect. A mixture of gases (e.g. Entonox) remains in a gaseous state, even though one component (N_2O) would normally be liquid at high storage pressures.

Humidification

Absolute humidity is the mass of water vapour present in a given volume of air. *Relative humidity* is the ratio of the mass of water vapour to the mass of water vapour when fully saturated, expressed as a percentage.

Saturation

- Fully saturated air – 44g/m^3
- Upper trachea – 34g/m^3
  >20 µm drops condense on breathing circuit
  5 µm drops settle on trachea
  1 µm drops reach alveoli.

Measurements

- Hair hygrometer
- Regnault's hygrometer – measures dew point
- Electrical resistance
- Mass spectrometer.

Methods of humidification

- *Heat and moisture exchanger* – also acts as bacterial filter. Can achieve levels of humidity in trachea of 20–25g/m^3. Cheap
- *Bubble humidifier* – fresh gas is bubbled through water. More efficient if bubbles are small, increasing their surface area. Heated water also improves efficiency by supplying energy for latent heat of vaporization. Bacterial multiplication is prevented by heating water to high temperatures, ≈60°C. This risks scalding of patient, so a thermistor is needed near the ETT. Can achieve levels of humidity of 40g/m^3
- *Venturi effect* – humidifies gas to 60g/m^3
- *Water dropped onto heated wire*
- *Ultrasonic* – can achieve levels of humidity >90g/m^3
- *Spinning plate* – can achieve levels of humidity >90g/m^3.

Electricity

Macroshock. Skin-to-skin contact:

- 1 mA – tingle
- 15 mA – let-go threshold

- 50 mA – respiratory arrest
- 100 mA – VF.

Microshock. Direct myocardial contact. Current $\geq 100\,\mu A$. Less effect at higher frequency, e.g. diathermy at 20 kHz.

Classification of electrical equipment

- *Class 1 equipment* – earthed metal casing
- *Class 2 equipment* – outer casing protected by double insulation with no exposed metal work; therefore an earth wire is not required
- *Class BF* – surface contact with patient. Maximum patient leak = $100\,\mu A$
- *Class CF* – may contact the heart directly. Maximum patient leak = $10\,\mu A$.

Bibliography

Parbrook GD, Davis PD, Parbrook EO: *Basic physics and measurement in anaesthesia*, Oxford, 1995, Butterworth-Heinemann.
Ward C, editor: Ward's Anaesthetic Equipment, ed 5, London, 2005, WB Saunders.

Reports | **13**

ANAESTHETIC GUIDELINES

Guidelines of the Association of Anaesthetists of Great Britain and Ireland

HIV AND OTHER BLOOD BORNE VIRUSES 1992

See 'General topics', p. 192.

IMMEDIATE POST-ANAESTHETIC RECOVERY 1993
Association of Anaesthetists of Great Britain and Ireland 1993

Basic recovery facilities

The patient should normally be placed in the left lateral position and transferred on to a tipping trolley to the recovery room. The recovery room should be fully staffed, available at all times and be able to give continuous individual nursing care to each patient. Handover should include pre-existing diseases, airway and cardiovascular problems, postoperative orders and analgesia.

Observations should include O_2 administration and saturation, respiratory rate, heart rate, blood pressure, level of consciousness, pain and i.v. infusions.

Patients should not be discharged to the ward until they can maintain their own airway and have protective reflexes, cardiovascular and respiratory stability, adequate analgesia and are normothermic.

Day-case patients on discharge should be accompanied by a responsible adult, be given written advice on analgesia and hospital contact number, and be warned against drinking alcohol and operating machinery for at least 24 h.

Recovery room

Effective emergency call system, defibrillator and anaesthetic machine must be available in the recovery room. The room must be well lit with waste gas scavenging and temperature of 21–22°C. Children should be segregated from adults.

Each bay should contain an O_2 source, breathing circuit (e.g. Mapleson C), pulse oximeter, ECG, suction and BP measuring equipment.

Each recovery trolley should contain an O_2 cylinder, be capable of tipping head-down, have suction equipment and have padded cot sides.

Training of recovery staff

Minimum standards of training for recovery room staff.

BLOOD BORNE VIRUSES AND ANAESTHESIA – AN UPDATE 1996

See 'General topics', p. 193.

THE ANAESTHESIA TEAM 1998
Association of Anaesthetists of Great Britain and Ireland, 1998

Recommendations

- A team-based approach to anaesthesia offers many advantages for the provision of a high-quality anaesthesia service.
- Pre-admission screening is a vital early component of pre-anaesthetic assessment. It reduces cancellations and promotes effective usage. It does not replace the need for the anaesthetist's preoperative visit.
- Anaesthetists must have dedicated, skilled assistance wherever anaesthesia is administered.
- Recovery areas must have trained staff available throughout all operating hours and until the last patient meets all the criteria for discharge.
- All acute hospitals providing in-patient surgical services must have an acute pain team led by a consultant anaesthetist.

ANAESTHESIA AND PERIOPERATIVE CARE OF THE ELDERLY 2001

See 'Anaesthesia for the elderly', p. 153.

PREOPERATIVE ASSESSMENT. THE ROLE OF THE ANAESTHETIST 2001

See 'Preoperative assessment', p. 216.

PROVISION OF ANAESTHETIC SERVICES IN MAGNETIC RESONANCE UNITS 2002

Summary

1. The continuous presence of a strong magnetic field, and restricted access to the patient, means that the provision of anaesthesia within MR units presents unique problems.
2. Whenever a new MR unit is planned, the possibility of managing sedated or anaesthetized patients should be considered.
3. In the planning process, adequate space should be made available for the provision of anaesthesia services.
4. A nominated consultant anaesthetist should be responsible for anaesthesia services in MR units.
5. The level of assistance for the anaesthetist must be equal to that expected in the operating theatre environment.
6. Immediate access from the scanning room to the anaesthetic preparation/resuscitation area is essential as in the event of an emergency, the patient must be removed from the magnetic field without delay.
7. Anaesthetic equipment that is used in the scanning room should be MR compatible.
8. The monitoring of patients in MR units during anaesthesia, sedation and recovery must comply with minimum monitoring standards.
9. It is essential that a remote monitoring facility is available to allow the anaesthetic team to remain outside the scanning room once the patient's condition is stable.
10. Only personnel, who have received appropriate training and are fully conversant with the local protocols, are allowed to enter the controlled area unsupervised.
11. Resources should be provided to minimize the risk of personal exposure to strong magnetic fields and noise levels.

POST-ANAESTHETIC RECOVERY 2002

See 'Post-Anaesthetic Recovery', p. 211.

CHECKING ANAESTHETIC EQUIPMENT 2004 (3E)

See 'Anaesthetic equipment', p. 399.

DAY SURGERY – REVISED EDITION 2005

See 'Day surgery', p. 184.

RECOMMENDATIONS FOR THE SAFE TRANSFER OF PATIENTS WITH BRAIN INJURY 2006

See 'Neuroanaesthesia', p. 83.

CONSENT FOR ANAESTHESIA 2006

Recommendations

- Information about anaesthesia, preferably in the form of a patient-friendly leaflet, should be provided to patients undergoing elective surgery before they meet their anaesthetist.
- The anaesthetic room immediately before induction is not an acceptable place or time to provide elective patients with new information other than in exceptional circumstances.
- The amount and the nature of information that should be disclosed to the patient should be determined by the question: 'What would this patient regard as relevant when coming to a decision about which of the available options to accept?'
- At the end of an explanation about a procedure, patients should be asked whether they have any questions; any such questions should be addressed fully and details recorded.
- Anaesthetists should record details of the elements of a discussion in the patient record, noting what risks, benefits and alternatives were explained.
- A separate formal consent form signed by the patient is not required for anaesthetic procedures that are done to facilitate another treatment or as part of an inter-related process.
- Adults should be presumed to have capacity to consent unless there is contrary evidence.
- The Mental Capacity Act 2005 (MCA) allows patients without capacity to express their previously-determined wishes by means of an Advance Decision or by means of a proxy using a Lasting Power of Attorney.
- When planning to allow trainees or others to use an opportunity presented by a patient for training in practical procedures, the anaesthetist should make every effort to minimize risk and maximize benefits, and should consider alternative ways of achieving the same end. Specific consent for such procedures may or may not be required depending on the circumstances.

RECOMMENDATIONS FOR STANDARDS OF MONITORING DURING ANAESTHESIA AND RECOVERY 2007 (4E)

See 'Monitoring', p. 410.

GUIDELINES FOR THE MANAGEMENT OF A MALIGNANT HYPERTHERMIA CRISIS 2007

See 'Malignant hyperthermia', p. 131.

PERIOPERATIVE MANAGEMENT OF THE MORBIDLY OBESE PATIENT 2007

See 'Anaesthesia for the morbidly obese patient', p. 137.

GUIDELINES FOR THE MANAGEMENT OF SEVERE LOCAL ANAESTHETIC TOXICITY 2007

See 'Pharmacology', p. 380.

SUSPECTED ANAPHYLACTIC REACTIONS ASSOCIATED WITH ANAESTHESIA 2009 (4E)

See 'Anaphylactic reactions', p. 158.

GOOD PRACTICE IN THE MANAGEMENT OF CONTINUOUS EPIDURAL ANALGESIA IN THE HOSPITAL SETTING 2004

Royal College of Anaesthetists & Association of Anaesthetists of Great Britain & Ireland (www.aagbi.org/publications/guidelines/docs/epidanalg04.pdf)

See 'Pain', p. 355.

OAA/AAGBI GUIDELINES FOR OBSTETRIC ANAESTHESIA SERVICES 2005

Association of Anaesthetics of Great Britain and Ireland and the Obstetric Anaesthetists Association. Revised Guidelines

See 'Obstetrics', p. 302.

MANAGEMENT OF ANAESTHESIA FOR JEHOVAH'S WITNESSES 2005 (2E)

See 'Blood', p. 170.

BLOOD TRANSFUSION AND THE ANAESTHETIST – BLOOD COMPONENT THERAPY 2005

See 'Blood', p. 166.

BLOOD TRANSFUSION AND THE ANAESTHETIST – RED CELL TRANSFUSION 2008

See 'Blood', p. 166.

INFECTION CONTROL IN ANAESTHESIA 2008

Summary

1. A named consultant in each department of anaesthesia should liaise with Trust Infection Control Teams and Occupational Health Departments to ensure that relevant specialist standards are established and monitored in all areas of anaesthetic practice.

2. Precautions against the transmission of infection between patient and anaesthetist or between patients should be a routine part of anaesthetic practice. In particular, anaesthetists must ensure that hand hygiene becomes an indispensable part of their clinical culture.

3. Anaesthetists must comply with local theatre infection control policies including the safe use and disposal of sharps.

4. Anaesthetic equipment is a potential vector for transmission of disease. Policies should be documented to ensure that nationally recommended decontamination practices are followed and audited for all reusable anaesthetic equipment.

5. Single use equipment should be utilized where appropriate but a sterile supplies department (SSD) should process reusable items.

6. An effective, new bacterial/viral breathing circuit filter should be used for every patient and a local policy developed for the re-use of breathing circuits in line with manufacturer's instructions. The AAGBI recommends that anaesthetic departments should consider changing anaesthetic circuits on a daily basis in line with daily cleaning protocols.

7. Appropriate infection control precautions should be established for each anaesthetic procedure, to include maximal barrier precautions for the insertion of central venous catheters, spinal and epidural procedures and any invasive procedures in high-risk patients.

BLOOD TRANSFUSION AND THE ANAESTHETIST – INTRAOPERATIVE CELL SALVAGE 2009

See 'Blood', p. 167.

National Institute for Health and Clinical Excellence Guidelines

GUIDANCE ON THE USE OF ULTRASOUND LOCATING DEVICES FOR PLACING CENTRAL VENOUS CATHETERS 2002

(www.nice.org.uk/nicemedia/pdf/49_English_patient.pdf)

Summary

- 2-D imaging ultrasound guidance should be the preferred method when inserting of central venous catheter into the internal jugular vein in adults and children in 'elective situations'.
- 2-D imaging ultrasound guidance should be considered in most clinical situations where CVC insertion is necessary, whether the situation is elective or an emergency.
- Everyone who uses 2-D imaging ultrasound guidance to insert central venous catheters should have appropriate training to ensure they are competent to use the technique.
- Audio-guided Doppler ultrasound guidance is not recommended for use when inserting central venous catheters.

OBESITY – GUIDANCE ON THE PREVENTION, IDENTIFICATION, ASSESSMENT AND MANAGEMENT OF OVERWEIGHT AND OBESITY IN ADULTS AND CHILDREN 2006

(www.nice.org.uk/CG043)

See 'Anaesthesia for the obese patient', p. 138.

ACUTELY ILL PATIENTS IN HOSPITAL: RECOGNITION OF AND RESPONSE TO ACUTE ILLNESS IN ADULTS IN HOSPITAL 2007

(www.nice.org.uk/nicemedia/pdf/CG50QuickRefGuide.pdf)

See 'Intensive Care', p. 252.

ATRIAL FIBRILLATION: THE MANAGEMENT OF ATRIAL FIBRILLATION 2006

(www.nice.org.uk/CG036NICEguideline)

See 'Cardiovascular system', p. 9.

ANTIMICROBIAL PROPHYLAXIS AGAINST INFECTIVE ENDOCARDITIS IN ADULTS AND CHILDREN UNDERGOING INTERVENTIONAL PROCEDURES 2008
(www.nice.org.uk/nicemedia/pdf/CG64PIEQRG.pdf)

See 'Cardiovascular system', p. 12.

ULTRASOUND-GUIDED REGIONAL NERVE BLOCK 2009
(www.nice.org.uk/Guidance/IPG285)

Summary

- Current evidence on the safety and efficacy of ultrasound-guided regional nerve block appears adequate to support the use of this procedure provided that normal arrangements are in place for clinical governance, consent and audit.
- Clinicians wishing to perform this procedure should be experienced in the administration of regional nerve blocks and trained in ultrasound guidance techniques.

ULTRASOUND-GUIDED CATHETERIZATION OF THE EPIDURAL SPACE 2008
(www.nice.org.uk/nicemedia/pdf/IPG249Guidance.pdf)

See 'Pain', p. 354.

INTRAOPERATIVE BLOOD CELL SALVAGE IN OBSTETRICS 2005
(www.nice.org.uk/IPG144distributionlist)

See 'Obstetrics', p. 307.

HEAD INJURY: TRIAGE, ASSESSMENT, INVESTIGATION AND EARLY MANAGEMENT OF HEAD INJURY IN INFANTS, CHILDREN AND ADULTS 2007
(www.nice.org.uk/nicemedia/pdf/CG56QuickRedGuide.pdf)

See 'Trauma', p. 240.

VENOUS THROMBOEMBOLISM: REDUCING THE RISK 2010
(http://guidance.nice.org.uk/CG92)

See 'Anaesthesia for orthopaedic surgery', p. 107.

INTRAOPERATIVE NERVE MONITORING DURING THYROID SURGERY 2008
(www.nice.org.uk/nicemedia/pdf/IPG255Guidance.pdf)

See 'Thyroid disease', p. 125.

INADVERTENT PERIOPERATIVE HYPOTHERMIA 2008
(www.nice.org.uk/nicemedia/pdf/CG65Guidance.pdf)

See 'Thermoregulation', p. 148.

Other guidelines

LOCAL ANAESTHESIA FOR INTRAOCULAR SURGERY
Royal College of Anaesthetists and Royal College of Ophthalmologists 2001

See 'Anaesthesia for ophthalmic surgery', p. 102.

GUIDELINES FOR AUTOLOGOUS BLOOD TRANSFUSION
British Committee for Standards in Haematology Blood Transfusion Task Force 1997

See 'Blood', p. 165.

GUIDELINES ON POST-EXPOSURE PROPHYLAXIS (PEP) FOR HEALTH CARE WORKERS OCCUPATIONALLY EXPOSED TO HIV
Department of Health 1997 (www.dh.gov.uk/prod_consum_dh/ groups/dh_digitalassets/@dh/@en/documents/digitalasset/ dh_4072980.pdf)

See 'Human immunodeficiency virus', p. 191.

CADAVERIC ORGANS FOR TRANSPLANTATION. A CODE OF PRACTICE FOR THE DIAGNOSIS OF BRAIN STEM DEATH
Department of Health 1998 (www.dh.gov.uk/prod_consum_dh/ groups/dh_digitalassets/@dh/@en/documents/digitalasset/ dh_4011718.pdf)

See 'Organ donation and transplantation', p. 204.

STANDARDS AND GUIDELINES FOR GENERAL ANAESTHESIA FOR DENTISTRY
Royal College of Anaesthetists 1999

See 'Dental anaesthesia', p. 88.

GUIDELINES FOR THE PREVENTION OF ENDOCARDITIS
Report of the Working Party of the British Society for Antimicrobial Chemotherapy 2006 (http://jac.oxfordjournals.org/cgi/reprint/ dkl121v1)

See 'Cardiovascular system', p. 13.

GUIDELINES ON THE PREVENTION OF POSTOPERATIVE VOMITING (POV) IN CHILDREN
The Association of Paediatric Anaesthetists of Great Britain and Ireland 2007 (www.apagbi.org.uk/docs)

See 'Paediatrics', p. 319.

CONSENSUS GUIDELINE ON PERIOPERATIVE FLUID MANAGEMENT IN CHILDREN V 1.1
Association of Paediatric Anaesthetists of Great Britain and Ireland 2007 (www.apagbi.org.uk/docs/Perioperative_Fluid_Management_2007.pdf)

See 'Paediatrics', p. 314.

BRITISH CONSENSUS GUIDELINES ON INTRAVENOUS FLUID THERAPY FOR ADULT SURGICAL PATIENTS 2008
(www.ics.ac.uk/downloads/2008112340_GIFTASUP\%20FINAL_31-10-08.pdf)

See 'Intensive care', p. 265.

BRITISH THORACIC SOCIETY GUIDELINE FOR EMERGENCY OXYGEN USE IN ADULT PATIENTS 2008
See 'Oxygen', p. 364.

BRITISH GUIDELINE ON THE MANAGEMENT OF ASTHMA
British Thoracic Society and Scottish Intercollegiate Guidelines Network 2009 (www.brit-thoracic.org.uk/ClinicalInformation/Asthma/AsthmaGuidelines/tabid/83/Default.aspx)

See 'Anaesthesia for asthmatics', p. 49.

Bibliography

Association of Anaesthetists of Great Britain and Ireland: *Checklist for anaesthetic machines*, London, 1990, AAGBI.

Association of Anaesthetists of Great Britain and Ireland: *HIV and other blood borne viruses – guidance for anaesthetists*, London, 1992, AAGBI.

Association of Anaesthetists of Great Britain and Ireland: *Immediate postanaesthetic recovery*, London, 1993, AAGBI.

Association of Anaesthetists of Great Britain and Ireland: *Recommendations for standards of monitoring during anaesthesia and recovery*, 4th ed, 2007. Reproduced with the kind permission of the Association of anaesthetists of Great Britain and Ireland.

Association of Anaesthetists of Great Britain and Ireland: *Peri-Operative Management of the Morbidly Obese Patient*, 2007. Reproduced with the kind permission of the Association of anaesthetists of Great Britain and Ireland.

Infection control in anaesthesia, 2008. Reproduced with the kind permission of the Association of anaesthetists of Great Britain and Ireland.

Association of Anaesthetists of Great Britain and Ireland: *Recommendations for the safe transfer of patients with brain injury*, 2006. Reproduced with the kind permission of the Association of anaesthetists of Great Britain and Ireland.

Association of Anaesthetists of Great Britain and Ireland: *Blood transfusion and the anaesthetist – red cell transfusion*, 2008. Reproduced with the kind permission of the Association of anaesthetists of Great Britain and Ireland.

Association of Anaesthetists of Great Britain and Ireland: *Blood transfusion and the anaesthetist – blood component therapy*, 2005. Reproduced with the kind permission of the Association of anaesthetists of Great Britain and Ireland.

Association of Anaesthetists of Great Britain and Ireland: *Post-anaesthetic recovery*, 2002. Reproduced with the kind permission of the Association of anaesthetists of Great Britain and Ireland.

Association of Anaesthetists of Great Britain and Ireland and the British Society of Allergy and Clinical Immunology: Revised guidelines. *Suspected anaphylactic reactions associated with anaesthesia*, 4th ed., 2009. Reproduced with the kind permission of the Association of anaesthetists of Great Britain and Ireland.

Association of Anaesthetists of Great Britain and Ireland: *A report received by Council of the Association of Anaesthetists on blood borne viruses and anaesthesia – an update*, London, 1996, AAGBI.

Association of Anaesthetists of Great Britain and Ireland: *Checking anaesthetic equipment 3*, 2004. Reproduced with the kind permission of the Association of anaesthetists of Great Britain and Ireland.

Consent for anaesthesia, 2006. Reproduced with the kind permission of the Association of anaesthetists of Great Britain and Ireland.

Association of Anaesthetists of Great Britain and Ireland: *Guidelines for the management of a malignant hyperthermia crisis*, 2007. Reproduced with the kind permission of the Association of anaesthetists of Great Britain and Ireland.

Association of Anaesthetists of Great Britain and Ireland: *Pre-operative assessment. The role of the anaesthetist*, 2001. Reproduced with the kind permission of the Association of anaesthetists of Great Britain and Ireland.

Association of Anaesthetists of Great Britain and Ireland: *The anaesthesia team*, London, 1998, AAGBI.

Association of Anaesthetists of Great Britain and Ireland: *Management of anaesthesia for Jehovah's witnesses*, 2nd ed., 2005. Reproduced with the kind permission of the Association of anaesthetists of Great Britain and Ireland.

Association of Anaesthetists of Great Britain and Ireland and the Obstetric Anaesthetists Association: Revised Guidelines, OAA/AAGBI *guidelines for obstetric anaesthesia services*, 2005. Reproduced with the kind permission of the Association of anaesthetists of Great Britain and Ireland.

Association of Anaesthetists of Great Britain and Ireland: *Peri-Operative Management of the Morbidly Obese Patient*, 2007. Reproduced with the kind permission of the Association of anaesthetists of Great Britain and Ireland.

Association of Anaesthetists of Great Britain and Ireland: *Peri-Operative Management of the Morbidly Obese Patient*, 2007. Reproduced with the kind permission of the Association of anaesthetists of Great Britain and Ireland.

Association of Anaesthetists of Great Britain and Ireland: Immediate postanesthetic recovery, 1993. Reproduced with the kind permission of the Association of anaesthetists of Great Britain and Ireland.

The anaesthesia team, 1998. Reproduced with the kind permission of the Association of anaesthetics of Great Britain and Ireland. www.aagbi.org/publications/guidelines/docs/epidanalg 04.pdf. Reproduced with the kind permission of the Association of anaesthetists of Great Britain and Ireland.

British Committee for Standards in Haematology Blood Transfusion Task Force: Autologous Transfusion Working Party, Napier J A, Bruce M, Chapman J, et al: Guidelines for autologous transfusion. II. Perioperative haemodilution and cell salvage, *Br J Anaesth* 78:768–771, 1997.

British Consensus Guidelines on Intravenous Fluid Therapy for Adult Surgical Patients, 2008. http://www.bapen.org.uk/pdfs/bapen_pubs/giftasup.pdf.

British National Formulary: Infective endocarditis prophylaxis, *British National Formulary* 37(5.1):1999.

Department of Health: *A code of practice for the diagnosis of brain stem death including guidelines for the identification and management of potential organ and tissue donors*, London, 1998, HMSO.

Department of Health: Guidelines on post-exposure prophylaxis (PEP) for health care workers occupationally exposed to HIV, 1997. www.dh.gov.uk/en/PublicationsAndStatistics/LettersAndCirculars/ProfessionalLetters/ChiefOfficerLetters/DH_4004143.

Neuroanaesthesia Society of Great Britain and Ireland and the Association of Anaesthetists of Great Britain and Ireland: *Recommendations for the transfer of patients with acute head injuries to neurosurgical units*, London, 1996, NSGBI/AAGBI.

NICE: Guidance on the use of ultrasound locating devices for placing central venous catheters, 2002. http://guidance.nice.org.uk/TA49/Guidance/pdf/English.

NICE: Atrial fibrillation: the management of atrial fibrillation, London, 2006, National Institute for Health and Clinical Excellence, 2006. www.nice.org.uk/CG036NICEguideline.

NICE: Obesity – Guidance on the prevention, identification, assessment and management of overweight and obesity in adults and children, London, 2006, National Institute for Health and Clinical Excellence, 2006. www.nice.org.uk/CG043.

NICE: Ultrasound guided catheterisation of the epidural space, 2008. http://guidance.nice.org.uk/IPG249/Guidance/pdf/English.

NICE: Antimicrobial prophylaxis against infective endocarditis in adults and children undergoing interventional procedures, London, 2008, National Institute for Health and Clinical Excellence, 2008. www.nice.org.uk/nicemedia/pdf/CG64PIEQRG.pdf.

NICE: Inadvertent perioperative hypothermia. NICE clinical guideline, 2008, www.nice.org.uk/CG065.

NICE: Ultrasound guided regional nerve block, London, 2009, National Institute for Health and Clinical Excellence, 2009. http://guidance.nice.org.uk/IPG285/PublicInfo/pdf/English.

O'Driscoll BR, Howard LS, Davison AG on behalf of the: British Thoracic Society: British Thoracic Society guideline for emergency oxygen use in adult patients, *Thorax* 63(Suppl VI):vi1–vi68, 2008.

Royal College of Anaesthetists & Association of Anaesthetist of Great Britain & Ireland: Good practice in the management of continuous epidural analgesia in the hospital setting, 2004. www.aagbi.org/publications/guidelines/docs/epidanalg04.pdf.

Royal College of Anaesthetists: Sedation and anaesthesia in radiology, *Report of a Joint Working Party*, London, 1992, RCA.

Royal College of Anaesthetists and College of Ophthalmologists: *Report of the Joint Working Party on Anaesthesia in Ophthalmic Surgery*, London, 1993, RCA and Co.

Royal College of Anaesthetists: *Standards and guidelines for general anaesthesia and dentistry*, London, 1999, RCA.

Royal College of Radiologists: *Making the best use of a department of clinical radiology. Guidelines for doctors*, 3, London, 1995, RCR.

NATIONAL CONFIDENTIAL ENQUIRIES INTO PERIOPERATIVE DEATHS (NCEPOD)

CEPOD was established in 1988 to review surgical and anaesthetic practice in the UK. The first report covered three areas, but it has been a national report (NCEPOD) since 1989. It involves all NHS and most private hospitals. The reports are anonymous and confidential and are peer-reviewed by consultants representing the medical colleges.

CEPOD 1987

Covered three areas (i.e. not national): N.E. Thames Health Authority (HA), Northern HA and South Western HA.

Recommendations

- Need for national assessment of clinical practice
- No SHO/registrar should undertake any emergency case without consultation with their consultant/SR
- Resources should be concentrated on a single site
- Neurological and neonatal surgery should be performed in specialist units
- Patients must be adequately resuscitated preoperatively if possible
- Moribund patients should be allowed to die with dignity.

NCEPOD 1989 – CHILDREN

Involved all hospitals, i.e. first national CEPOD. Covered deaths in children ≤10 years occurring within 30 days of surgery, of which there were 115 non-cardiac deaths and 160 cardiac deaths.

Recommendations

- Anaesthetists should not undertake occasional paediatric anaesthesia
- No trainee should anaesthetize a child without discussion with the consultant
- Neonates should be transferred to a paediatric centre.

NCEPOD 1990 – DEATHS

Random sample of 20% of adult postoperative deaths; 19 000 deaths, mostly within 5 days of surgery; 59% of anaesthetists were working without assistance.

Recommendations

- All essential services should be on one site
- Surgeon and anaesthetist should be in agreement about need for surgery
- Proper pain relief needs a high-dependency unit
- Provision of daytime emergency theatre is needed to prevent delays
- All grades of anaesthetist should be involved in audit and continuing education.

NCEPOD 1991/2 – SPECIFIC PROCEDURES

Reviewed 15 specific surgical procedures from all specialities.

Recommendations

- Surgical and anaesthetic skills should be more matched to the condition of the patient
- 42% of deaths after total hip replacement were found to have a pulmonary embolus. Therefore a local policy on prophylaxis must be determined and followed
- Some patients with GI obstruction had no NG tube, resulting in aspiration
- Stresses importance of fluid balance in the elderly
- Patients about to die should not be subjected to surgery
- Capnography and ventilator disconnect alarms are underused.

NCEPOD 1992/3

Reviewed 19 816 deaths in patients aged 6–70 years.

Recommendations

- Trainees with less than 3 years' training should not anaesthetize without appropriate supervision
- Practitioners should recognize their limitations and not hesitate to consult a more experienced colleague
- The skills of the anaesthetist and surgeon should be appropriate for the physiological and pathological status of the patient
- Appropriately trained staff must accompany all patients with life-threatening conditions during transfer between and within hospitals
- The medical profession must develop and enforce standards of practice for the management of many common acute conditions (e.g. head injury, aortic aneurysm, GI bleeding).

NCEPOD 1993/4 – POSTOPERATIVE DEATHS

Reviewed one death per consultant surgeon or gynaecologist.

Recommendations

- Surgical operations should not be started in hospitals without appropriate critical care services
- Anaesthetist must have appropriately skilled and dedicated non-medical assistants
- Consultation between surgeons and anaesthetists needs to be more frequent in order to promote a team approach
- The use of protocols in the management of certain clinical conditions needs to be increased.

NCEPOD 1994/5 – POSTOPERATIVE DEATHS

Reviewed 1818 deaths within 3 days of surgery.

Recommendations

- High-dependency and ICU beds are still inadequate and resources need to be increased to correct deficiencies
- Communication between specialists and between grades needs to be more frequent and more effective
- Patients >90 years of age, those with aortic stenosis, those who need radical pelvic surgery and those in for emergency vascular operations require individual attention by consultant anaesthetists and consultant surgeons
- Clinical records and data collection need to be improved.

NCEPOD 1995/6 – OUT-OF-HOURS OPERATING

Reviewed 53 162 'out-of-hours' cases performed over a period equal to 1 week's work for each participating hospital.

Key points

- Decision-making – too many decisions were taken by juniors; the decision to operate should be made by consultants
- Preoperative management – guidance from experienced staff was needed, including preoperative ICU admission if necessary
- Management of intravenous fluids – was sometimes poor
- Records and charts – were often poorly kept.

Recommendations

- All hospitals admitting emergency surgical patients must be of sufficient size to provide 24-hour operating rooms. There should also be sufficient medical staff to perform these functions
- These provisions should be continuous throughout the year: trauma and acute surgical emergencies do not recognize weekends or public holidays
- Patients expect to be treated and managed by trained and competent staff. Patients assume trainees to be taught appropriately and supervised as necessary. Consultants should acknowledge these facts and react accordingly.

NCEPOD 1996/7 – SPECIFIC SURGICAL PROCEDURES

Reviewed 2541 deaths following specific surgical operations.

Recommendations

Obstructed airway in head and neck surgery. Management should be planned between surgical and anaesthetic staff. Awake fibreoptic intubation and tracheostomy using LA should be considered among the options. A fibreoptic intubating laryngoscope should be readily available for use in all surgical hospitals.

Anaesthesia for carotid endarterectomy. Invasive arterial pressure monitoring should be routine and perioperative BP control needs to be excellent.

Oesophageal surgery. Preoperative resuscitation was often inadequate. One-lung ventilation should be performed by anaesthetists with appropriate experience in the technique. Attention to postoperative respiratory care is essential to achieve a good outcome.

CVP monitoring during anaesthesia and surgery. May be indicated for patients with acute or chronic medical conditions. CVP is a core anaesthetic skill that needs regular practice.

Non-steroidal anti-inflammatory drugs. Must be used with caution in patients with renal impairment, hypertension and cardiac failure, GI ulceration and asthma.

Other recommendations. Morbidity/mortality meetings should take place in all anaesthetic departments. Surgeons need to recognize the limits of surgical procedures; a decision to operate may not be in the best interests of the patient.

NCEPOD 1997/8 – DEATHS AT THE EXTREMES OF AGE

Reviewed 19 643 deaths occurring within 30 days of surgery in children ($\leq$15 years) and elderly ($\geq$90 years).

Recommendations: Paediatric surgery

- Anaesthetic and surgical trainees need to know when they must inform their consultants before undertaking any paediatric procedures
- The death of any child within 30 days of surgery should be subjected to peer review
- The concentration of paediatric surgical services would increase expertise and reduce occasional practice.

Recommendations: Surgery for the elderly

- Fluid management is often poor and should be accorded the same status as drug prescription. Multidisciplinary reviews to develop good working practices are required
- A team of senior physicians, surgeons and anaesthetists need to be closely involved with these patients who have poor physical status and high intraoperative risk
- Pain management must be provided by those with appropriate specialized experience
- The decision to operate must be accompanied by a decision to provide appropriate postoperative care
- No elderly patient requiring an urgent operation, once fit for surgery, should wait more than 24 hours.

NCEPOD 1998/9 – ONE IN TEN SAMPLE OF DEATH

Will allow comparison with the 1992 NCEPOD report which considered one in five deaths. Will be available on NCEPOD website (www.ncepod. org.uk).

Bibliography

Buck N, Devlin HB, Lunn JN: *The Report of a Confidential Enquiry into Perioperative Deaths*, London, 1987, Nuffield Provincial Hospitals Trust and the King Edward's Hospital Fund for London.

Callum KG, Gray AJG, Hoile RW, et al: *Extremes of Age: The Report of the National Confidential Enquiry into Perioperative Deaths 1999*, London, 1999, NCEPOD.

Campling EA, Devlin HB, Lunn JN: *The Report of the National Confidential Enquiry into Perioperative Deaths 1989*, London, 1990, NCEPOD.

Campling EA, Devlin HB, Hoile RW, et al: *The Report of the National Confidential Enquiry into Perioperative Deaths 1990*, London, 1992, NCEPOD.

Campling EA, Devlin HB, Hoile RW, et al: *The Report of the National Confidential Enquiry into Perioperative Deaths 1991/2*, London, 1993, NCEPOD.

Campling EA, Devlin HB, Hoile RW, et al: *The Report of the National Confidential Enquiry into Perioperative Deaths 1992/3*, London, 1995, NCEPOD.

Campling EA, Devlin HB, Hoile RW, et al: *The Report of the National Confidential Enquiry into Perioperative Deaths 1995/6*, London, 1997, NCEPOD.

Gallimore SC, Hoile RW, Ingram GS, et al: *The Report of the National Confidential Enquiry into Perioperative Deaths 1994/5*, London, 1997, NCEPOD.

Gray AJG, Hoile RW, Ingram GS, et al: *The Report of the National Confidential Enquiry into Perioperative Deaths 1996/7*, London, 1998, NCEPOD.

Lunn JN, Devlin HB, Hoile RW: *The Report of the National Confidential Enquiry into Perioperative Deaths 1993/4*, London, 1996, NCEPOD.

SUMMARY OF THE REVISED GUIDELINES FOR THE MANAGEMENT OF MASSIVE OBSTETRIC HAEMORRHAGE

Report on Confidential Enquiries into Maternal Deaths in the United Kingdom 1994

- Summon all the extra staff required, particularly the duty anaesthetic registrar
- Inform haematology and blood transfusion
- Take blood for cross-matching and coagulation studies. Order a minimum of 6 units, only using group O Rh D-negative blood if transfusion must be given immediately. Use of packed cells requires additional colloid (gelatins or hydroxyethylstarch solutions, not dextrans) once >40% blood volume is lost
- Insert at least two 14G intravenous cannulae. CVP measurement should be continuously displayed and invasive BP is extremely useful
- Perform regular Hb, platelet and coagulation studies. Restoring normovolaemia is a priority. Consider FFP, cryoprecipitate and platelets

- Pressure bags ensure rapid fluid administration. Blood filters are rarely necessary and slow down infusion rates. Administer all fluids, and in particular blood, through a blood warmer
- Additional calcium is only necessary if there is evidence of Ca^{2+} deficiency. Use 10% calcium chloride in preference to gluconate
- Regular monitoring of pulse, BP, CVP, blood gases and urinary output. Consider early transfer to an intensive care unit.

SUMMARY OF GUIDELINES FOR THE TREATMENT OF OBSTETRIC HAEMORRHAGE IN WOMEN WHO REFUSE BLOOD TRANSFUSION

Report on Confidential Enquiries into Maternal Deaths in the United Kingdom 1996

- Mostly Jehovah's Witnesses, of which there are 125000 in the UK
- Massive obstetric haemorrhage may occur rapidly, and in patients who may refuse blood transfusion, the management of massive haemorrhage should be considered in advance
- Patients who refuse blood transfusions should be managed in a unit which has facilities for prompt management of haemorrhage, including hysterectomy
- Hb and ferritin should be monitored closely during pregnancy and haematinics used throughout pregnancy to maximize iron stores. Donation of blood for subsequent autotransfusion is inappropriate, because the amount of blood required to treat massive obstetric haemorrhage is far in excess of the amount that could be donated during pregnancy
- Extra vigilance is required in managing these patients, to detect early bleeding and clotting abnormalities. Prompt and early intervention is necessary, particularly with regard to surgery
- The consultant anaesthetist and haematologist should be informed as soon as abnormal bleeding has been detected
- Dextrans should be avoided for fluid replacement because of their possible effects on haemostasis. Intravenous crystalloid and plasma expanders such as Haemaccel should be used. Intravenous vitamin K should be given if bleeding is severe. Desmopressin, methylprednisolone and fibrinolytic inhibitors such as aprotinin and tranexamic acid should be considered
- The use of hyperbaric oxygen therapy has enabled survival with a haemoglobin concentration of 2.6 g/dl, although it is recognized that it is unrealistic to book women only where this facility is available

- If the patient refuses to accept blood or blood products, her wishes must be respected. Any adult patient (over 18 years old) who has the necessary mental capacity to do so is entitled to refuse treatment, even if the refusal is likely to result in death
- If the woman survives the acute episode, erythropoietin, parenteral iron therapy and adequate protein for haemoglobin synthesis should be given.

REPORTS ON CONFIDENTIAL ENQUIRIES INTO MATERNAL AND CHILD HEALTH

Definitions of maternal deaths

Maternal deaths. Deaths of women while pregnant or within 42 days of termination of pregnancy, from any cause related to or aggravated by the pregnancy or its management, but not accidental or incidental causes.

Direct. Deaths resulting from obstetric complications of the pregnant state, from interventions, omissions, incorrect treatment, or from a chain of events resulting from any of the above.

Indirect. Deaths resulting from previous existing disease, or disease that developed during pregnancy and which was not due to direct obstetric causes, but which was aggravated by the physiological effects of pregnancy.

Table 13.1 Direct deaths attributed to anaesthesia – United Kingdom: 1985–2005

	Number of direct deaths directly associated with anaesthesia	Rate per million maternities	Percentage of maternal deaths
1985–1987	6	2.6	4.3
1988–1990	4	1.7	2.8
1991–1993	8	3.5	6.3
1994–1996	1	0.5	0.7
1997–1999	3	1.4	2.8
2000–2002	6	3.0	5.7
2003–2005	6	2.8	4.5

Lewis, G. (ed.), 2007. The Confidential Enquiry into Maternal and Child Health (CEMACH). Saving Mothers' Lives: Reviewing Maternal Deaths to Make Motherhood Safer—2003-2005. The Seventh Report on Confidential Enquiries into Maternal Deaths in the United Kingdom. CEMACH, London.

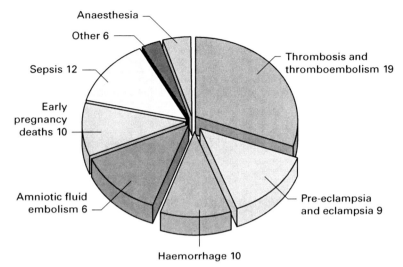

Figure 13.1 Percentage of direct deaths assessed as having substandard care by cause of death—United Kingdom: 2003–2005.

WHY MOTHERS DIE 2000–2002
Confidential Enquiries into Maternal and Child Health (CEMACH) 2005

There were 261 maternal deaths in 2000–2002, of which seven were directly attributable to anaesthesia and a further 20 in which perioperative/ anaesthesia management contributed to the death.

Key recommendations:

Service provision

Dedicated obstetric anaesthesia services should be available in all consultant obstetric units to provide high dependency care, epidural analgesia, anaesthesia and postoperative recovery. Difficult cases requiring special skills may require the assistance of anaesthetic colleagues in other subspecialties, as well as colleagues in other disciplines.

Anaesthesia training must ensure competence in airway management, especially the recognition and management of oesophageal intubation.

Obese pregnant women (BMI >35) are at greater risk from anaesthesia and should be referred to the anaesthetist early.

Supportive counselling of anaesthetic personnel involved in a maternal death is essential.

Individual practitioners

Invasive monitoring should be used, particularly in the presence of haemodynamic instability (e.g. haemorrhage). Samples for arterial blood gas estimation should be taken early and any metabolic acidosis should be taken seriously.

Care of women at high risk of, or with, major haemorrhage must involve a consultant obstetric anaesthetist at the earliest possible time. Early critical are referral and early institution of intensive therapy should be considered where appropriate.

Women with suspected raised intracranial pressure require expert neurological assessment and consultant with all appropriate specialties to determine the optimal mode of delivery.

SAVING MOTHERS' LIVES: REVIEWING MATERNAL DEATHS TO MAKE MOTHERHOOD SAFER 2003–2005
Confidential Enquiries into Maternal and Child Health (CEMACH) 2007

There were 150 maternal deaths in 2003–2005, of which six were directly attributable to anaesthesia and a further 31 in which perioperative/anaesthesia management contributed to the death.

Learning points:

Management of obstetric haemorrhage. Women with placenta praevia who have had a previous caesarean section are at risk of massive haemorrhage and should be managed in units with immediate access to blood transfusion and intensive care. These cases require consultant anaesthetist involvement.

The earlier recognition of hypovolaemia would be helped by the routine use of an early warning score system. Blood pressure parameters may need adjusting in patients with pregnancy-induced hypertension. Where there is a possibility of bleeding, a near-patient method of haemoglobin estimation may be life-saving and should be available in all obstetric units.

High volume infusions of intravenous fluid must be warmed beforehand. Women who are being resuscitated should be insulated and actively warmed. Hypothermia at temperatures <33.8°C produces a significant coagulopathy, despite the presence of normal clotting factor levels. In the situation of hypothermia and dilutional coagulopathy, both rewarming and administration of coagulation factors are required. If tachycardia persists after intraoperative haemorrhage, the woman must remain in theatre until both surgeon and anaesthetist are satisfied that her condition is stable. Invasive monitoring should be used when the cardiovascular system is compromised by haemorrhage or disease.

Uterine atony may be prevented by slow i.v. syntocinon. However, syntocinon causes hypotension, particularly in the hypovolaemic patient when it should be given slowly.

Anaesthesia and sepsis. Cardiovascular collapse can happen suddenly in septic patients. Circulatory support requires invasive monitoring and careful fluid resuscitation in a Critical Care unit or operating theatre environment.

Anaesthesia and obesity. All obstetric units should develop protocols for the management of morbidly obese women. These should include pre-assessment clinics, special ward and theatre equipment such as large blood pressure cuffs, beds and operating tables and long regional block needles. Management by consultant anaesthetists is essential and difficulties with airway management and intubation should be anticipated. Invasive arterial blood pressure measurement should be considered in morbidly obese women where NIBP is often inaccurate. All morbidly obese women in childbirth should be given prophylactic low molecular weight heparin.

Bibliography

Confidential Enquiries into Maternal and Child Health (CEMACH). Why mothers die 2000–2002: *The 6th Report of the Confidential Enquiries into Maternal Deaths in the United Kingdom*, 2005. December www.cemach.org.uk.

Confidential Enquiries into Maternal and Child Health (CEMACH). Saving mothers' lives: Reviewing maternal deaths to make motherhood safer 2003–2005: *The 7th Report of the Confidential Enquiries into Maternal Deaths in the United Kingdom*, 2007. December www.cemach.org.uk.

Appendix

SYLLABUS FOR THE PRIMARY FRCA EXAMINATION

The exams syllabus has been replaced by the 'Knowledge' sections of the Competency Based Training document for Specialty Training (ST) years 1 and 2.

The CCT in anaesthetics – Basic level syllabus

1. Preoperative assessment	II – C - 2
2. Premedication	II – C - 5
3. Anaesthesia and HDU and ICU equipment: monitoring and safety	II – C - 6
4. Induction of general anaesthesia	II – C - 8
5. Intraoperative care (including sedation)	II – C - 10
6. Postoperative and recovery care	II – C - 12
7. Intensive and high dependency care	II – C - 14
8. Regional anaesthesia	II – C - 16
9. Management of trauma, stabilization and transfer of patients	II – C - 18
10. Obstetric anaesthesia and analgesia	II – C - 20
11. Paediatric anaesthesia	II – C - 21
12. Anaesthesia and the elderly	II – C - 24
13. Pain medicine	II – C - 25
14. Infection control	II – C - 26
15. Critical incidents	II – C - 27
16. Management of respiratory and cardiac arrest	II – C - 29
17. Anatomy	II – C - 30
18. Physiology and biochemistry	II – C - 32
19. Pharmacology	II – C - 35
20. Physics and clinical measurement	II – C - 37
21. Statistical methods	II – C - 39

1: Preoperative assessment

1.1: Knowledge

B:1.1.1 Implications for anaesthesia of commoner elective conditions requiring gynaecological, abdominal, orthopaedic, ENT, dental, urological and body surface surgery. Knowledge of special interest practice and specialized techniques is not required unless specified elsewhere.

B:1.1.2 The relevance of trauma, intestinal obstruction and acute abdominal emergencies

B:1.1.3 The ASA classification and other scoring systems such as Glasgow coma scale (GCS)

B:1.1.4 The interpretation of relevant preoperative investigations

B:1.1.5 Restriction of food and fluid by mouth, cessation of smoking, correction of dehydration

B:1.1.6 Assessment of difficulties in airway management and the importance of the 'shared airway'

B:1.1.7 Implications for anaesthesia of common medical conditions (ischaemic heart disease, hypertension, diabetes, asthma, rheumatoid arthritis, etc.)

B:1.1.8 Anaesthetic implications of current drug therapy and whether it should be continued, modified stopped or changed perioperatively

B:1.1.9 Need for and methods of perioperative antithrombotic treatment

B:1.1.10 The importance of an anaesthetic history and genetic diseases in anaesthesia with respect to suxamethonium apnoea, anaphylaxis and malignant hyperpyrexia

B:1.1.11 Assessment of postoperative analgesic needs

B:1.1.12 Assessment of whether ICU or HDU care will be required postoperatively

B:1.1.13 The importance of consent and the issues surrounding it

B:1.1.14 Dangers of repeat anaesthesia

B:1.1.15 Assessment of cardiopulmonary exercise tests for the prediction of postoperative outcomes

1.2: Skills

History taking

B:1.2.1 Anaesthetic history: personal and familial

B:1.2.2 Previous airway/intubation difficulties

B:1.2.3 Medication: current and past

B:1.2.4 Allergies and previous drug reactions

B:1.2.5 Previous anaesthetic exposure and surgery

B:1.2.6 Respiratory status and symptoms (especially asthma and COPD)

B:1.2.7 Cardiovascular status and symptoms (especially IHD and hypertension)

B:1.2.8 Neurological status and symptoms (especially epilepsy, CVAs, conscious level and including mental state)

B:1.2.9 Gastrointestinal problems (especially reflux, obstruction, potentially delayed gastric emptying)

B:1.2.10 Arthropathies and other musculo-skeletal problems (especially rheumatoid arthritis)

B:1.2.11 Renal conditions

B:1.2.12 Hepatic conditions (especially jaundice, cirrhosis)

B:1.2.13 Endocrine conditions (especially diabetes, steroid therapy)

B:1.2.14 Skin conditions

B:1.2.15 Obstetric conditions

B:1.2.16 Congenital disorders affecting anaesthesia

B:1.2.17 Hereditary disorders affecting anaesthesia

B:1.2.18 Haemoglobinopathies

B:1.2.19 Coagulopathies

B:1.2.20 Nutritional abnormalities (especially obesity)

B:1.2.21 Social problems and identification of high risk groups for infection

Physical examination

B:1.2.22 Teeth/airway/cervical spine/intubation assessment

B:1.2.23 Cardiovascular system (IHD, hypertension, LVF)

B:1.2.24 Respiratory system (asthma, COPD)

B:1.2.25 Nutritional state (obesity)

B:1.2.26 Neurological system (GCS: any acute or residual effects of CVA)

B:1.2.27 Abdomen and GI tract

B:1.2.28 Anaemia

B:1.2.29 Jaundice

B:1.2.30 Sequelae of diabetes and steroids

B:1.2.31 Musculo-skeletal problems (including relevance to positioning, neck stability, regional blockade)

Data interpretation

B:1.2.32 Clinical:

B:1.2.33 Respiratory function tests

B:1.2.34 Electrocardiographs

B:1.2.35 Central venous pressure measurement

B:1.2.36 Systolic, diastolic and mean arterial pressure

B:1.2.37 Exercise tests of the cardiac and respiratory function

B:1.2.38 Interpreting fluid balance and other charts

B:1.2.39 Radiological (showing clear abnormalities):

B:1.2.40 Chest radiographs

B:1.2.41 Films showing long bone, skull, vertebral and rib fractures

B:1.2.42 Simple CAT and MRI scans of head demonstrating fractures/haemorrhage

B:1.2.43 Neck and thoracic inlet films

B:1.2.44 Films showing abdominal fluid levels/air

B:1.2.45 Laboratory:

B:1.2.46   Haematology (including coagulation and sickle tests)

B:1.2.47   Urea and electrolytes

B:1.2.48   pH and blood gases

B:1.2.49   Liver function tests

B:1.2.50   Thyroid function

Factors in special groups

B:1.2.51 Children (aged 5 years and over)

B:1.2.52 The elderly

B:1.2.53 Day-case patients

Planning

B:1.2.54 Deciding on the appropriate preoperative assessment

B:1.2.55 Deciding on an anaesthetic technique appropriate to the patient

B:1.2.56 Ensuring the necessary resources are available for safe patient care

1.3: Attitudes and behaviour

Communication

B:1.3.1 Consent for:

B:1.3.2   general anaesthesia (including a discussion of the risks)

B:1.3.3   epidural/caudal/spinal/regional/local blocks ((including a discussion of the risks)

B:1.3.4 Explanation of need for preoperative routine and specialized tests (including hepatitis screening, HIV testing and sickle cell status)

B:1.3.5 Explanation of pain management, side-effects and complications of:

B:1.3.6   oral/sublingual/rectal/subcutaneous/IM/IV/nasal/transdermal drugs

B:1.3.7   epidural/regional techniques/local blocks

B:1.3.8   inhalational analgesia

B:1.3.9   patient controlled analgesia

B:1.3.10 Discussion of preoperative medication choices

B:1.3.11 Explanation of postoperative expectations and care

B:1.3.12 Communication with other professionals

Other attitudes

B:1.3.13 Care and compassion for patients

B:1.3.14 Ability to achieve appropriate information transfer

B:1.3.15 Ethical behaviour

B:1.3.16 Professional, unemotional approach

B:1.3.17 Reassurance

B:1.3.18 Attention to detail

B:1.3.19 Punctuality

B:1.3.20 Clean neat appearance and politeness

B:1.3.21 Proper interaction with other professions and professionals

B:1.3.22 Helpfulness

1.4: *Workplace training objectives*

B:1.4.1 Able to assess the airway for potential difficulties with airway management

B:1.4.2 Able to take a relevant history

B:1.4.3 Able to interpret preoperative investigations and respond to them

B:1.4.4 Able to recognize when senior advice or assistance is required

B:1.4.5 Able to assess and plan the anaesthetic management of ASA I & II patients

B:1.4.6 Able to recognize ASA III, IV & V patients, and have a knowledge of the implications of this for anaesthesia

B:1.4.7 Able to assess the impact of the presenting surgical condition on the patient's physiological status

B:1.4.8 Able to assess suitability of patients for day-case surgery

B:1.4.9 Able to identify patients at a high risk of nausea and vomiting

B:1.4.10 Able to explain risks and options of routine anaesthesia to patients and to obtain their consent

B:1.4.11 Have a knowledge of how to deal with emergencies arising before anaesthesia and how to stabilize a patient's condition until senior assistance can arrive (see also Section 13)

2: Premedication

2.1: *Knowledge*

B:2.1.1 Rationale for use of premedicant drugs

B:2.1.2 Choice of drugs, advantages and disadvantages

B:2.1.3 Rationale for antacid, and prokinetic premedication

B:2.1.4 Rationale for antithrombotic therapy

B:2.1.5 Understanding of causes of delayed gastric emptying

2.2: *Skills*

B:2.2.1 Assessment of level of anxiety and address patient's concerns

B:2.2.2 Recognition of situations leading to delayed gastric emptying

B:2.2.3 Checking a patient prior to premedication and on arrival in the anaesthetic room/theatre

2.3: *Attitudes and behaviour*

B:2.3.1 Able to reassure patient and allay anxiety

B:2.3.2 Explain (as appropriate) problems/complications to patients/ relatives concerning:

B:2.3.3 • difficult intubation and dentition

B:2.3.4 • sore throat, nausea and vomiting

B:2.3.5 • thrombophlebitis

B:2.3.6 • post-spinal headache

B:2.3.7 • suxamethonium apnoea and pains

B:2.3.8 • anaphylaxis

B:2.3.9 • malignant hyperpyrexia

2.4: Workplace training objectives

B:2.4.1 To become practised at answering patients questions in the most appropriate way

B:2.4.2 To always try to alleviate anxiety

B:2.4.3 To ensure thromboprophylaxis is considered

B:2.4.4 To gain a knowledge of the properties and effects of premedicant drugs

3: Anaesthesia, HDU and ICU equipment: monitoring and safety

3.1: Knowledge

B:3.1.1 Physical principles underlying the function of the anaesthetic machine, pressure regulators, flowmeters, vaporizers, breathing systems

B:3.1.2 Chemistry of absorption of carbon dioxide

B:3.1.3 Principles of lung ventilators, disconnection monitors

B:3.1.4 Manufacture and storage of oxygen, nitrous oxide, carbon dioxide, compressed air

B:3.1.5 Pipeline and suction systems, gas cylinders

B:3.1.6 Minimum monitoring requirements

B:3.1.7 Basis for pre-use checks of anaesthetic machine, breathing systems and monitoring apparatus

B:3.1.8 Airways, tracheal tubes, tracheostomy tubes, emergency airways, laryngeal masks, fixed and variable performance oxygen therapy equipment, self-inflating bags

B:3.1.9 The content of an anaesthetic record

B:3.1.10 **Function and use of resuscitation equipment, transfusion devices**

B:3.1.11 Humidification devices

B:3.1.12 Environmental control of the operating theatre including temperature, humidity, air changes and scavenging systems for waste anaesthetic gases and vapours

B:3.1.13 Sterilization and cleaning of equipment

B:3.1.14 Electrical safety

B:3.1.15 Characteristics of intravenous cannulae, spinal and epidural needles

3.2: Skills

B:3.2.1 Checking the anaesthetic machine

B:3.2.2 Checking pipelines

B:3.2.3 Changing and checking cylinders

B:3.2.4 Connecting up breathing systems

B:3.2.5 Checking breathing systems

B:3.2.6 Setting up/checking/monitoring lung ventilators

B:3.2.7 Setting up/checking alarm limits for monitoring equipment

B:3.2.8 Collecting data from monitors

B:3.2.9 Record-keeping

B:3.2.10 Checking resuscitation equipment

B:3.2.11 Assembling resuscitation equipment

B:3.2.12 Selecting defibrillator settings

B:3.2.13 Recognizing machine, breathing system and equipment errors: miss-assembly and disconnections

B:3.2.14 Composing equipment checklists for:

B:3.2.15 • resuscitation equipment

B:3.2.16 • difficult and failed intubation

B:3.2.17 • CVP monitoring

B:3.2.18 • arterial pressure monitoring

B:3.2.19 • epidural/spinal packs

B:3.2.20 • paediatric intubation set

3.3: Attitudes and behaviour

B:3.3.1 Recognition that anaesthetic equipment comprises anaesthesia tool kit

B:3.3.2 Shared responsibility for equipment with theatre staff

B:3.3.3 Commitment to understand as fully as possible the working principles of all anaesthetic equipment

B:3.3.4 Determination to maximize safety, and not to compromise it by accepting substandard equipment both as to range and quality

3.4: Workplace training objectives

B:3.4.1 To check anaesthesia machine

B:3.4.2 To assemble and check breathing systems

B:3.4.3 To set up and check ventilator

B:3.4.4 To describe the requirements for minimal monitoring

B:3.4.5 To decide when additional monitoring (e.g. CVP, arterial line) is needed

B:3.4.6 To set up and check monitoring equipment and alarm limits

B:3.4.7 To check resuscitation equipment

B:3.4.8 To keep a good anaesthetic record

4: Induction of general anaesthesia

4.1: Knowledge

B:4.1.1 Intravenous and inhalational induction of anaesthesia; advantages and disadvantages of each technique

B:4.1.2 Indications for tracheal intubation

B:4.1.3 Selection of tube type (oral, nasal, armoured, etc.), diameter and length

B:4.1.4 Management of difficult intubation and failed intubation

B:4.1.5 Methods of confirming placement of the endotracheal tube; oesophageal and endobronchial intubation, complications

B:4.1.6 Insertion and use of oral airways, face masks and laryngeal mask airway

B:4.1.7 Causes of regurgitation and vomiting during induction, prevention and management of pulmonary aspiration

B:4.1.8 Cricoid pressure

B:4.1.9 Induction of anaesthesia in special circumstances (head injury, full stomach, upper airway obstruction, shock)

B:4.1.10 Drugs: pharmacology and dosages of induction agents, relaxants, analgesics, and inhalational agents and types of drug error: wrong drug, dose, route; use of safe practice to minimize risks

B:4.1.11 Side-effects of drugs used and their interactions

B:4.1.12 Monitoring during induction

B:4.1.13 Recognition and management of anaphylactic and anaphylactoid reactions including follow-up and patient information

B:4.1.14 Management of intra-arterial injection of harmful substances (e.g. antibiotics, thiopental)

B:4.1.15 Management of asthma, COPD, hypertension, IHD, rheumatoid arthritis

B:4.1.16 Problems of the obese patient

4.2: Skills

B:4.2.1 i.v. and inhalational induction of anaesthesia in patients with elective and urgent conditions requiring gynaecological, abdominal, orthopaedic, ENT, dental, urological and body surface surgery. (Knowledge of special interest practice and specialized techniques is not required unless specified elsewhere.)

B:4.2.2 Checking patient in the anaesthetic room

B:4.2.3 Safety checking of equipment (see Section 7)

B:4.2.4 Obtaining vascular access – suitability of sites and technique of intravenous injection

B:4.2.5 Airway assessment and optimizing the patient's position for airway management

B:4.2.6 Airway management with mask and oral/nasal airways

B:4.2.7 Introduction and checking correct placement of laryngeal mask airway

B:4.2.8 Appropriate choice and passage of oral and nasal endotracheal tubes

B:4.2.9 Intubation up to grade II Cormack–Lehane

B:4.2.10 Use of gum elastic bougie and stilette

B:4.2.11 Identifying correct/incorrect placement of tube (oesophagus/main bronchus)

B:4.2.12 Interpretation of capnograph trace

B:4.2.13 Failed intubation drill

B:4.2.14 Rapid sequence induction/cricoid pressure

B:4.2.15 Checking difficult intubation kit and paediatric intubation set

B:4.2.16 Use of monitoring equipment, including application of ECG electrodes

B:4.2.17 Managing of cardiovascular and respiratory changes during and after induction of general anaesthesia

B:4.2.18 Appropriate safe practice in selecting, checking, drawing up, diluting, labelling and administration of drugs

4.3: Attitudes and behaviour

B:4.3.1 Safety first

B:4.3.2 Always knowing the whereabouts of senior assistance

B:4.3.3 Being clear in explanations to patient and staff

B:4.3.4 Being reassuring to patients during induction of anaesthesia

B:4.3.5 Being polite, calm and having a professional approach

4.4: Workplace training objectives

B:4.4.1 To perform routine intravenous induction of anaesthesia

B:4.4.2 To perform routine gaseous induction of anaesthesia

B:4.4.3 To identify the correct placement of the endotracheal tube after intubation

B:4.4.4 To rehearse failed intubation drill

B:4.4.5 To discuss induction of general anaesthesia in difficult airways, shocked patients and others of ASA>II

B:4.4.6 To manage the cardiovascular and respiratory complications of induction of general anaesthesia

B:4.4.7 To describe the management of aspiration, anaphylaxis, failed intubation and malignant hyperpyrexia

5: Intraoperative care (including sedation)

5.1: Knowledge

B:5.1.1 Techniques of maintenance of general anaesthesia involving both spontaneous and controlled ventilation (except special interest and highly specialized practice)

B:5.1.2 Definition of and methods of sedation

B:5.1.3 Management of the shared airway

B:5.1.4 Effects and hazards of the pneumoperitoneum induced for laparoscopic surgery

B:5.1.5 Drugs: pharmacology, uses and dosages of induction agents used for i.v. maintenance, relaxants, analgesics, inhalational agents

B:5.1.6 Methods of producing muscle relaxation

B:5.1.7 Choice of spontaneous and controlled ventilation and methods of monitoring them

B:5.1.8 Minimum monitoring standards

B:5.1.9 Additional monitoring for sick patients (e.g. CVP, urine flow)

B:5.1.10 Detection and prevention of awareness

B:5.1.11 Management of important critical incidents occurring during anaesthesia

B:5.1.12 Diagnosis and treatment of pneumothorax

B:5.1.13 Principles of fluid balance

B:5.1.14 Blood and blood products; synthetic colloids; crystalloids

B:5.1.15 Management of massive haemorrhage, volume expansion, blood transfusion (hazards including incompatibility reaction)

B:5.1.16 Correct intraoperative positioning on theatre table, care of pressure points, avoidance of nerve injury: complications of supine and prone positions

B:5.1.17 Management of asthma, COPD, hypertension, IHD, rheumatoid arthritis, jaundice, steroid therapy, diabetes

B:5.1.18 Content of the anaesthetic record

B:5.1.19 Modification of technique in repeat anaesthesia

B:5.1.20 Understanding basic surgical operations

5.2: Skills

B:5.2.1 Maintenance of appropriate levels of anaesthesia with inhalational and intravenous agents in patients with elective and urgent conditions requiring gynaecological, abdominal, orthopaedic, ENT, dental, urological and body surface surgery. (Knowledge of special interest practice and specialized techniques is not required unless specified elsewhere.)

B:5.2.2 Transferring the patient from trolley to operating table

B:5.2.3 Positioning the patient

B:5.2.4 Airway control: recognition and correction of problems

B:5.2.5 Laryngoscopy and intubation and its problems

B:5.2.6 Detection and correction of airway obstruction

B:5.2.7 Use of oral airways, facemasks and laryngeal mask airway

B:5.2.8 Sharing the airway

B:5.2.9 Management of appropriate intermittent positive pressure ventilation

B:5.2.10 Methods of pain relief during maintenance

B:5.2.11 Management of effects of drugs used during anaesthesia

B:5.2.12 Management of hypo- and hypertension

B:5.2.13 Provision of intraoperative fluids; transfusion of blood and blood products

B:5.2.14 Management of diabetes

B:5.2.15 Methods of detection of awareness

B:5.2.16 Management of appropriate muscle relaxation

B:5.2.17 Management of any critical incidents which occur during anaesthesia

B:5.2.18 Interpretation and limitations of monitoring equipment

5.3: *Attitudes and behaviour*

B:5.3.1 Vigilance

B:5.3.2 Attention to detail

B:5.3.3 Attention to multiple sources of data continuously

B:5.3.4 Recognition of need to communicate with colleagues

5.4: *Workplace training objectives*

B:5.4.1 To manage anaesthetized spontaneously breathing patients

B:5.4.2 To manage anaesthetized ventilated patients

B:5.4.3 To manage sedated patients

B:5.4.4 To manage diabetes perioperatively

B:5.4.5 To manage steroid cover

B:5.4.6 To check blood and blood products

B:5.4.7 To apply and interpret appropriate monitoring

B:5.4.8 To know how to deal with emergencies as they occur in anaesthesia and how to stabilize a patient's condition until senior assistance arrives

B:5.4.9 To plan ahead with the surgeon any unusual requirements of anaesthesia

6. Postoperative and recovery care

6.1: *Knowledge*

B:6.1.1 Causes and treatment of failure to breathe at end of operation

B:6.1.2 Distinguishing between opiate excess, continued anaesthetic effect and/or residual paralysis

B:6.1.3 Care of the unconscious patient

B:6.1.4 Monitoring the patient in recovery

B:6.1.5 Interpretation of nerve stimulator patterns

B:6.1.6 Oxygen therapy, indications and techniques

B:6.1.7 Management of cyanosis, hypo- and hypertension, shivering and stridor

B:6.1.8 Postoperative fluid balance and prescribing

B:6.1.9 Assessment of pain and methods of pain management

B:6.1.10 Methods of treating of postoperative nausea and vomiting

B:6.1.11 Causes and management of postoperative confusion

B:6.1.12 Management of asthma, COPD, hypertension, IHD, rheumatoid arthritis, jaundice, steroid therapy, diabetes

B:6.1.13 Management of the obese patient

B:6.1.14 Recovery room equipment

B:6.1.15 Prevention, diagnosis and management of postoperative pulmonary atelectasis, deep vein thrombosis and pulmonary embolus

B:6.1.16 Criteria for discharge of day-stay patients

6.2: Skills

B:6.2.1 Recovery from anaesthesia in patients with elective and urgent conditions requiring gynaecological, abdominal, orthopaedic, ENT, dental, urological and body surface surgery. (Knowledge of special interest practice and specialized techniques is not required unless specified elsewhere.)

B:6.2.2 Clear instructions during handover of patient to recovery staff

B:6.2.3 Assessment of full return of protective reflexes

B:6.2.4 Assessment of adequacy of ventilation/reversal

B:6.2.5 Recognition of residual relaxant action

B:6.2.6 Use of nerve stimulator

B:6.2.7 Extubation and airway protection in presence of potentially full stomach

B:6.2.8 Prescription of postoperative fluids

B:6.2.9 Assessment of fluid balance and need for urethral catheterization

B:6.2.10 Evaluation and management of postoperative confusion

B:6.2.11 Assessment of postoperative pain

B:6.2.12 Prescription of postoperative pain regimen

B:6.2.13 Treatment of nausea and vomiting

B:6.2.14 Stabilization before discharge from Recovery

B:6.2.15 Continuation of care until discharge from Recovery, and beyond as appropriate

B:6.2.16 Criteria for discharge of patients to ward

B:6.2.17 Criteria for discharge of day-stay patients

6.3: Attitudes and behaviour

B:6.3.1 Clear communication

B:6.3.2 Responding rapidly to calls for help

B:6.3.3 Follow-up of sick patients on the ward before going home

6.4: Workplace training objectives

B:6.4.1 To achieve a smooth, controlled return of vital functions and reflexes

B:6.4.2 To practice giving clear instructions to recovery staff

B:6.4.3 To be able to discharge patients safely back to the ward

B:6.4.4 To know the criteria for discharge of day-stay patients

B:6.4.5 To recognize and treat common recovery room complications

B:6.4.6 To recognize and treat conditions and circumstances requiring HDU or ICU care

B:6.4.7 To know the equipment requirements of a recovery room

7: Intensive and high dependency care

During ST Years 1 and 2 trainees in anaesthesia are required to spend a total of 3 months in intensive care training. The basic level knowledge, skills and attitudes lists below are compatible with the recommendations of the Intercollegiate

Board for Training in Intensive Care Medicine (IBTICM) for this level of training in intensive care medicine. Because these are reproduced in full, there is obviously repetition of material that appears in other sections. There is, in addition, guidance on assessment for ICM.

7.1: Knowledge

B:7.1.1 An understanding of the potential benefits of high dependency and intensive care

B:7.1.2 Common causes of admission to high dependency and intensive care

B:7.1.3 Method of examination of the unconscious patient

B:7.1.4 The principles of brainstem death diagnosis

B:7.1.5 An understanding of sepsis and the basic patterns of failure of the major organs

B:7.1.6 The common causes of cardiac and respiratory arrest

B:7.1.7 The anatomy of the oropharynx, larynx, trachea and bronchial tree

B:7.1.8 Basic anatomy of neck, upper thorax, arms, wrists, inguinal region and foot relevant to insertion of venous and arterial access

B:7.1.9 Method of inserting a chest drain and relief of tension pneumothorax

B:7.1.10 Understanding of the choice of intravenous fluids appropriate for use in major fluid loss, and their pharmacology

B:7.1.11 The recognition of basic cardiac dysrhythmias and the current therapies (physical (carotid sinus massage), electrical (defibrillation and countershock), electrolytic (Mg^{++}, Ca^{++}), and pharmacological (adrenaline (epinephrine), atropine, lidocaine and 2nd line drugs))

B:7.1.12 Pharmacology of the common inotropic agents used in the critically ill (adrenaline (epinephrine), noradrenaline (norepinephrine))

B:7.1.13 Pharmacology of major analgesics used as respiratory depressants (morphine, fentanyl series), and common side-effects and contraindications

B:7.1.14 Pharmacology of common muscle relaxants (depolarizing and non-depolarizing) and common side-effects and contraindications

B:7.1.15 Pharmacology of intravenous sedative and anaesthetic induction agents used in the critical care unit

B:7.1.16 Thromboprophylaxis in intensive and high dependency patients

B:7.1.17 Choice of antibiotics

B:7.1.18 Use of diuretics for cardiac and respiratory failure and to maintain urine output

B:7.1.19 The basic cardiac and respiratory physiology

B:7.1.20 The basic physiology of respiration and the consequences of positive pressure ventilation

B:7.1.21 An understanding of common blood gas abnormalities

B:7.1.22 An understanding of the use of ventilation in use on critically ill patients, with a knowledge of the vocabulary

B:7.1.23 An understanding of the uses and limitations of monitoring equipment

B:7.1.24 The content of an ICU record

B:7.1.25 An insight into likely outcome based upon severity scoring

B:7.1.26 The grief response

7.2: Skills

B:7.2.1 Cardiopulmonary resuscitation

B:7.2.2 Maintenance of a clear airway using bag and mask

B:7.2.3 Insertion of an endotracheal tube, via the oral route

B:7.2.4 Change of tracheostomy tube

B:7.2.5 Examination and care of the unconscious patient

B:7.2.6 Insertion of adequate peripheral venous access sufficient to manage major haemorrhage

B:7.2.7 Insertion of central venous and arterial cannulae

B:7.2.8 Institution and maintenance of controlled mechanical ventilation in a critically ill patient

B:7.2.9 Ability to summarize and provide a succinct analysis of the patient's medical history, ongoing therapies and expected problems to medical and nursing colleagues

B:7.2.10 Good communication with patients, relatives and staff

B:7.2.11 Ability to explain and discuss the nature of the patient's illness with relatives

7.3: Attitudes and behaviour

B:7.3.1 Understanding of the needs and behaviour of worried and grieving relatives

B:7.3.2 Commitment to good communication

B:7.3.3 Willingness to accept failures of therapy

B:7.3.4 Involving others with specialist skills

B:7.3.5 Recognition of team approach

7.4: Workplace training objectives

B:7.4.1 To gain the skills and confidence to resuscitate adult patients following cardio-pulmonary arrest

B:7.4.2 To care for the unconscious patient

B:7.4.3 To recognize of an adult critically ill patient and begin resuscitation with appropriate urgency

B:7.4.4 To communicate well with the nursing staff in the ICU, patients, relatives and other hospital staff

B:7.4.5 To recognize one's own limitations and the nature and importance of team working

B:7.4.6 To make clear presentations of patients to other medical and nursing staff

B:7.4.7 To offer comfort to patient and relatives when there is no prospect of survival

Assessment guidelines
- Ward based assessment of interaction with relatives by feedback from senior nursing staff
- Ward based assessment of interaction with nursing staff
- Ward based observation of skills in airway control and vascular access
- Training room based assessment of resuscitation skills (unless having completed ALS course within the last 12 months). This could be undertaken by a Resuscitation Training Officer
- Oral assessment of pharmacology and physiology in ICU setting
- Observation during presentation of assignment during weekly seminar/ teaching session

8: Regional anaesthesia

Regional techniques are integral components of anaesthesia in the UK, but the College recognizes that it is inappropriate to expect that every trainee will become competent in every possible block technique, although they must be competent in all the generic aspects of block performance. All trainee anaesthetists are expected to be able to perform both spinal and lumbar epidural block, but Schools of Anaesthesia will vary in the range of other blocks to which trainees can be exposed. The basic level curriculum thus indicates which other blocks might be learned at this stage, but only if appropriate opportunities are available. Assessments should be as outlined in Section 1.2, for spinal and lumbar epidural blocks, and trainees must recognize that they should not attempt blocks until they have received supervised training, and passed the relevant assessment.

8.1: Knowledge

B:8.1.1 Pharmacology of local anaesthetics and spinal opioids

B:8.1.2 Anatomy of spine, nerve roots, cauda equina, intercostal nerves, brachial plexus, femoral nerve, inguinal canal, nerves at wrist and ankle, nerve supply of larynx

B:8.1.3 Dermatomes and levels for common operations (e.g. inguinal hernia, haemorrhoids)

B:8.1.4 Technique of spinal and epidural (including caudal) anaesthesia: single shot and catheter techniques

B:8.1.5 Management of the complications of spinal and epidural (including caudal) analgesia (associated hypotension, shivering, nausea and anxiety)

B:8.1.6 Management of accidental total spinal blockade

B:8.1.7 Management of dural tap

B:8.1.8 Techniques and complications of intravenous regional anaesthesia (IVRA)

B:8.1.9 Toxicity of local anaesthetic agents and its management

B:8.1.10 Management of failed/deteriorating regional block

B:8.1.11 Methods of sedation

B:8.1.12 Absolute and relative contraindications to regional blockade

B:8.1.13 Dangers of accidental intravenous administration of local anaesthetic drugs

8.2: Skills

B:8.2.1 Technique of spinal and epidural (including caudal) analgesia in any suitable patients

B:8.2.2 Recognition of contraindicated or unsuitable patients or those in whom a block would be difficult to perform

B:8.2.3 Management of hypotension, nausea, anxiety and shivering induced by spinal or epidural blockade

B:8.2.4 Postoperative care following spinal or epidural block (including urinary retention)

B:8.2.5 Prescription of continuous epidural infusions

B:8.2.6 Use of epidural techniques for postoperative pain management

B:8.2.7 Checking epidural/spinal packs

B:8.2.8 Technique of intravenous regional anaesthesia (IVRA)

B:8.2.9 Performance of some simple peripheral nerve blocks

B:8.2.10 Use of drugs to provide sedation

B:8.2.11 Combined general and regional anaesthesia

B:8.2.12 Appropriate safe practice in selecting, checking, drawing up, diluting, labelling and administration of local anaesthetic agents

8.3: Attitudes and behaviour

B:8.3.1 Safety first

B:8.3.2 Considering views of patient and surgeon

B:8.3.3 Management of theatre environment with awake patient

B:8.3.4 Planning list to allow block to take effect

B:8.3.5 Communication and reassurance

B:8.3.6 Consent for regional blockade

8.4: Workplace training objectives

B:8.4.1 To obtain consent from patients

B:8.4.2 To create a safe and supportive environment in theatre

B:8.4.3 To position patients and to instruct and use assistants properly

B:8.4.4 To establish spinal and epidural blockade

B:8.4.5 To maintain epidural blockade using top up and continuous techniques with local anaesthetics and opioids

B:8.4.6 To perform IVRA

B:8.4.7 To perform some simple peripheral nerve blocks

B:8.4.8 To know the criteria for the safe discharge of patients from recovery

9: Management of trauma, stabilization and transfer of patients

9.1 Knowledge

B:9.1.1 Performance and interpretation of the primary and secondary survey

B:9.1.2 Emergency airway management

B:9.1.3 Anatomy and technique of cricothyrotomy/tracheostomy/mini-tracheotomy

B:9.1.4 Establishing i.v. access: interosseous cannulation

B:9.1.5 Immediate specific treatment of life-threatening illness or injury, with special reference to thoracic and abdominal trauma

B:9.1.6 Recognition and management of hypovolaemic shock

B:9.1.7 Effects of trauma on gastric emptying

B:9.1.8 Central venous access: anatomy and techniques

B:9.1.9 Central venous pressure monitoring

B:9.1.10 Arterial pressure monitoring

B:9.1.11 Pleural drain insertion

B:9.1.12 Peritoneal lavage

B:9.1.13 Principles of the management of head injury

B:9.1.14 Mechanisms and effects of raised intracranial pressure: coup and contra-coup injuries

B:9.1.15 Methods of preventing the 'second insult' to the brain

B:9.1.16 Principles of anaesthesia in the presence of a recent head injury

B:9.1.17 Management of cervical spine injuries

B:9.1.18 Principles of the safe transfer of patients

B:9.1.19 Understanding portable monitoring systems

B:9.1.20 Recognition and management of dilutional coagulopathy

B:9.1.21 Factors affecting intraocular pressure

9.2: Skills

B:9.2.1 Assessment and immediate management of trauma patient: primary and secondary survey

B:9.2.2 Glasgow coma scale

B:9.2.3 Recognition of need for appropriate investigations (Hb, cross-match, chest X-ray, etc.)

B:9.2.4 Assessment and management of circulatory shock

B:9.2.5 Emergency airway management, oxygen therapy and ventilation

B:9.2.6 Chest drain insertion and management: emergency relief of tension pneumothorax

B:9.2.7 Cannulation of major vessels for resuscitation and monitoring

B:9.2.8 Care and immobilization of cervical spine

B:9.2.9 Transfers within and between hospitals of adults who do not have life-threatening conditions or a severe head injury

B:9.2.10 Analgesia for trauma victim

B:9.2.11 Urinary catheterization in traumatized patient

B:9.2.12 Establishing central venous pressure monitoring: interpretation of readings

B:9.2.13 Establishing arterial pressure monitoring: interpretation of readings

B:9.2.14 Anaesthesia in the presence of a recent head injury (which itself does not require surgery)

B:9.2.15 Anaesthesia for a penetrating eye injury

B:9.2.16 Ability to deal with emergencies before, during and after anaesthesia and the ability to stabilize a patient's condition until senior assistance arrives

9.3: Attitudes and behaviour

B:9.3.1 Trauma matters: importance of speed of response and proper resuscitation

B:9.3.2 Try to offer the best chance of survival

B:9.3.3 Focus on the golden hour

B:9.3.4 Communication with appropriate specialists

B:9.3.5 Ability to take control when either appropriate or necessary

B:9.3.6 Insist on stabilization before transfer

B:9.3.7 Pretransfer checking of kit and personnel

B:9.3.8 Communication with relatives

9.4: Workplace training objectives

B:9.4.1 To perform assessment, immediate care and management of the traumatized patient (including the principles of managing a head injury)

B:9.4.2 To stabilize a patient's condition until senior assistance arrives

B:9.4.3 To know when to get senior or other specialist help

B:9.4.4 To know how to deal with emergencies related to trauma before, during and after anaesthesia

B:9.4.5 To transfer a *stable* ventilated patient safely to another site, either in the same or in a different hospital

10: Obstetric anaesthesia and analgesia

10.1: Knowledge

B:10.1.1 Physiological changes associated with a normal pregnancy

B:10.1.2 Functions of the placenta: placental transfer: feto-maternal circulation

B:10.1.3 The fetus: fetal circulation: changes at birth

B:10.1.4 Pain pathways relevant to labour

B:10.1.5 Methods of analgesia during labour: indications and contraindications

B:10.1.6 Effect of pregnancy on the technique of general and regional anaesthesia

B:10.1.7 Principles of anaesthesia for incidental surgery during pregnancy

10.2: Skills (to observe or perform)

B:10.2.1 Preoperative assessment of pregnant patient

B:10.2.2 Anaesthesia for retained products of conception

B:10.2.3 Analgesia for labour

B:10.2.4 Management of APH and PPH

B:10.2.5 Management of dilutional coagulopathy

B:10.2.6 Intubation problems in the full-term mother

B:10.2.7 Anaesthesia/analgesia for instrumental delivery

B:10.2.8 Anaesthesia for retained placenta

B:10.2.9 Anaesthesia for caesarean section

10.3: Attitudes and behaviour

B:10.3.1 Attempt by conscientious care to recognize problems early

B:10.3.2 Seek senior help early

B:10.3.3 Good communication with mother, partner and other family members

B:10.3.4 Calmness under pressure

B:10.3.5 Timely assistance and prompt response to requests for analgesia and help

B:10.3.6 Reassurance to the mother

B:10.3.7 Compassion and kindness when the outcome of labour has been poor

10.4: Workplace training objectives

B:10.4.1 All trainees should have an attachment to an obstetric service to observe and preferably perform the listed skills. Before progressing to indirect supervision trainees must successfully complete the workplace assessment of the basic competences for obstetric anaesthesia described in Section 1.2 of *The CCT in Anaesthetics II*. If a trainee repeatedly fails to pass the assessment of basic competency they may not be signed off for the competences listed in Sections 10.1 to 10.3 above, and such a trainee must not work on an obstetric unit without direct supervision

11: Paediatric anaesthesia

11.1: Knowledge (infants and children)

B:11.1.1 Anatomical differences in the airway, head, and spinal cord from the adult

B:11.1.2 Deciduous and permanent dentition

B:11.1.3 Physiological differences from the adult

B:11.1.4 Haematological and biochemical changes with age

B:11.1.5 Estimation of blood volume, replacement of fluid loss

B:11.1.6 Modification of drug dosages

B:11.1.7 Analgesia for children

B:11.1.8 Premedication, including local anaesthesia for venepuncture

B:11.1.9 Calculation of tube sizes, selection of masks and airways

B:11.1.10 Choice of breathing system

B:11.1.11 Upper respiratory tract infections and when to cancel operations

B:11.1.12 Psychological aspects of sick children

11.2: Skills (aged 5 and above, unless otherwise stated)

B:11.2.1 Preoperative assessment of the previously fit child

B:11.2.2 Anaesthesia in fit children for elective and urgent general, ENT, and ophthalmic surgery, minor trauma and other non-specialist procedures

B:11.2.3 Venous access (including local anaesthesia premedication)

B:11.2.4 Airway management, selection of correct sized tubes and masks, etc.

B:11.2.5 i.v. and gaseous induction of general anaesthesia

B:11.2.6 Spontaneous and ventilated maintenance of anaesthesia

B:11.2.7 Caudal and other simple blocks

B:11.2.8 Management and stabilization of the injured child (excluding neonates and infants) until senior help arrives

B:11.2.9 Paediatric resuscitation (practised in a resuscitation teaching session) as described by the Resuscitation Council (UK)

11.3: Attitudes and behaviour

B:11.3.1 Communication with the child and parents

B:11.3.2 Reassurance for the child and parents

B:11.3.3 Issues of consent

B:11.3.4 Management of the environment during induction of anaesthesia

11.4: Workplace training objectives

B:11.4.1 The variation in paediatric exposure will vary greatly among trainees during ST Years 1 and 2. Trainees should take whatever opportunities they can to obtain the skills in the list above. It is accepted that not all trainees will have sufficient clinical opportunity to progress beyond direct supervision

11.5: Training in child protection

Anaesthetists of all grades may encounter children who have suffered physical and/or sexual abuse in various situations:

1. Resuscitation of a critically ill child who has sustained an injury under circumstances that cannot wholly be explained by natural circumstances or is consistent with intentional trauma or abuse

2. In the paediatric intensive care unit, e.g. following severe head injury, where the above needs to be considered

3. When called upon to anaesthetize a child for a formal forensic examination, possibly involving colposcopy, sigmoidoscopy and the collection of specimens. This may also include medical photography/video records

4. Rarely a child may tell the anaesthetist about abuse ('disclosure')

5. During the course of a routine preoperative examination or surgical procedure, the anaesthetist or surgeon notes unusual or unexplained signs which may be indicative of physical or sexual abuse

In all these situations, it is essential that healthcare professionals, including the anaesthetist, act in the best interests of the child.

11.5.1: Knowledge
B:11.5.1.1 Situations in which abuse of children may present

B:11.5.1.2 Signs indicative of a possible need to safeguard the infant or child

B:11.5.1.3 Awareness of local CP procedures

11.5.2: Skills
B:11.5.2.1 Clearly communicate concerns (includes documentation)

B:11.5.2.2 Ability to manage the child and their parents in a sensitive, appropriate manner

11.5.3: Attitudes and behaviour
B:11.5.3.1 Understands need to communicate concerns within team

B:11.5.3.2 Asks for senior and/or paediatrician support when appropriate

11.5.4: Workplace and training objectives
B:11.5.4.1 Demonstrates knowledge of local safeguarding children procedures

11.5.5: Additional notes
It is suggested that this training can be achieved in a 1 hour scenario based discussion or PBL format. In addition, all trainees should be familiar with the RCoA/APA/RCPCH Guideline *Child Protection and the Anaesthetist: Safeguarding Children in the Operating Theatre.*

General principles – What to do if child abuse or neglect is suspected

- *Good communication is essential.* Anaesthetists are advised not to intervene alone, and suspicions should be discussed with the individual identified in the local guideline. In particular it would *not* be appropriate to institute or initiate formal *examination* while the child is anaesthetized, as separate consent is required
- Further management needs to be agreed in conjunction with the paediatrician, surgeon and anaesthetist. Consideration needs to be given to:
  - Informing the parents (except in the case of fabricated or fictitious illness and child sexual abuse)
  - Further assessment
  - Informing social services and/or the police
- Full documentation is essential
- The paediatrician should lead this process, and may seek advice from the Named or Designated doctor for child protection

Duties of the anaesthetist
- To act in the best interests of the child
- To be aware of the child's rights to be protected
- To respect the rights of the child to confidentiality
- To contact a paediatrician with experience of child protection for advice (on-call paediatrician for Named or Designated doctor/nurse)
- To be aware of the local chid protection mechanisms
- To be aware of the rights of those with parental responsibility

12: Anaesthesia and the elderly

12.1: Knowledge

B:12.1.1 Physiological changes with age

B:12.1.2 Altered pharmacological response

B:12.1.3 Erosion of physiological reserve

B:12.1.4 Frequent co-morbidities

B:12.1.5 Positioning difficulties

B:12.1.6 Communication difficulties (eyesight, hearing, CVAs)

B:12.1.7 Mental clarity, memory loss

B:12.1.8 Causes of postoperative confusion

B:12.1.9 Importance of social circumstances

12.2: Skills

B:12.2.1 Modifications necessary when anaesthetizing the elderly

B:12.2.2 Management of postoperative confusion

12.3: Attitudes and behaviour

B:12.3.1 Special efforts to communicate clearly (NB deafness and blindness)

B:12.3.2 Old people have feelings too

B:12.3.3 Respect for the social norms of older people

B:12.3.4 Problems of consent in mental infirmity

B:12.3.5 Recognizing the limitations of therapy

B:12.3.6 Ethics of 'do not resuscitate' orders

12.4: Workplace training objectives

B:12.4.1 When anaesthetizing elderly patients to be aware of the special problems they pose

13: Pain medicine

13.1: Knowledge

B:13.1.1 Afferent nociceptive pathways, dorsal horn, peripheral and central mechanisms, neuromodulatory systems, supraspinal mechanisms

B:13.1.2 Nociceptive pain, visceral pain, neuropathic pain

B:13.1.3 Influence of therapy on nociceptive mechanisms

B:13.1.4 The analgesic ladder

B:13.1.5 Simple analgesics: drugs and mechanisms

B:13.1.6 Opioids: drugs and mechanisms

B:13.1.7 Non-steroidal anti-inflammatory agents: drugs and mechanisms

B:13.1.8 Local anaesthetic agents: drugs and mechanisms

B:13.1.9 Measurement of pain

B:13.1.10 Organization and objectives of an acute pain service

13.2: Skills

B:13.2.1 Assessment and management of postoperative pain and nausea

B:13.2.2 Monitoring acute pain and pain relieving methods

B:13.2.3 Use of simple analgesics: paracetamol: NSAIDs

B:13.2.4 Opioids: intramuscular, intravenous infusion, intravenous PCA, subcutaneous PCA, epidural, intrathecal

B:13.2.5 Regional local anaesthetic techniques: lumbar epidural, caudal epidural, simple peripheral nerve blocks

B:13.2.6 Inhalational analgesia

B:13.2.7 Specific clinical groups: children, elderly, impaired consciousness, intensive care

B:13.2.8 Contributing to an acute pain service

13.3: Attitudes and behaviour

B:13.3.1 Communication with patients, relatives, staff

B:13.3.2 Rapid response to unrelieved pain

B:13.3.3 Management tempered by awareness of potential complications and side-effects

B:13.3.4 Awareness of limitations in pain management

B:13.3.5 Making efforts to follow patients up on the wards

B:13.3.6 Recognition of need for team approach and partnerships in a pain team

13.4: Workplace training objectives

B:13.4.1 To prescribe appropriately for patients in pain awaiting surgery

B:13.4.2 To prescribe pain management for patients after common surgical procedures

B:13.4.3 To institute appropriate action to relieve pain quickly in recovery

B:13.4.4 To become familiar and technically proficient with a variety of therapeutic methods listed above in the skills list

14: Infection control

14.1: Knowledge

B:14.1.1 Universal precautions and good working practices (hand washing, gloves, etc.)

B:14.1.2 Cross infection: modes and common agents

B:14.1.3 Emergence of resistant strains: antibiotic policies in a hospital

B:14.1.4 Common surgical infections: antibiotic choice and prophylaxis

B:14.1.5 Infections from contaminated blood

B:14.1.6 Hepatitis and HIV infections: modes of infection: natural history: at risk groups

B:14.1.7 Immunization policy

B:14.1.8 Sterilization of equipment

B:14.1.9 Strategy if contaminated

14.2: Skills

B:14.2.1 Preoperative assessment: awareness of at risk groups
B:14.2.2 Recognition of the immunocompromised patient
B:14.2.3 Administration of i.v. antibiotics: risk of allergy and anaphylaxis
B:14.2.4 Aseptic techniques
B:14.2.5 Use of disposable filters and breathing systems
B:14.2.6 Use of protective clothing/gloves/masks, etc.

14.3: Attitudes and behaviour

B:14.3.1 Every patient entitled to the best care available
B:14.3.2 Prevention of self-infection
B:14.3.3 Prevention of cross infection

14.4: Workplace training objectives

B:14.4.1 To think about and apply the skills and attitudes listed above to all patients
B:14.4.2 To wash hands between patients

15: Critical incidents

15.1: Knowledge

Common causes of critical incidents
Principles of the causes, detection and management of:
B:15.1.1 Cardiac and/or respiratory arrest
B:15.1.2 Unexpected hypoxia with or without cyanosis
B:15.1.3 Unexpected increase in peak airway pressure
B:15.1.4 Progressive fall in minute volume during spontaneous respiration or IPPV
B:15.1.5 Fall in end tidal CO_2
B:15.1.6 Rise in end tidal CO_2
B:15.1.7 Rise in inspired CO_2
B:15.1.8 Unexpected hypotension
B:15.1.9 Unexpected hypertension
B:15.1.10 Sinus tachycardia
B:15.1.11 Arrhythmias (ST segment changes; sudden tachydysrhythmia; sudden bradycardia; ventricular ectopics – ventricular tachycardia – ventricular fibrillation)
B:15.1.12 Convulsions
Management of the following specific conditions:
B:15.1.13 Aspiration of vomit
B:15.1.14 Laryngospasm
B:15.1.15 Bronchospasm
B:15.1.16 Tension pneumothorax

B:15.1.17 Gas/fat/pulmonary embolus

B:15.1.18 Adverse drug reactions

B:15.1.19 Anaphylaxis

B:15.1.20 Transfusion of mismatched blood or blood products

B:15.1.21 Malignant hyperpyrexia

B:15.1.22 Inadvertent intra-arterial injection of irritant fluids

B:15.1.23 High spinal block

B:15.1.24 Local anaesthetic toxicity

B:15.1.25 Failed intubation

B:15.1.26 Difficulty with IPPV and sudden or progressive loss of minute volume

15.2: Skills

B:15.2.1 Early recognition of deteriorating situation by careful monitoring

B:15.2.2 Practice response protocols in resuscitation room or in simulation with other relevant healthcare professionals when appropriate

B:15.2.3 Respond appropriately if any of them happen

B:15.2.4 Ability to obtain the attention of others when a crisis is occurring

15.3: Attitudes and behaviour

B:15.3.1 Vigilance

B:15.3.2 Awareness of the importance and process of critical incident reporting

B:15.3.3 Acceptance that it can happen to you: the unexpected happens to everybody

B:15.3.4 Following through a critical incident with warning flags, presentation at morbidity meetings, proper reporting, etc.

B:15.3.5 Information to patient and where necessary, counselling and advice

15.4: Workplace training objectives

B:15.4.1 To have management plans for the listed critical incidents

B:15.4.2 To practise whenever possible in mock-up situations or simulation with other relevant healthcare professionals when appropriate

B:15.4.3 To respond appropriately if a critical incident occurs

16: Management of respiratory and cardiac arrest

Trainees can be regarded as achieving the necessary competences if they have successfully completed an ALS course in the last 12 months.

16.1: Knowledge

B:16.1.1 Patient assessment: diagnosis of causes of cardio-respiratory arrest

B:16.1.2 Causes of cardio-respiratory arrest during induction, maintenance and recovery from anaesthesia

B:16.1.3 Importance of considering non-cardiac causes of cardio-respiratory arrest

B:16.1.4 Methods of airway management (mouth-mouth/nose, bag-mask, LMA, intubation)

B:16.1.5 Recognition and management of life-threatening arrhythmias including defibrillation and drug therapy

B:16.1.6 Recognition and management of non-cardiac causes of cardio-respiratory arrest

B:16.1.7 Knowledge of specific problems of paediatric resuscitation

B:16.1.8 Ethical aspects of resuscitation

16.2: Skills

B:16.2.1 Recognition of cardiac and respiratory arrest

B:16.2.2 Resuscitation equipment checklist

B:16.2.3 ABC

B:16.2.4 Practical life support – following current algorithm

B:16.2.5 Managing the airway

B:16.2.6 External chest compression

B:16.2.7 Vascular access, suitability of sites

B:16.2.8 Arrhythmia recognition and management (drugs/defibrillators/pacemakers)

B:16.2.9 Defibrillation and defibrillator settings

B:16.2.10 Deciding when further resuscitation is futile

B:16.2.11 Diagnosis of death

B:16.2.12 Fluid balance assessment/management

16.3: Attitudes and behaviour

B:16.3.1 Always resuscitate unless certain it is inappropriate

B:16.3.2 Not to resuscitate orders

B:16.3.3 Recognize need for team leader

B:16.3.4 Desire to offer the best possible chance of survival

B:16.3.5 Recognition of futility

B:16.3.6 Dealing sensitively and honestly with relatives

B:16.3.7 Medico-legal aspects of resuscitation (police reports, etc.)

16.4: Workplace training objectives

B:16.4.1 To resuscitate adults (and know the principles of resuscitating children) from cardio-respiratory arrest to the standards set by the Resuscitation Council (UK)

B:16.4.2 To discuss ethical aspects of resuscitation

17: Anatomy

Trainees should be able to demonstrate a good understanding of human anatomy relevant to the practice of anaesthesia at basic level and to support progress to intermediate level training.

17.1: Knowledge

Respiratory system

B:17.1.1 Mouth, nose, pharynx, larynx, trachea, main bronchi, segmental bronchi, structure of bronchial tree: differences in the child

B:17.1.2 Airway and respiratory tract, blood supply, innervation and lymphatic drainage

B:17.1.3 Pleura, mediastinum and its contents

B:17.1.4 Lungs, lobes, microstructure of lungs

B:17.1.5 Diaphragm, other muscles of respiration, innervation

B:17.1.6 The thoracic inlet and 1st rib

B:17.1.7 Interpretation of a normal chest X-ray

Cardiovascular system

B:17.1.8 Heart, chambers, conducting system, blood and nerve supply

B:17.1.9 Pericardium

B:17.1.10 Great vessels, main peripheral arteries and veins

B:17.1.11 Fetal and materno-fetal circulation

Nervous system

B:17.1.12 Brain and its subdivisions

B:17.1.13 Spinal cord, structure of spinal cord, major ascending and descending pathways

B:17.1.14 Spinal meninges, subarachnoid and extradural space, contents of extradural space

B:17.1.15 CSF and its circulation

B:17.1.16 Spinal nerves, dermatomes

B:17.1.17 Brachial plexus, nerves of arm

B:17.1.18 Intercostal nerves

B:17.1.19 Nerves of abdominal wall

B:17.1.20 Nerves of leg and foot

B:17.1.21 Autonomic nervous system

B:17.1.22 Sympathetic innervation, sympathetic chain, ganglia and plexuses

B:17.1.23 Parasympathetic innervation

B:17.1.24 Stellate ganglion

B:17.1.25 Cranial nerves: base of skull: trigeminal ganglion

B:17.1.26 Innervation of the larynx

B:17.1.27 Eye and orbit

Vertebral column

B:17.1.28 Cervical, thoracic, and lumbar vertebrae

B:17.1.29 Sacrum, sacral hiatus

B:17.1.30 Ligaments of vertebral column

B:17.1.31 Surface anatomy of vertebral spaces, length of cord in child and adult

Surface anatomy

B:17.1.32 Structures in antecubital fossa

B:17.1.33 Structures in axilla: identifying the brachial plexus

B:17.1.34 Large veins and anterior triangle of neck

B:17.1.35 Large veins of leg and femoral triangle

B:17.1.36 Arteries of arm and leg

B:17.1.37 Landmarks for tracheostomy, cricothyrotomy

B:17.1.38 Abdominal wall (including the inguinal region): landmarks for suprapubic urinary and peritoneal lavage catheters

17.2: Objectives for trainees

This knowledge base will be tested in the Primary Examination. Some clinical aspects may be asked in the workplace assessments.

18: Physiology and biochemistry

Trainees should have a good general understanding of human physiology, be able to apply physiological principles and knowledge to clinical practice at basic level and to support progress to intermediate level training.

18.1: Knowledge

General

B:18.1.1 Organization of the human body and control of internal environment

B:18.1.2 Variations with age

B:18.1.3 Function of cells; genes and their expression

B:18.1.4 Cell membrane characteristics; receptors

B:18.1.5 Protective mechanisms of the body

Biochemistry

B:18.1.6 Acid–base balance and buffers

B:18.1.7 Ions, e.g. Na^+, K^+, Ca^{++}, Cl^-, $HCO3^-$

B:18.1.8 Cellular metabolism

B:18.1.9 Enzymes

Body fluids and their functions and constituents

B:18.1.10 Capillary dynamics and interstitial fluid

B:18.1.11 Osmolarity: osmolality, partition of fluids across membranes

B:18.1.12 Lymphatic system

B:18.1.13 Special fluids especially cerebrospinal fluid: also pleural, pericardial

B:18.1.14 and peritoneal fluids

Haematology and immunology

B:18.1.15 Red blood cells: haemoglobin and its variants

B:18.1.16 Blood groups

B:18.1.17 Haemostasis and coagulation

B:18.1.18 White blood cells

B:18.1.19 The inflammatory response
B:18.1.20 Immunity and allergy
Muscle
B:18.1.21 Action potential generation and its transmission
B:18.1.22 Neuromuscular junction and transmission
B:18.1.23 Muscle types
B:18.1.24 Skeletal muscle contraction
B:18.1.25 Smooth muscle contraction: sphincters
B:18.1.26 Motor unit
Heart/circulation
B:18.1.27 Cardiac muscle contraction
B:18.1.28 The cardiac cycle: pressure and volume relationships
B:18.1.29 Rhythmicity of the heart
B:18.1.30 Regulation of cardiac function; general and cellular
B:18.1.31 Control of cardiac output (including the Starling relationship)
B:18.1.32 Fluid challenge and heart failure
B:18.1.33 Electrocardiogram and arrhythmias
B:18.1.34 Neurological and humoral control of systemic blood pressures, blood volume and blood flow (at rest and during physiological disturbances, e.g. exercise, haemorrhage and Valsalva manoeuvre)
B:18.1.35 Peripheral circulation: capillaries, vascular endothelium and arteriolar smooth muscle
B:18.1.36 Characteristics of special circulations including: pulmonary, coronary, cerebral, renal, portal and fetal
Renal tract
B:18.1.37 Blood flow and glomerular filtration and plasma clearance
B:18.1.38 Tubular function and urine formation
B:18.1.39 Assessment of renal function
B:18.1.40 Regulation of fluid and electrolyte balance
B:18.1.41 Regulation of acid–base balance
B:18.1.42 Micturition
B:18.1.43 Pathophysiology of acute renal failure
Respiration
B:18.1.44 Gaseous exchange: O_2 and CO_2 transport, hypoxia and hyper- and hypocapnia, hyper- and hypobaric pressures
B:18.1.45 Functions of haemoglobin in oxygen carriage and acid–base equilibrium
B:18.1.46 Pulmonary ventilation: volumes, flows, dead space
B:18.1.47 Effect of IPPV on lungs
B:18.1.48 Mechanics of ventilation: ventilation/perfusion abnormalities
B:18.1.49 Control of breathing, acute and chronic ventilatory failure, effect of oxygen therapy
B:18.1.50 Non-respiratory functions of the lungs

Nervous system

B:18.1.51 Functions of nerve cells: action potentials, conduction and synaptic mechanisms

B:18.1.52 The brain: functional divisions

B:18.1.53 Intracranial pressure: cerebrospinal fluid, blood flow

B:18.1.54 Maintenance of posture

B:18.1.55 Autonomic nervous system: functions

B:18.1.56 Neurological reflexes

B:18.1.57 Motor function: spinal and peripheral

B:18.1.58 Senses: receptors, nociception, special senses

B:18.1.59 Pain: afferent nociceptive pathways, dorsal horn, peripheral and central mechanisms, neuromodulatory systems, supraspinal mechanisms, visceral pain, neuropathic pain, influence of therapy on nociceptive mechanisms

B:18.1.60 Spinal cord: anatomy and blood supply, effects of spinal cord section

Liver

B:18.1.61 Functional anatomy and blood supply

B:18.1.62 Metabolic functions

Gastrointestinal

B:18.1.63 Gastric function; secretions, nausea and vomiting

B:18.1.64 Gut motility, sphincters and reflex control

B:18.1.65 Digestive functions

Metabolism

B:18.1.66 Nutrients: carbohydrates, fats, proteins, vitamins and minerals

B:18.1.67 Metabolic pathways, energy production and enzymes; metabolic rate

B:18.1.68 Hormonal control of metabolism: regulation of plasma glucose, response to trauma

B:18.1.69 Physiological alterations in starvation, obesity, exercise and the stress response

B:18.1.70 Body temperature and its regulation

Endocrinology

B:18.1.71 Mechanisms of hormonal control: feedback mechanisms, effect on membrane and intracellular receptors

B:18.1.72 Hypothalamic and pituitary function

B:18.1.73 Adrenocortical hormones

B:18.1.74 Adrenal medulla: adrenaline (epinephrine) and noradrenaline (norepinephrine)

B:18.1.75 Pancreas: insulin, glucagon and exocrine function

B:18.1.76 Thyroid and parathyroid hormones and calcium homeostasis

Pregnancy

B:18.1.77 Physiological changes associated with normal pregnancy

B:18.1.78 Materno-fetal, fetal and neonatal circulation

B:18.1.79 Functions of the placenta: placental transfer

B:18.1.80 Fetus: changes at birth

18.2: Objectives for trainees

This knowledge base will be tested in the Primary Examination. Some clinical aspects may be asked in the workplace assessments.

19: Pharmacology

Trainees should have a good understanding of general pharmacological principles, together with knowledge of drugs likely to be encountered in (a) anaesthetic practice and (b) current treatment of patients presenting for anaesthesia. The level of knowledge should be sufficient to enable clinical practice at basic level and to support progress to intermediate level training.

19.1: Knowledge

Applied chemistry

B:19.1.1 Types of intermolecular bonds

B:19.1.2 Laws of diffusion. Diffusion of molecules through membranes

B:19.1.3 Solubility and partition coefficients

B:19.1.4 Ionization of drugs

B:19.1.5 Drug isomerism

B:19.1.6 Protein binding

B:19.1.7 Oxidation and reduction

Mode of action of drugs

B:19.1.8 Dynamics of drug-receptor interaction

B:19.1.9 Agonists, antagonists, partial agonists, inverse agonists

B:19.1.10 Efficacy and potency. Tolerance

B:19.1.11 Receptor function and regulation

B:19.1.12 Metabolic pathways; enzymes; drug: enzyme interactions; Michaelis–Menten equation

B:19.1.13 Enzyme inducers and inhibitors

B:19.1.14 Mechanisms of drug action

B:19.1.15 Ion channels: types: relation to receptors. Gating mechanisms

B:19.1.16 Signal transduction: cell membrane/receptors/ion channels to intracellular molecular targets, second messengers

B:19.1.17 Action of gases and vapours

B:19.1.18 Osmotic effects. pH effects. Adsorption and chelation

B:19.1.19 Mechanisms of drug interactions:

B:19.1.20 Inhibition and promotion of drug uptake. Competitive protein binding. Receptor interactions

B:19.1.21 Effects of metabolites and other degradation products

Pharmacokinetics and pharmacodynamics

B:19.1.22 Drug uptake from: gastrointestinal tract, lungs, transdermal, subcutaneous, i.m., i.v., epidural, intrathecal routes

B:19.1.23 Bioavailability

B:19.1.24 Factors determining the distribution of drugs: perfusion, molecular size, solubility, protein binding

B:19.1.25 The influence of drug formulation on disposition

B:19.1.26 Distribution of drugs to organs and tissues: body compartments

B:19.1.27 Influence of specialized membranes: tissue binding and solubility

B:19.1.28 Materno-fetal distribution

B:19.1.29 Distribution in CSF and extradural space

B:19.1.30 Modes of drug elimination:

B:19.1.31   Direct excretion

B:19.1.32   Metabolism in organs of excretion: phase I and II mechanisms

B:19.1.33   Renal excretion and urinary pH

B:19.1.34   Non-organ breakdown of drugs

B:19.1.35 Pharmacokinetic analysis:

B:19.1.36   Concept of a pharmacokinetic compartment

B:19.1.37   Apparent volume of distribution

B:19.1.38   Clearance

B:19.1.39   Clearance concepts applied to whole body and individual organs

B:19.1.40   Simple 1 and 2 compartmental models: concepts of wash-in and wash-out curves

B:19.1.41   Physiological models based on perfusion and partition coefficients

B:19.1.42   Effect of organ blood flow: Fick principle

B:19.1.43   Pharmacokinetic variation: influence of body size, sex, age, disease, pregnancy, anaesthesia, trauma, surgery, smoking, alcohol and other drugs

B:19.1.44 Effects of acute organ failure (liver, kidney) on drug elimination

B:19.1.45 Pharmacodynamics: concentration-effect relationships: hysteresis

B:19.1.46 Pharmacogenetics: familial variation in drug response

B:19.1.47 Adverse reactions to drugs: hypersensitivity, allergy, anaphylaxis, anaphylactoid reactions

Systematic pharmacology

B:19.1.48 Anaesthetic gases and vapours

B:19.1.49 Hypnotics, sedatives and intravenous anaesthetic agents

B:19.1.50 Simple analgesics

B:19.1.51 Opioids and other analgesics; and opioid antagonists

B:19.1.52 Non-steroidal anti-inflammatory drugs

B:19.1.53 Neuromuscular blocking agents (depolarizing and non-depolarizing), and anticholinesterases

B:19.1.54 Drugs acting on the autonomic nervous system: cholinergic and adrenergic agonists and antagonists

B:19.1.55 Drugs acting on the heart and cardiovascular system (including inotropes, vasodilators, vasoconstrictors, antiarrhythmics, diuretics)

B:19.1.56 Drugs acting on the respiratory system (including respiratory stimulants and bronchodilators)

B:19.1.57 Antihypertensives
B:19.1.58 Anticonvulsants
B:19.1.59 Anti-diabetic agents
B:19.1.60 Diuretics
B:19.1.61 Antibiotics
B:19.1.62 Corticosteroids and other hormone preparations
B:19.1.63 Antacids. Drugs influencing gastric secretion and motility
B:19.1.64 Antiemetic agents
B:19.1.65 Local anaesthetic agents
B:19.1.66 Plasma volume expanders
B:19.1.67 Antihistamines
B:19.1.68 Antidepressants
B:19.1.69 Anticoagulants
B:19.1.70 Vitamin K, B_{12} and thiamine

19.2: Objectives for trainees

This knowledge base will be tested in the Primary Examination. Some clinical aspects may be asked in the workplace assessments.

20: Physics and clinical measurement

Candidates should have a good understanding of the principles of physics and clinical measurement with an emphasis on the function of monitoring equipment safety and measurement techniques.

20.1: Knowledge

B:20.1.1 Mathematical concepts: relationships and graphs
B:20.1.2 Concepts only of exponential functions and logarithms: wash-in, wash-out and tear away
B:20.1.3 Basic measurement concepts: linearity, drift, hysteresis, signal: noise ratio, static and dynamic response
B:20.1.4 SI units: fundamental and derived units
B:20.1.5 Other systems of units where relevant to anaesthesia (e.g. mmHg, bar, atmospheres)
B:20.1.6 Simple mechanics: mass, force, work and power
B:20.1.7 Heat: freezing point, melting point, latent heat
B:20.1.8 Conduction, convection, radiation
B:20.1.9 Mechanical equivalent of heat: laws of thermodynamics
B:20.1.10 Measurement of temperature and humidity
B:20.1.11 Colligative properties: osmometry
B:20.1.12 Physics of gases and vapours
B:20.1.13 Absolute and relative pressure
B:20.1.14 The gas laws; triple point; critical temperature and pressure
B:20.1.15 Density and viscosity of gases

B:20.1.16 Laminar and turbulent flow; Poiseuille's equation, the Bernoulli principle

B:20.1.17 Vapour pressure: saturated vapour pressure

B:20.1.18 Measurement of volume and flow in gases and liquids

B:20.1.19 The pneumotachograph and other respirometers

B:20.1.20 Principles of surface tension

B:20.1.21 Basic concepts of electricity and magnetism

B:20.1.22 Capacitance, inductance and impedance

B:20.1.23 Amplifiers: band width, filters

B:20.1.24 Amplification of biological potentials: ECG, EMG, EEG

B:20.1.25 Sources of electrical interference

B:20.1.26 Processing, storage and display of physiological measurements

B:20.1.27 Bridge circuits

B:20.1.28 Basic principles and safety of lasers

B:20.1.29 Basic principles of ultrasound and the Doppler effect

B:20.1.30 Principles of cardiac pacemakers and defibrillators

B:20.1.31 Electrical hazards: causes and prevention

B:20.1.32 Electrocution, fires and explosions

B:20.1.33 Diathermy and its safe use

B:20.1.34 Principles of pressure transducers

B:20.1.35 Resonance and damping, frequency response

B:20.1.36 Measurement and units of pressure

B:20.1.37 Direct and indirect methods of blood pressure measurement

B:20.1.38 Principles of pulmonary artery and wedge pressure measurement

B:20.1.39 Cardiac output: Fick principle, thermodilution

B:20.1.40 Measurement of gas and vapour concentrations (oxygen, carbon dioxide, nitrous oxide, and volatile anaesthetic agents) using infra-red, paramagnetic, fuel cell, oxygen electrode and mass spectrometry methods

B:20.1.41 Measurement of pH, pCO_2, pO_2

B:20.1.42 Measurement CO_2 production/oxygen consumption/respiratory quotient

B:20.1.43 Simple tests of pulmonary function, e.g. peak flow measurement, spirometry

B:20.1.44 Capnography

B:20.1.45 Pulse oximetry

B:20.1.46 Measurement of neuromuscular blockade

B:20.1.47 Measurement of pain

20.2: Objectives for trainees

This knowledge base will be tested in the Primary Examination. Some clinical aspects of safety and measurement will probably be asked in the workplace assessments.

21: Statistical methods

Trainees will be required to demonstrate understanding of basic statistical concepts, but will not be expected to have practical experience of statistical methods. Emphasis will be placed on methods by which data may be summarized and presented, and on the selection of statistical measures for different data types. Candidates will be expected to understand the statistical background to measurement error and statistical uncertainty.

21.1: Knowledge

Data collection
B:21.1.1 Simple aspects of study design
B:21.1.2 Defining the outcome measures and the uncertainty of measuring them
B:21.1.3 The basic concept of meta-analysis and evidence based medicine
Descriptive statistics
B:21.1.4 Types of data and their representation
B:21.1.5 The normal distribution as an example of parametric distribution
B:21.1.6 Indices of central tendency and variability
Deductive and inferential statistics
B:21.1.7 Simple probability theory and the relation to confidence intervals
B:21.1.8 The null hypothesis
B:21.1.9 Choice of simple statistical tests for different data types
B:21.1.10 Type I and type II errors

21.2: Objectives for trainees

This knowledge base will be tested in the Primary Examination. Some clinical aspects may be asked in the workplace assessments.

Table A1.1 Blueprint of workplace-based assessments mapped against basic level competences

Basic level competences	Workplace-based assessments			
	DOPS	Anaes-CEX	CBD	MSF
Anaesthesia, HDU and ICU equipment: monitoring and safety	X	X		
Anaesthesia and the elderly	X	X	X	X
Anatomy			X	
Critical incidents	X	X	X	X
Day surgery	X	X	X	X

Table A1.1 Blueprint of workplace-based assessments mapped against basic level competences—cont'd

Basic level competences	Workplace-based assessments			
	DOPS	Anaes-CEX	CBD	MSF
ENT	X	X	X	X
General surgery/gynaecology/urology (± transplantation)	X	X	X	X
Induction of general anaesthesia	X	X	X	
Initial assessment of competency	X			
Infection control	X	X	X	
Intensive and high dependency care	X	X	X	X
Intraoperative care (including sedation)	X	X	X	
Management of respiratory and cardiac arrest	X	X	X	X
Management of trauma, stabilization and transfer of patients	X	X	X	
Obstetric anaesthesia and analgesia	X	X	X	X
Orthopaedic anaesthesia	X	X	X	X
Paediatric anaesthesia	X	X	X	X
Pain medicine		X	X	X
Pharmacology			X	
Physics and clinical measurement			X	
Physiology and biochemistry			X	
Postoperative and recovery care	X	X	X	
Preoperative assessment	X	X	X	X
Pre-medication	X	X	X	X
Regional anaesthesia	X	X	X	X
Statistical methods			X	
Trauma and accidents	X	X	X	X
Vascular anaesthesia	X	X	X	X

SYLLABUS FOR THE FINAL FRCA EXAMINATION

The CCT in anaesthetics – Intermediate level syllabus

The exams syllabus has been replaced by the 'Knowledge' sections of the Competency Based Training document for ST years 3 and 4.

Index

1: Generic knowledge and skills

Listed here are generic aspects of knowledge and skills that may or may not have been covered within the various other units of training, but which should not be omitted. Knowledge and skills relating to the airway are particularly emphasized. As with other aspects of competence at intermediate level, these will generally represent a further development of the basic competencies in ST Years 1 and 2.

1.1: Knowledge

In:1.1.1 Anaesthetic and monitoring equipment:

In:1.1.2   standards

In:1.1.3   care, cleaning, disinfecting and sterilization (particularly airway equipment)

In:1.1.4   potential defects and problems

In:1.1.5   safety precautions and checking

In:1.1.6 Anaesthesia in abnormal environments:

In:1.1.7   altitude

In:1.1.8   in pressure chambers/at depth

In:1.1.9   low temperature

In:1.1.10 Problems for patients and staff of:

In:1.1.11   age (anaesthesia and the elderly)

In:1.1.12   obesity

In:1.1.13   smoking

In:1.1.14   alcoholism

In:1.1.15   drug dependency and addiction

In:1.1.16   hepatitis B and C carriers

In:1.1.17   HIV and AIDS

In:1.1.18   variant CJD

In:1.1.19   pacemakers

In:1.1.20 Hazards for patients and staff of:

In:1.1.21   anaesthetic drugs and pregnancy

In:1.1.22   electricity and electrocution

In:1.1.23   diathermy

In:1.1.24   sharps injury

In:1.1.25   pollution by anaesthetic gases

In:1.1.26   fires and explosions

In:1.1.27 Intravenous fluid replacement:

In:1.1.28   blood transfusion

In:1.1.29   Jehovah's Witnesses

In:1.1.30   blood substitutes

In:1.1.31   disseminated intravascular coagulation

In:1.1.32   colloid/crystalloid

In:1.1.73 The obstructed airway:
In:1.1.74   recognition
In:1.1.75   immediate treatment of acute obstruction
In:1.1.76   anaesthetic management of acute and chronic obstruction
In:1.1.77   flexible nasendoscopy and imaging
In:1.1.78 Emergency cricothyrotomy:
In:1.1.79   needle
In:1.1.80   purpose built cannula >4 mm ID
In:1.1.81   surgical
In:1.1.82 Extubation strategies – routine, predicted and unexpected difficulty
In:1.1.83 Complications of difficult airway management
In:1.1.84 Follow-up care of patient, documentation and patient information
In:1.1.85 Surgical approach to the airway – indications, techniques, conduct
In:1.1.86 Percutaneous cricothyrotomy and tracheostomy

1.2: Skills

In:1.2.1 Recognition of the difficult airway:
In:1.2.2   when to ask for help
In:1.2.3 Failed rapid sequence intubation:
In:1.2.4   performance of recognized 'drills' for failed intubation/ventilation
In:1.2.5 Alternative methods of intubation:
In:1.2.6   other laryngoscopy blades and bougies
In:1.2.7   low skill fibreoptic intubation, e.g. via laryngeal mask or specialized airway
In:1.2.8 Placement and checking of double lumen tubes
In:1.2.9 Anaesthetic techniques for laryngoscopy, bronchoscopy and tracheostomy
In:1.2.10 Extubation in abnormal airway
In:1.2.11 Clinical review of patient to detect and treat airway instrumentation damage
In:1.2.12 Interpretation of CT, MRI imaging and flow-volume loops

Additional desirable clinical skills to be learnt primarily in the non-clinical environment (skills laboratory/manikin/simulator) but supplemented by some clinical experience. The availability of equipment to display the fibreoptic image on a screen will also extend the opportunities for clinical teaching.

In:1.2.13 Awake intubation:
In:1.2.14   indications
In:1.2.15   use with the compromised airway
In:1.2.16 Fibreoptic intubation through the nose and mouth with and without concurrent ventilation
In:1.2.17 Fibre-endoscopy skills to:
In:1.2.18   visualize tracheo-bronchial tree

In:1.2.19 confirm placement of single and double lumen tubes

In:1.2.20 intubate through the laryngeal mask

In:1.2.21 Blind and fibreoptic assisted intubation via the intubating laryngeal mask

In:1.2.22 Elective trans-tracheal ventilation to aid difficult intubation

In:1.2.23 Retrograde intubation – blind and fibreoptic assisted

In:1.2.24 Placement bronchial blockers

In:1.2.25 Specialized bougies and airway exchange catheters

In:1.2.26 Use of the Combitube or other supraglottic balloon device

In:1.2.27 Emergency cricothyrotomy:

In:1.2.28 landmarks

In:1.2.29 insertion of needle/cannula

In:1.2.30 confirmation of position within trachea

In:1.2.31 fixation

In:1.2.32 pressures required for adequate gas flows

In:1.2.33 ventilation through cannula/catheter

In:1.2.34 complications

In:1.2.35 Application of 30 N cricoid force

2: Academic/research

An understanding of the scientific basis of anaesthetic practice is essential. This unit of training effectively underwrites the understanding and education of trainees in all the other aspects of the training that they will receive during intermediate level training. Even if separate time is not allocated, the concepts identified here should be fundamental to the education of trainees at this stage of training.

2.1: Knowledge

In:2.1.1 The scientific basis of clinical practice

In:2.1.2 The methodology and processes of clinical and laboratory research including the ethical considerations raised by research, the importance of study design in clinical research and the importance of statistical analyses

In:2.1.3 The audit cycle

In:2.1.4 The major national audit processes, including National Confidential Enquiry into Patient Outcomes and Deaths (NCEPOD)

In:2.1.5 Critical Incident Reporting:

In:2.1.6 purpose and value

In:2.1.7 methods – local/national

In:2.1.8 anonymity – pros and cons

2.2: Skills

In:2.2.1 Able to locate published research in a systematic manner

In:2.2.2 Critically interpret and evaluate the value of published clinical research

In:2.2.3 Plan and prepare a presentation and present to a live audience

2.3: Attitudes and behaviour

In:2.3.1 Maintain an inquisitive, questioning approach to clinical practice

In:2.3.2 Cultivate an evidence-based practice

In:2.3.3 Awareness of and detachment from vested interests or entrenched views

In:2.3.4 Develop a readiness to both listen and explain

In:2.3.5 Demonstrate a willingness to teach and learn

In:2.3.6 Develop an informed critical approach to the scientific literature

2.4: Workplace training objectives

In:2.4.1 Trainees should gain competency in the critical interpretation and evaluation of published clinical research and be able to assess the benefit of applying the results of research to clinical practice

Recommended local requirements to support training

* A suitably experienced consultant or clinical academic
* Library and computing facilities
* Regular academic meetings

3: Cardiac/thoracic anaesthesia

This is an intermediate level 'Key Unit of Training' in which trainees should spend the equivalent of at least 1 month of training and, normally, not more than 3 months. It is recognized that for intermediate level training there will, due to the distribution of specialist units, be considerable variability in the degree of experience available to individual trainees. Through attachments and links between Schools of Anaesthesia, it is expected that the majority of trainees will receive at least 1 month of experience in this anaesthetic special interest area. However, where experience in this special interest is more freely available, a unit of training should be limited to 3 months within the intermediate level training programme.

3.1: Knowledge

Cardiac anaesthesia

In:3.1.1 Preoperative assessment and perioperative care of patients with cardiac disease

In:3.1.2 Induction and maintenance of anaesthesia for high risk cardiac procedures, including valve replacement

In:3.1.3 Antibiotic prophylaxis against subacute bacterial endocarditis

In:3.1.4 Problems of cardiopulmonary bypass

In:3.1.5 Postoperative cardiac critical care, including analgesia, sedation and ventilatory management

In:3.1.6 Significance of cardiac tamponade

In:3.1.7 Interpretation of ECG and CXR

In:3.1.8 Interpretation of invasive and non-invasive cardiovascular monitoring

In:3.1.9 Temperature control and patient rewarming methods

In:3.1.10 Coagulopathy

In:3.1.11 Cardiac pacing modes

In:3.1.12 Intra-aortic balloon counter pulsation

In:3.1.13 Understanding of the adult patient with congenital heart disease

In:3.1.14 A working knowledge of the following investigations:

In:3.1.15   stress testing

In:3.1.16   cardiac catheterization

In:3.1.17   echocardiography – transthoracic/transoesophageal

In:3.1.18   radionuclide scan

Thoracic anaesthesia

In:3.1.19 Preoperative pulmonary function tests

In:3.1.20 Local and general anaesthesia for bronchoscopy including techniques of ventilation

In:3.1.21 Understanding of fibreoptic bronchoscopic techniques for airway management

In:3.1.22 Principles of one-lung anaesthesia

In:3.1.23 Management of a pneumothorax

In:3.1.24 Principles of underwater seals on chest drains

In:3.1.25 Postoperative care and analgesia after thoracic surgery

3.2: Skills

Generic

In:3.2.1 Internal jugular and subclavian venous cannulation

In:3.2.2 Arterial cannulation

In:3.2.3 Invasive pressure monitoring, including pulmonary artery catheters and interpretation of derived indices

In:3.2.4 Postoperative analgesia by appropriate methods including local techniques

In:3.2.5 Cardiopulmonary resuscitation and appropriate use of defibrillators

Cardiac anaesthesia

In:3.2.6 Preoperative assessment of patients with valvular and with ischaemic heart disease

In:3.2.7 Induction and maintenance of anaesthesia for elective coronary bypass

In:3.2.8 Management of the patient during cardiopulmonary bypass

In:3.2.9 Use of inotropes and vasodilators

In:3.2.10 Anaesthesia for procedures in intensive care including emergency re-sternotomy, re-intubation, tracheostomy or cardioversion

Thoracic anaesthesia

In:3.2.11 Preoperative assessment, preparation of patients with pulmonary disease

In:3.2.12 Preoperative assessment, preparation of patients for thoracic surgery

In:3.2.13 Induction and maintenance of anaesthesia for minor thoracic procedures, in particular, bronchoscopy and the use of the Sanders injector

In:3.2.14 Use of single and double lumen endobronchial intubation

In:3.2.15 Fibreoptic endoscopic confirmation of tube placement

In:3.2.16 Induction and maintenance of anaesthesia for major thoracic procedures

In:3.2.17 One lung ventilation

3.3: Attitudes and behaviour

In:3.3.1 To communicate effectively with surgical colleagues/other members of the theatre team

In:3.3.2 To be able to summarize a case to critical care staff

In:3.3.3 Understand how to communicate with the intubated patient in intensive care

In:3.3.4 To be able to recognize the need for senior help when appropriate

In:3.3.5 Maintain accurate clinical records

In:3.3.6 Presentation of material to departmental meetings and participation in clinical audit

3.4: Workplace training objectives

In:3.4.1 By gaining experience in cardiothoracic anaesthesia, the trainee should also develop competency in the management of cardiovascular and pulmonary problems arising in non-cardiac surgical patients

Cardiac surgery

In:3.4.2 The trainee should develop the ability to assess the circulation and have experience in the use of inotropes and vasoactive agents to support of the circulation in patients with cardiac disease. They should also develop an understanding of the problems of extracorporeal circulation

Thoracic surgery

In:3.4.3 The trainee should understand the problems of one lung anaesthesia and develop experience in the placement of double-lumen tubes

Recommended local requirements to support training
Cardiac surgery

- Cardiac surgery must take place in theatres equipped to a high standard for anaesthesia and monitoring with facilities for cardiopulmonary bypass and mechanical support of the circulation
- Rapid access to biochemistry and haematology services
- Each cardiac unit must have a consultant anaesthetist with dedicated responsibility for cardiac anaesthetic services

- There must be appropriate support facilities provided
- Extensive patient monitoring is required
- Adequate critical care facilities must be provided
- There must be resident medical staff cover of the intensive care unit
- There must be an ongoing, adequately resourced, audit programme

Thoracic surgery

- On-site pulmonary function laboratory facilities must be available
- Patients must be managed in an area equipped and staffed to a high standard
- Patients may routinely return to a high dependency care facility; however, supporting intensive care facilities should also be easily accessible
- Pain relief and other clinical protocols must be clearly defined

4: Intensive care medicine

This is an intermediate level 'Key Unit of Training'. 'Step 1' (previously Intermediate) Training in ICM requires 6 months of training within the specialty. All trainees in anaesthesia must receive a minimum of 3 months training in ICM during ST Years 3 and 4.

This requirement is based on the recognition that knowledge and skills gained in critical care underpin the trainees' ability to gain competency in aspects of anaesthesia later in their training. The training should be to the IBTICM's standards for Step 1 Training. The second 3 months training in ICM would normally be obtained in ST Year 5. However, provided other 'units of training' in the ST Years 3 and 4 are not compromised, this second period can also be completed during this time. It is expected, however, that this will be the exception rather than the rule.

4.1: Knowledge

General

In:4.1.1 Trainees should have a good understanding of the diagnosis and management of the critically ill patient. All trainees should be familiar with the monitoring and life support equipment used in the treatment of critically ill patients. Trainees must be able to demonstrate their knowledge of practical invasive procedures, with an understanding of the principles and hazards involved and the interpretation of data from such procedures.

In:4.1.2 Transport of the critically ill:

In:4.1.3 assessment and organization of transfer

In:4.1.4 physiological consequences of acceleration

In:4.1.5 problems of working in isolated environments

In:4.1.6 Outreach care:

In:4.1.7 early warning signs and symptoms

In:4.1.8 infection and multiple organ failure

In:4.1.9 Sepsis and endotoxaemia:

In:4.1.10 nosocomial infections

In:4.1.11 assessment and management of oxygen delivery

In:4.1.12 antibiotics and immunotherapy

In:4.1.13 reperfusion injury and antioxidants

In:4.1.14 Cardiovascular system to include:

In:4.1.15 pathophysiology and management of cardiogenic and hypovolaemic shock

In:4.1.16 pulmonary embolism

In:4.1.17 investigation and management of cardiac failure

In:4.1.18 investigation and management of arrhythmias

In:4.1.19 Respiratory system to include:

In:4.1.20 airway care, including tracheal intubation and clearance of secretions

In:4.1.21 humidification

In:4.1.22 management of tracheostomy and decannulation

In:4.1.23 ventilators and modes of pulmonary ventilation (including non-invasive ventilation)

In:4.1.24 management of acute and chronic respiratory failure

In:4.1.25 management of severe asthma

In:4.1.26 Nervous system to include:

In:4.1.27 central nervous system infection

In:4.1.28 acute polyneuropathy

In:4.1.29 traumatic and non-traumatic coma

In:4.1.30 encephalopathies

In:4.1.31 cerebral ischaemia

In:4.1.32 status epilepticus

In:4.1.33 brainstem death

In:4.1.34 Renal, electrolyte and metabolic disorders to include:

In:4.1.35 diagnosis, prevention and management of acute renal failure

In:4.1.36 fluid, electrolyte and acid–base disorders

In:4.1.37 body temperature

In:4.1.38 adrenal and thyroid dysfunction

In:4.1.39 Haematological disorders to include:

In:4.1.40 coagulopathies

In:4.1.41 immunocompromised patients

In:4.1.42 Gastrointestinal disorders:

In:4.1.43 acute liver failure – diagnosis and management

In:4.1.44 acute pancreatitis

In:4.1.45 gut ischaemia

In:4.1.46 gastrointestinal ulceration and bleeding

In:4.1.47 translocation and absorption disorders

In:4.1.48 Nutrition:

In:4.1.49   enteral and parenteral nutrition: methods, nutrients, and complications

In:4.1.50 Analgesia, anxiolysis and sedation

In:4.1.51 Trauma:

In:4.1.52   management of multiple injuries

In:4.1.53   near-drowning

In:4.1.54   burns and smoke inhalation

In:4.1.55 Cardiopulmonary resuscitation

In:4.1.56 Management of acute poisoning:

In:4.1.57   paracetamol

In:4.1.58   aminophylline

In:4.1.59   digoxin

In:4.1.60   Ecstasy

In:4.1.61   tricyclics

In:4.1.62 Organ donation

In:4.1.63 Scoring systems and audit

In:4.1.64 Ethics

Paediatric (for optional 3-month module)

In:4.1.65 Principal anatomical and physiological differences in neonates and infants

In:4.1.66 Principal pharmacological differences in neonates and infants

In:4.1.67 Sedation and analgesia in children

In:4:1.68 Fluid management of medical and surgical emergencies

In:4.1.69 Respiratory management: nasal CPAP, pressure controlled ventilation, high frequency oscillatory ventilation

In:4.1.70 Differential diagnosis of the collapsed neonate (cardiac, sepsis, metabolic, non-accidental injury)

In:4.1.71 Common presentations of paediatric cardiac anomalies

In:4.1.72 Management of paediatric medical conditions requiring critical care: septicaemia, bronchiolitis, epilepsy, diabetic ketoacidosis and basic working knowledge of other metabolic emergencies

In:4.1.73 Principal psychological aspects of critically ill children

4.2: Skills

General

In:4.2.1 Arterial and central venous access

In:4.2.2 Insertion of thoracic drain

In:4.2.3 Insertion of oro- or nasogastric tube

Specific

In:4.2.4 Recognition of the critically ill patient

In:4.2.5 Insertion of flow-directed pulmonary artery catheter

In:4.2.6 Insertion of transvenous pacemaker

In:4.2.7 Insertion of oesophageal Doppler probe

In:4.2.8 Ultrasound visualization of main veins

In:4.2.9 Percutaneous tracheostomy

In:4.2.10 Fibreoptic bronchoscopic clearance of sputum

In:4.2.11 Peritoneal lavage

In:4.2.12 Set up ventilator for adult suffering from severe ARDS

In:4.2.13 Assist in prone positioning patient

In:4.2.14 Assist in weaning patient from IPPV via assist/CPAP

Paediatric (for optional 3 month module)

In:4.2.15 Transferring critically ill children and working knowledge of specific relevant equipment

In:4.2.16 Resuscitation of infants and children, including intubation and insertion of arterial and venous catheters and intra-osseous needles

In:4.2.17 Selection of age and size appropriate materials for the above procedures

4.3: Attitudes and behaviour

In:4.3.1 An awareness of the importance of communication skills and interpersonal relationships will be expected

In:4.3.2 Obtaining consent/assent for procedures in the critical care unit

In:4.3.3 Breaking bad news

In:4.3.4 Requesting post mortem investigation

In:4.3.5 Explaining need for unexpected/early discharge

In:4.3.6 Introducing the concept of organ donation

Paediatric (optional 3 month module)

In:4.3.7 Importance of parental roles and family dynamics in paediatric intensive care

In:4.3.8 Early initiation of child protection measures

In:4.3.9 'Listening to the child' and 'Fraser Competence'

4.4: Workplace training objectives

In:4.4.1 There will be variation in the experience and degree of competence that individual trainees will achieve in this initial period of ICM training. However, for example, they should be able to admit and manage a patient who has undergone major emergency for instance in vascular surgery or to admit and organize the early management of a patient suffering from severe respiratory failure complicated by acute renal failure

Recommended local requirements to support training

- There should be a separate designated facility (the Intensive Care Unit) for the care of the critically ill patient
- There must be a sufficient number of intensive care and high dependency beds available to serve the designated population

- The Critical Care Unit must be properly staffed and equipped for the care of such patients
- All staff providing Critical Care, medical, nursing and paramedical must be appropriately trained
- Critical Care services should be subject to clinical audit using the Intensive Care National Audit and Research Centre Case Mix Program
- Information on the provision of intensive care and high dependency care within a Trust (Augmented Care Period Dataset) must now be collected as part of the Contract Minimum Dataset

5: Neuroanaesthesia

This is an intermediate level 'Key Unit of Training' in which trainees should spend the equivalent of at least 1 month of training and, normally, not more than 3 months.

Anaesthetic training for Neurosurgery and Neuroradiology will take place within designated specialist centres with the appropriate critical care facilities.

5.1: Knowledge

In:5.1.1 Preoperative assessment and management of patients with neurological disease

In:5.1.2 Anaesthesia for imaging relevant to the CNS

In:5.1.3 Anaesthesia for MRI including problems of magnetic fields

In:5.1.4 Anatomy of the skull and skull base

In:5.1.5 Anatomy, physiological control and effect of drugs on cerebral blood volume and flow, ICP, $CMRO_2$

In:5.1.6 Principles of anaesthesia for craniotomy, to include vascular disease, cerebral tumours and posterior fossa lesions

In:5.1.7 Anaesthetic implications of pituitary disease including endocrine effects (acromegaly) and trans-sphenoidal surgery

In:5.1.8 Perioperative management of interventional neuroradiological procedures

In:5.1.9 Anaesthesia for spinal column surgery and anaesthetic implications of spinal cord trauma

In:5.1.10 Principles of immediate postoperative management including pain relief and special considerations with narcotics

In:5.1.11 Principles of neurological monitoring

In:5.1.12 Implications of prion diseases for the anaesthetist and other staff

In:5.1.13 Anaesthetic and critical care implications of neuromedical diseases:

In:5.1.14   Guillain–Barré syndrome

In:5.1.15   myasthenia gravis – pharmacological management/thymectomy

In:5.1.16   myasthenic syndrome

In:5.1.17   dystrophia myotonica

In:5.1.18   muscular dystrophy

In:5.1.19   paraplegia and long-term spinal cord damage

In:5.1.20   control of convulsions including status epilepticus

In:5.1.21   tetanus

In:5.1.22   trigeminal neuralgia including thermocoagulation

5.2: Skills

In:5.2.1 The trainee will be supervised during the provision of anaesthesia for:

In:5.2.2 Planned

In:5.2.3   intracranial surgery

In:5.2.4   spinal surgery

In:5.2.5 Emergency neurosurgery for:

In:5.2.6   head trauma

In:5.2.7 Safe patient positioning – prone, park-bench (lateral)

In:5.2.8 The trainee will be instructed in the non-surgical management of the head trauma patient

In:5.2.9 Resuscitation and patient transfer

In:5.2.10 Monitoring:

In:5.2.11   insertion of arterial lines

In:5.2.12   insertion of CVP lines

In:5.2.13   techniques for detection and management of air embolism

In:5.2.14   EEG and evoked potentials

In:5.2.15   intracranial pressure measurement

In:5.2.16   spinal drainage

In:5.2.17 Critical care:

In:5.2.18   indications for ventilation

In:5.2.19   the role of drugs

In:5.2.20   management of raised intracranial pressure and manipulation of cerebral perfusion pressure

In:5.2.21   fluid and electrolyte balance in neurocritical care

In:5.2.22   complications

In:5.2.23   treatment of raised intracranial pressure

In:5.2.24   cerebral protection and prevention of cerebral ischaemia

In:5.2.25   management of patients for organ donation

In:5.2.26 Neuroradiology:

In:5.2.27   practical aspects of patient management for CT and MRI

In:5.2.28   anaesthetic considerations in interventional radiology

5.3: Attitudes and behaviour

In:5.3.1 To understand the problems of obtaining consent in patients with impaired consciousness

In:5.3.2 To appreciate the limits of medical intervention

In:5.3.3 To gain the ability to establish a rapport with the operating neurosurgeon and exchange information during surgery on aspects of changes in the patient's vital signs which are relevant to the operative procedure

In:5.3.4 To communicate well with the nursing staff in the ICU, patients, relatives and other hospital staff

In:5.3.5 To offer comfort to the patient and relatives when there is no prospect of survival

In:5.3.6 To understand the requirements for organ donation

5.4: Workplace training objectives

In:5.4.1 Trainees should gain an understanding of the principles of neuroanaesthesia and the associated neuro-critical care in order to manage, with safety, patients for routine operations on the brain and spinal cord. For patients with head injury, trainees should be able to manage their resuscitation, stabilization and transfer

Recommended local requirements to support training

- Neuroanaesthesia should only take place in Neuroscience Centres
- Staffing levels in the operating theatre should be sufficient to allow anaesthetists to work in teams during long operations
- Interventional neuroradiology requires full neuroanaesthesia cover by consultants
- Neuro-critical care is a joint responsibility between neuroanaesthesia and neurosurgery; there should be specific sessions for neuroanaesthetists in critical care
- The provision of beds for neurocritical care must be adequate, the ventilation of patients in other areas should only occur in exceptional circumstances
- Operating theatres, intensive care units (ICU) and neuroradiology facilities including scanners should all be in close proximity

For patients with head injuries
- The care of head injured patients is an integral part of neuroanaesthesia. Specialist units accepting these patients need to make specific arrangements including protocols, staff training and rapid availability of facilities. Optimal management will improve outcome and save resources in the long term
- Local guidelines on the transfer of patients with head injuries should be drawn up between the referring hospital trusts and the neurosurgical unit which should be consistent with established national guidelines. Details of the transfer of the responsibility for patient care should also be agreed
- Only in exceptional circumstances should a patient with a significantly altered conscious level requiring transfer for neurosurgical care not be intubated

6: Obstetric anaesthesia

This is an intermediate level 'Key Unit of Training' in which trainees should spend the equivalent of at least 1 month of training and, normally, not more than 3 months.

Obstetric anaesthesia and analgesia is the only area of anaesthetic practice where two patients are cared for simultaneously. Pregnancy is a physiological rather than a pathological state. Patient expectations are high and the mother expects full involvement in her choices of care. The majority of the workload is the provision of analgesia in labour and anaesthesia for delivery. Multidisciplinary care for the sick mother is increasingly important and highlighted.

6.1: Knowledge

In:6.1.1 Anatomy and physiology of pregnancy

In:6.1.2 Physiology of labour

In:6.1.3 Placental structure and mechanisms affecting drug transfer across the placenta

In:6.1.4 Basic knowledge of obstetrics

In:6.1.5 Gastrointestinal physiology and acid aspiration prophylaxis

In:6.1.6 Pharmacology of drugs relevant to obstetric anaesthesia

In:6.1.7 Pain and pain relief in labour

In:6.1.8 Emergencies in obstetric anaesthesia:

In:6.1.9   pre-eclampsia, eclampsia, failed intubation, major haemorrhage,

In:6.1.10   maternal resuscitation, amniotic fluid embolus, total spinal

In:6.1.11 Use of magnesium sulphate

In:6.1.12 Incidental surgery during pregnancy

In:6.1.13 Assessment of fetal wellbeing in utero

In:6.1.14 Thromboprophylaxis

In:6.1.15 Feeding/starvation policies

In:6.1.16 Influence of common concurrent medical diseases

In:6.1.17 Management of twin pregnancy

In:6.1.18 Management of premature delivery

In:6.1.19 Maternal morbidity and mortality

In:6.1.20 Management of difficult or failed intubation

In:6.1.21 Maternal and neonatal resuscitation

In:6.1.22 Legal aspects related to fetus

6.2: Skills

In:6.2.1 Assessment of pregnant woman presenting for anaesthesia/analgesia

In:6.2.2 Epidural/subarachnoid analgesia for labour

In:6.2.3 Management of complications of regional block and of failure to achieve adequate block

In:6.2.4 Epidural and subarachnoid anaesthesia for caesarean section, and other operative deliveries

In:6.2.5 Conversion of analgesia for labour to that for operative delivery

In:6.2.6 General anaesthesia for caesarean section

In:6.2.7 Airway management

In:6.2.8 Management of the awake patient during surgery

In:6.2.9 Ability to ventilate the newborn with bag and mask

In:6.2.10 Anaesthesia for interventions other than delivery

In:6.2.11 Post-delivery pain relief

In:6.2.12 Management of accidental dural puncture and post-dural puncture headache

In:6.2.13 Recognition of sick mother

In:6.2.14 High dependency care of obstetric patients

In:6.2.15 Optimization for the 'at risk' baby

6.3: Attitudes and behaviour

In:6.3.1 To be aware of local guidelines in the obstetric unit

In:6.3.2 To communicate a balanced view of the advantages, disadvantages, risks and benefits of various forms of analgesia and anaesthesia appropriate to individual patients

In:6.3.3 To communicate effectively with partner and relatives

In:6.3.4 To help deal with disappointment

In:6.3.5 To be involved in the initial management of complaints

In:6.3.6 To communicate effectively with midwives

In:6.3.7 To obtain consent appropriately

In:6.3.8 To keep good records

In:6.3.9 To identify priorities

In:6.3.10 To attempt by conscientious care to recognize problems early

In:6.3.11 To allocate resources and call for assistance appropriately

In:6.3.12 To be aware of local audits and self audit

6.4: Workplace training objectives

In:6.4.1 Within the obstetric team, the trainee should play a full part; communicating effectively about anaesthetic and analgesic techniques used in obstetrics and developing organizational skills. They should consolidate clinical management of common obstetric practice but recognize and treat common complications exercising proper judgement in calling for help

Recommended local requirements to support training

- Training should normally be provided in units carrying out at least 2000 deliveries annually
- There should be at least one consultant anaesthetic session allocated for every 500 deliveries. (In units with a frequent turnover of inexperienced trainees, with a higher than average epidural or caesarean section rate and/or a substantial number of high risk cases, sessions above this minimum will be required)
- Local protocols should be available to guide trainees in the management of common obstetric emergencies based on the individual units staffing and local support
- Appropriately trained assistance for the anaesthetist (to NVQ level 3 in Operating Department Practice or in possession of the appropriate ENB qualification) must be locally available whenever a trainee anaesthetist

is required to manage a patient during an operative delivery. The person providing this assistance to the anaesthetist should have no other duties at that time

- Access for patients to critical care facilities must be immediately available at all times
- Appropriate anaesthetic 'bench books' should be available within the delivery suite

7: Paediatric anaesthesia

This is an intermediate level 'Key Unit of Training' in which trainees should spend the equivalent of at least 1 month of training and, normally, not more than 3 months.

Paediatric anaesthesia and pain management includes everything from healthy children in DGHs to the sickest premature babies in tertiary referral centres and in paediatric intensive care units (PICU). It is not expected that all trainees will be able to gain experience with neonates and preterm babies during ST Years 3 and 4. In considering the listed competencies required, it should be recognized that these will generally relate more to *Knowledge* rather than to *Skills*. However, those who intend to progress to a post with an interest in paediatric anaesthesia may be able to gain access to more paediatric training during these years, when their *Skills* should begin to include those areas listed under *Knowledge: Neonates*.

7.1: Knowledge

General

In:7.1.1 Anatomical and physiological characteristics which affect anaesthesia and the changes which take place during growth from neonate to a young child

In:7.1.2 Paediatric medical and surgical problems including major congenital abnormalities, congenital heart disease and syndromes, e.g. Down's and their implications for anaesthesia

In:7.1.3 Starvation and hypoglycaemia

In:7.1.4 Preoperative assessment and psychological preparation for surgery

In:7.1.5 Anaesthetic equipment and the differences from adult practice

Children and infants

In:7.1.6 Anaesthetic management of children for minor operations and major elective and emergency surgery

In:7.1.7 Management of recovery

In:7.1.8 Management of postoperative pain, and nausea and vomiting in children

In:7.1.9 Management of acute airway obstruction including croup and epiglottitis

Neonates

In:7.1.10 Anatomical, physiological and pharmacological differences to the older child/adult

In:7.1.11 Preoperative assessment

In:7.1.12 Anaesthetic techniques and thermoregulation

In:7.1.13 Analgesia

In:7.1.14 Neonatal equipment and monitoring

In:7.1.15 Anaesthetic problems and management of important congenital anomalies including those requiring surgical correction in the neonatal period (tracheo-oesophageal fistula, diaphragmatic hernia, exomphalos, gastroschisis, intestinal obstruction, pyloric stenosis)

In:7.1.16 Special problems of the premature and ex-premature neonate

In:7.1.17 Resuscitation of the newborn

PICU

In:7.1.18 Principles of paediatric intensive care: management of the commoner problems, ventilatory and circulatory support, multi-organ failure

In:7.1.19 Principles of safe transport of critically ill children and babies

7.2: Skills

Children and infants

In:7.2.1 Resuscitation – basic life support (BLS) and advanced life support (ALS) at all ages

In:7.2.2 Preoperative assessment and preparation

In:7.2.3 Techniques of induction, maintenance and monitoring for elective and emergency anaesthesia

In:7.2.4 Selection, management and monitoring of children for diagnostic and therapeutic procedures carried out under sedation

In:7.2.5 Maintenance of physiology: glucose, fluids, temperature

In:7.2.6 Strategies and practice for the management of anaesthetic emergencies in children: loss of airway, laryngospasm, failed venous access, suxamethonium apnoea and anaphylaxis including latex allergy

In:7.2.7 Postoperative pain management including the use of local and regional anaesthetic techniques, simple analgesics, NSAIDs and use of opioids (including infusions and PCA)

In:7.2.8 Communication with paediatric patients and their family

7.3: Attitudes and behaviour

In:7.3.1. To understand consent in children: the law, research, restraint

In:7.3.2. To communicate with parents (carers) and children throughout the surgical episode

7.4: Workplace training objectives

In:7.4.1 The trainee should develop a wide knowledge of the anaesthetic needs of children and neonates. By the end of intermediate level training they should be able to organize and manage safely a list of straightforward paediatric cases over the age of 3 years with available consultant cover. They should understand the potential hazards of paediatric anaesthesia and have had as much practical training as is possible in planning for the management of such events

Recommended local requirements to support training

- Trainers for the initial period of training should be spending not less than the equivalent of one full operating session a week in paediatric anaesthesia
- Anaesthesia for children requires specially trained staff and special facilities
- Provision should be made for parents to be involved in the care of their children
- Adequate assistance for the anaesthetist by staff with paediatric training and skill should be available
- Paediatric anaesthetic equipment must be available where children are treated

7.5: Training in child protection

Anaesthetists of all grades may encounter children who have suffered physical and/or sexual abuse in various situations:

1. Resuscitation of a critically ill child who has sustained an injury under circumstances that cannot wholly be explained by natural circumstances or is consistent with intentional trauma or abuse
2. In the paediatric intensive care unit, e.g. following severe head injury, where the above needs to be considered
3. When called upon to anaesthetize a child for a formal forensic examination, possibly involving colposcopy, sigmoidoscopy and the collection of specimens. This may also include medical photography/video records
4. Rarely a child may tell the anaesthetist about abuse ('disclosure')
5. During the course of a routine preoperative examination or surgical procedure, the anaesthetist or surgeon notes unusual or unexplained signs which may be indicative of physical or sexual abuse

In all these situations, it is essential that healthcare professionals, including the anaesthetist, act in the best interests of the child.

7.5.1 Knowledge
In:7.5.1.1 Situations in which abuse of children may present
In:7.5.1.2 Signs indicative of a possible need to safeguard the infant or child
In:7.5.1.3 Awareness of local CP procedures

7.5.2 Skills
In:7.5.2.1 Clearly communicates concerns (including documentation)
In:7.5.2.2 Ability to manage the child and their parents in a sensitive, appropriate manner

7.5.3 Attitudes and behaviour
In:7.5.3.1 Understands need to communicate concerns within team
In:7.5.3.2 Asks for senior and/or paediatrician support when appropriate

7.5.4 Workplace and training objectives
In:7.5.4.1 Demonstrates knowledge of local safeguarding children procedures

7.5.5 *Additional notes*

It is suggested that this training can be achieved in a 1 hour scenario based discussion or PBL format. In addition all trainees should be familiar with the RCoA/APA/RCPCH Guideline *Child Protection and the Anaesthetist: Safeguarding Children in the Operating Theatre.*

General principles – What to do if child abuse or neglect is suspected

- *Good communication is essential.* Anaesthetists are advised not to intervene alone, and suspicions should be discussed with the individual identified in the local guideline. In particular it would *not* be appropriate to institute or initiate formal *examination* while the child is anaesthetized, as separate consent is required
- Further management needs to be agreed in conjunction with the paediatrician, surgeon and anaesthetist. Consideration needs to be given to:
  - informing the parents (except in the case of fabricated or fictitious illness and child sexual abuse)
  - further assessment
  - informing social services and/or the police
- Full documentation is essential
- The paediatrician should lead this process, and may seek advice from the Named or Designated doctor for child protection.

Duties of the anaesthetist

- To act in the best interests of the child
- To be aware of the child's rights to be protected
- To respect the rights of the child to confidentiality
- To contact a paediatrician with experience of child protection for advice (on-call paediatrician for Named or Designated doctor/nurse)
- To be aware of the local chid protection mechanisms
- To be aware of the rights of those with parental responsibility

8: Pain management, acute and chronic

This is an intermediate level 'Key Unit of Training' in which trainees should spend the equivalent of at least 1 month of training and, normally, not more than 3 months.

The recommendations for training are in addition to the knowledge, skills, attitudes and workplace training objectives described for basic level training. Topics that are already included in the lists for basic level training are treated in greater depth during intermediate level training.

8.1 *Knowledge*

In:8.1.1 Anatomy, physiology, pharmacology and basic psychology relevant to pain management

In:8.1.2 Mechanisms of pain: somatic, visceral and neuropathic pain

In:8.1.3 Consequences of peripheral nerve injury, spinal cord injury and deafferentation

In:8.1.4 Assessment and measurement of acute pain

In:8.1.5 Techniques for control of acute pain: postoperative and post-traumatic - including children and neonates, the elderly, and patients who are handicapped, unconscious or receiving critical care

In:8.1.6 Application of pharmacological principles to the pain control: conventional analgesics and adjuvant analgesics; side effects; problems of drug dependency and addiction

In:8.1.7 Opioid and non-opioid medication, opioid infusions, patient controlled analgesia

In:8.1.8 Other medication used to manage chronic pain: antidepressants, anticonvulsants, antiarrhythmics and other adjuvant medication

In:8.1.9 Pharmacology of local anaesthetics

In:8.1.10 Principles of neural blockade for pain management: peripheral nerve, plexus, epidural and subarachnoid blocks; sympathetic blocks including stellate, coeliac plexus and lumbar sympathetic blocks; neurolytic agents and procedures; implanted catheters and pumps for drug delivery

In:8.1.11 Non-pharmacological methods of pain control. The principles of stimulation induced analgesia: transcutaneous electrical nerve stimulation and acupuncture

In:8.1.12 The role of other treatment modalities; physical therapy, surgery, psychological approaches, rehabilitation approaches, pain management programmes

In:8.1.13 Assessment of patients with chronic pain and of pain in patients with cancer

In:8.1.14 Understanding of the principles of chronic pain management in the pain clinic setting

In:8.1.15 Understanding of the importance of psychology and pain

In:8.1.16 Management of severe pain and associated symptoms in palliative care

In:8.1.17 Principles and ethics of pain research

8.2: Skills

In:8.2.1 Assessment and management of acute pain: postoperative, post-traumatic and non-surgical acute pain

In:8.2.2 Management of acute pain including special clinical groups: infants, patients with opioid dependence or tolerance, non-surgical acute pain (e.g. sickle cell disease crisis), patients who are handicapped or with impaired consciousness

In:8.2.3 Explanation of analgesic methods: oral; sublingual; subcutaneous, i.m.; i.v.; inhalational analgesia, patient controlled analgesia, epidural; regional techniques and local blocks; possible side-effects and complications

In:8.2.4 Neural blockade: brachial plexus blocks, paravertebral nerve block, intrathecal and epidural drug administration for acute and cancer pain

In:8.2.5 Management of side-effects of pain relieving medication and procedures

In:8.2.6 Basic assessment of patients with chronic pain

In:8.2.7 Recognition of neuropathic pain

In:8.2.8 Prescription of medication for chronic pain including antidepressants and anticonvulsants

In:8.2.9 Use of stimulation induced analgesia: transcutaneous electrical nerve stimulation

In:8.2.10 Basic assessment and management of pain in patients with cancer

8.3: Attitudes and behaviour

In:8.3.1 Listens to patients and their relatives

In:8.3.2 Provides explanations in a way that patients and relatives can understand

In:8.3.3 Appropriate communication with staff

In:8.3.4 Enlists help/advice from other professionals when appropriate

In:8.3.5 Awareness of role in a multi-professional team

In:8.3.6 Awareness of ethnic, cultural and spiritual issues in pain

In:8.3.7 Keeps adequate records

8.4: Workplace training objectives

In:8.4.1 Able to assess and manage acute pain for patients after most types of surgery including cardiothoracic, neurosurgery and paediatric surgery

In:8.4.2 Able to provide explanation of analgesic methods: oral, sublingual, subcutaneous, i.m., i.v. drugs, inhalational analgesia, patient controlled analgesia, epidural and regional techniques; possible side-effects and complications

In:8.4.3 Able to institute appropriate action for patients with unrelieved pain in the immediate postoperative period and unrelieved non-surgical acute pain on the wards

In:8.4.4 Able to establish priorities and formulate a treatment plan

In:8.4.5 Able to diagnose and institute initial management for neuropathic pain

In:8.4.6 Able to demonstrate technical proficiency with procedures from the skills list

In:8.4.7 Able to work as a part of a multiprofessional team

Recommended local requirements to support training

- Pain Management Services should be planned as an integrated programme although staffing and equipment resources for acute and non-acute pain may differ
  - Acute and non-acute pain management in all hospitals requires:
  - appropriate facilities, consultant sessional allocation and equipment
  - responsibility for the management of pain to be undertaken by appropriately trained consultants
  - liaison between pain management, palliative care services and other specialties to provide an inter-disciplinary approach in all areas

- ongoing education in the understanding of pain, its presentation and management, for all grades and disciplines caring for patients
- the provision of inter-disciplinary programmes which will improve patient rehabilitation while reducing pain and use of other healthcare resources
- Specific arrangements must be made for the treatment of children
- The services of investigation departments must be readily available and information concerning their services easily available to both staff and patients

9: Vascular anaesthesia

This is an intermediate level 'General Unit of Training' in which it is expected that all trainees will gain appropriate training.

Developments in interventional radiology are changing the range of elective vascular procedures taking place in the operating theatre. However, the demands for the anaesthesia and critical care of patients undergoing emergency vascular procedures, make it highly desirable that trainees receive appropriate training in this special interest if at all possible.

9.1: Knowledge

In:9.1.1 Resuscitation and management of major vascular accidents

In:9.1.2 Management of the patient with atherosclerotic disease

In:9.1.3 Management of the patient for major vascular surgery

In:9.1.4 Management of patients for endovascular radiological procedures (stenting, etc.)

In:9.1.5 Management of carotid artery surgery

In:9.1.6 Management of phaeochromocytoma

In:9.1.7 Sympathectomy

In:9.1.8 Postoperative management and critical care

In:9.1.9 Postoperative analgesia

In:9.1.10 Anaesthesia for non-cardiac surgery in patients with cardiac disease

In:9.1.11 Effects of smoking on health

In:9.1.12 Morbidity and mortality of vascular surgery

In:9.1.13 Massive blood transfusion, strategies for blood conservation, red cell salvage

In:9.1.14 Consequences of aortic cross-clamping and renal protection

9.2: Skills

In:9.2.1 Preoperative assessment

In:9.2.2 Insertion of invasive monitoring

In:9.2.3 Interpretation of information from monitoring

In:9.2.4 Management of massive blood loss

In:9.2.5 Maintenance of normothermia

In:9.2.6 Recognition and management of complications

In:9.2.7 Postoperative care

9.3: Attitudes and behaviour

In:9.3.1 Sympathetic explanation of risks and benefits of surgery and anaesthesia

In:9.3.2 Preoperative optimization

In:9.3.3 Teamwork with surgeons throughout perioperative period

In:9.3.4 Anticipation of problems

In:9.3.5 Recognition of need for help

In:9.3.6 Clarity of instructions for postoperative care

9.4: Workplace training objectives

In:9.4.1 Trainees should demonstrate competency in assessing cardiac and pulmonary function in patients with limited exercise tolerance, in the management of significant blood loss and in the use of drugs to support the heart and circulation

Recommended local requirements to support training

- Investigative facilities for cardiac and pulmonary function must be available
- Surgeons must be available with vascular expertise
- Anaesthetist with regular vascular list
- Vascular emergencies dealt with routinely
- Intensive Care/HDU facilities must be available

10: Day surgery

This is an intermediate level 'General Unit of Training' in which it is expected that all trainees will gain appropriate training.

Training should take place within a dedicated Day Surgery Unit where the management of cases as an outpatient is not compromised by elective or other operations taking place for in-patients.

10.1: Knowledge

In:10.1.1 Anaesthetic pre-assessment clinics

In:10.1.2 Instructions to patients, anaesthetic and social

In:10.1.3 Regional analgesia appropriate to day cases

In:10.1.4 General anaesthesia appropriate to day cases

In:10.1.5 Appropriate drugs for day cases

In:10.1.6 Recovery assessment

In:10.1.7 Postoperative analgesia

10.2: Skills

In:10.2.1 Instructions to patient:

In:10.2.2 Transport:

In:10.2.3   accompanying person who can drive if in own car

In:10.2.4   home not more than 1 hour away from day stay unit

In:10.2.5   level of care overnight

In:10.2.6 • telephone availability

In:10.2.7 Anaesthesia:

In:10.2.8   regional or local anaesthesia

In:10.2.9   local topical anaesthesia or sedation

In:10.2.10   general anaesthesia

In:10.2.11   recognize those unsuitable for day case management

In:10.2.12 General anaesthesia:

In:10.2.13   to limit the loss of physiological stability and to achieve rapid recovery

In:10.2.14   to select where appropriate analgesics and muscle relaxants used during outpatient GA to recognize when a patient is sufficiently recovered to return home supervised

In:10.2.15 Use of protocols or guidelines

10.3: Attitudes and behaviour

In:10.3.1 Good communication with nursing staff, patients, relatives and other hospital staff

In:10.3.2 The development of a professional and reassuring manner in order to allay patient anxieties

10.4: Workplace training objectives

In:10.4.1 The trainee must understand and apply agreed protocols with regard to patient selection and other aspects of care, and also appreciate the importance of minimizing postoperative complications such as nausea and pain, in patients who are returning home the same day

Recommended local requirements to support training

- Clear guidelines must exist for appropriate patient selection for day case surgery; these will include consideration of social factors
- Day surgery units will have a consultant in charge who chairs a multi-disciplinary management team
- Specific arrangements must be made for the treatment of children
- All patients must be assessed during the recovery phase for the adequacy of analgesia and fitness for discharge
- Clear written discharge criteria must be established
- Full written records must be maintained
- Specific instructions and information must be available for patients, their relatives and community services

11: Ear, nose and throat (otorhinolaryngology)

This is an intermediate level 'General Unit of Training' in which it is expected that all trainees will gain appropriate training.

11.1: Knowledge

In:11.1.1 Preoperative assessment, particularly prediction of a difficult intubation

In:11.1.2 Management of patients of all ages to include patients with: stridor; intubation difficulties; sleep apnoea; concomitant diseases

In:11.1.3 Local techniques and surface analgesia

In:11.1.4 Acute ENT emergencies (e.g. bleeding tonsils, croup, epiglottitis, foreign bodies). Laryngoscopy and bronchoscopy

In:11.1.5 Knowledge of special tubes, gags and equipment for microlaryngoscopy, bronchoscopy, laser surgery (e.g. Venturi devices, ventilating bronchoscope and fibreoptic bronchoscopy)

In:11.1.6 Middle ear surgery including hypotensive techniques

In:11.1.7 Major head and neck surgery (including laryngectomy)

In:11.1.8 Emergency airway management including tracheostomy

In:11.1.9 Use of helium

In:11.1.10 Postoperative management

11.2: Skills

Preoperative

In:11.2.1 Recognize the importance of preoperative assessment with particular attention to:

In:11.2.2   age (paediatric/adult/elderly)

In:11.2.3   concomitant disease GI tract

In:11.2.4   patients with sleep apnoea, stridor and intubation difficulties

In:11.2.5 Discuss the anaesthetic procedures with the patient and/or relatives (if a child is involved)

In:11.2.6 Discuss special requirements with the surgical team

In:11.2.7 Acute ENT emergencies such as bleeding tonsil bed, croup/epiglottitis

In:11.2.8 Prepare all appropriate drugs, appropriate masks, airways, tracheal tubes, bougies, laryngoscopes, throat packs

In:11.2.9 Use of appropriate disposable equipment to prevent transmission of nvCJD

Perioperative

In:11.2.10 Provide smooth anaesthesia/analgesic/surgical operating conditions

In:11.2.11 Cope with parental presence in the anaesthetic room

In:11.2.12 Use the appropriate tracheal tube or laryngeal mask

In:11.2.13 Use of special tubes, gags and goggles (laser surgery)

In:11.2.14 Techniques available for microlaryngoscopy and bronchoscopy (Venturi devices and ventilating bronchoscope)

In:11.2.15 Hypotensive anaesthetic techniques, when appropriate

In:11.2.16 To use invasive monitoring (arterial, CVP, urinary) for major surgical procedures on the head and neck

Postoperative

In:11.2.17 Extubation procedures to avoid laryngospasm

In:11.2.18 Oxygen therapy

In:11.2.19 Appropriate postoperative analgesia

In:11.2.20 Postoperative fluid balance

In:11.2.21 Maintain venous access after operation, if required

In:11.2.22 Postoperative anti-emetics

11.3: Attitudes and behaviour

In:11.3.1 Develop an understanding of the needs of the surgeon when operating on a shared airway but the absolute importance of not compromising patient safety

In:11.3.2 To support and guide recovery and other staff taking responsibility for the unconscious patient who has undergone surgery to the airway

11.4: Workplace training objectives

In:11.4.1 To develop confidence in the anaesthetic management of adults and children undergoing surgery to the airway

Recommended local requirements to support training

- Surgery is undertaken on patients of all ages from neonates to the elderly. Ear Nose and Throat units must have a paediatric facility with trained paediatric nurses
- Upper airway problems are commonplace, equipment and expertise for fibreoptic intubation must be available
- Rapid access to an experienced and efficient emergency service is required
- Access to beds for intensive or high dependency care must be available when required

12: General surgery/gynaecology/urology (± transplantation)

This is a 'General Unit of Training' in which it is expected that all trainees will gain appropriate intermediate level training.

Anaesthesia for general surgical procedures forms the backbone of specialist anaesthesia. Knowledge skills and attitudes learned during basic level training should be enhanced and refined as increased responsibility is taken by the trainee.

12.1: Knowledge

General surgery
In:12.1.1 Relevant anatomy and physiology for common surgical procedures

In:12.1.2 Anaesthesia for complex GI surgery including intrathoracic procedures

In:12.1.3 Emergency anaesthesia for general surgery

In:12.1.4 Carcinoid syndrome/tumours

In:12.1.5 Endocrinology; diseases relevant to hepatobiliary, pancreatic, splenic surgery

In:12.1.6 Management of thyroid (and parathyroid) surgery

In:12.1.7 Starvation/obesity

In:12.1.8 Metabolism; nutrients, carbohydrates, fats, proteins, vitamins, minerals

Gynaecology
In:12.1.9 Relevant anatomy and physiology

In:12.1.10 Endocrinology relating to gynaecology

In:12.1.11 Preoperative assessment

In:12.1.12 Laparoscopic surgery

In:12.1.13 Gynaecological procedures during pregnancy

Urology
In:12.1.14 Anatomy of the renal tract

In:12.1.15 Blood flow, GFR, plasma clearance

In:12.1.16 Tubular function, urine formation and micturition

In:12.1.17 Assessment of renal function

In:12.1.18 Disturbances of fluid balance, oedema and dehydration

In:12.1.19 Management of acid–base abnormalities

In:12.1.20 Renal failure and its management

In:12.1.21 Plasma electrolyte disturbances

In:12.1.22 Anaesthesia on spinal injuries patients for urological procedures

In:12.1.23 TUR syndrome

Transplantation
In:12.1.24 Principles and complications of immunosuppression

In:12.1.25 Specific anaesthetic problems associated with renal transplantation

In:12.1.26 Anaesthetic management of patients with transplanted organs

12.2: Skills

General surgery
In:12.2.1 Preoperative assessment and resuscitation of emergency surgical patient, e.g. trauma, obstruction and perforation

In:12.2.2 Postoperative analgesia, e.g. regional and field blocks

In:12.2.3 Assessment of need for ICU and HDU admission

In:12.2.4 Assessment of the elderly and children

In:12.2.5 Laparoscopic surgery

In:12.2.6 TIVA

Gynaecology

In:12.2.7 Regional techniques

In:12.2.8 Laparoscopic surgery

Urology

In:12.2.9 Regional techniques

In:12.2.10 Major procedures, e.g. nephrectomy, cystectomy

12.3: Attitudes and behaviour

General surgery

In:12.3.1 Can assess preoperative patients effectively and resuscitate appropriately

In:12.3.2 Links with other staff showing ability to coordinate a team

Gynaecology

In:12.3.3 Shows appropriate attitude and behaviour to the female patient

Transplantation

In:12.3.4 Understands the ethical implications of transplantation

12.4: Workplace training objectives

In:12.4.1 The trainee should demonstrate the required professional judgement in assessing and managing the risk of aspiration, in deciding the urgency of a case against any delay necessary for resuscitation and in assessing the requirement for postoperative critical care

13: Orthopaedic anaesthesia

This is an intermediate level 'General Unit of Training' in which it is expected that all trainees will gain appropriate training.

13.1: Knowledge

In:13.1.1 Preoperative assessment with particular reference to the problems of children, the elderly and patients with co-existing disease or injury such as congenital syndromes, rheumatoid arthritis or vertebral fractures

In:13.1.2 Special airway problems especially in the rheumatoid patient and those with cervical spine injury or pathology

In:13.1.3 Emergency anaesthesia for fractures

In:13.1.4 Resuscitation and management of patients with multiple injuries

In:13.1.5 Routine anaesthesia for joint replacement surgery, arthroscopy, fractured bones, dislocations and tendon repair

In:13.1.6 The problems that may result from the use of tourniquets and of cement

In:13.1.7 Problems of operations in the prone position

In:13.1.8 Anaesthesia for spinal surgery (including scoliosis)

In:13.1.9 Perioperative analgesia, including use of regional analgesia

In:13.1.10 Prevention, recognition and management of potential postoperative complications, including prophylaxis, recognition and management of deep venous thrombosis and pulmonary embolus, and fat embolus

In:13.1.11 Other specific complications of orthopaedic surgery including continuing blood loss, compartment syndromes, neurovascular deficit, complications due to difficulty of access to patients who may be on traction, in hip spicas, plaster jackets, and the problems of pressure areas

13.2: Skills

In:13.2.1 Airway assessment and management in the patient with rheumatoid arthritis

In:13.2.2 Safe positioning of patient, particularly in lateral and prone positions

In:13.2.3 Assessment and management of major blood loss

In:13.2.4 Correct application and use of tourniquets

13.3: Attitudes and behaviour

In:13.3.1 Provides explanations of anaesthesia for orthopaedic surgery in a way that patients can understand

In:13.3.2 Gentle handling of patient during positioning and performance of general or regional anaesthesia

In:13.3.3 Enlists help/advice from other professionals when appropriate

13.4: Workplace training objectives

In:13.3.4 Anaesthesia for orthopaedic lists enables trainees to attain competency in ensuring the smooth and efficient running of an operating list; liaising with other staff, avoiding delays and reassuring patients. They should demonstrate their ability to employ safe but effective methods for postoperative pain relief. In addition they should develop awareness of the potential hazards and complications of orthopaedic surgery

Recommended local requirements to support training

As well as the requirements for adequately staffed and equipped operating theatres, there must be provision of adequate recovery facilities, and access to an HDU if there is massive blood loss, severe hypothermia, or postoperative compromised lung function. An ICU will be needed if ventilation is required.

14: Regional anaesthesia

Regional techniques are integral components of anaesthesia in the UK now, but the College recognizes that it is inappropriate to expect that every trainee will become competent in every possible block technique, although they must be competent in all the generic aspects of block performance. Schools of Anaesthesia will vary in the range of blocks to which trainees can be exposed, but the basic level curriculum has indicated that all trainees should become competent in spinal and epidural block, with training in certain other blocks being appropriate at that stage if possible. During intermediate level training

1–2, trainees should increase their experience of regional techniques and, where opportunities allow, should increase the range of block techniques in which they become competent. The skills section below indicates the techniques which are considered most appropriate for this stage of training, experience of the various techniques normally being gained during relevant special interest attachments. Assessments should be as outlined in Section 1.2 for spinal and lumbar epidural blocks, and trainees must recognize that they should not attempt blocks until they have received supervised training, and passed the relevant assessment.

If training in these blocks is not available, it should be deferred to ST Years 3/4/5, or even until after achievement of CCT if an individual subsequently wishes to practice them.

14.1: Knowledge

In:14.1.1 Basic sciences applied to regional anaesthesia: anatomy, physiology and pharmacology

In:14.1.2 Advantages/disadvantages, risks/benefits and indications/ contraindications

In:14.1.3 Assessment, preparation and management of the patient for regional anaesthesia

In:14.1.4 The principles of minor and major peripheral nerve blocks (including cranial nerve blocks) and central neural blocks

In:14.1.5 Desirable effects, possible side-effects and complications of regional anaesthesia

In:14.1.6 Management of effects and complications

14.2: Skills

In:14.2.1 Assessment and preparation of the patient for regional anaesthesia, to include discussion of anaesthetic options (i.e. regional versus general)

In:14.2.2 Management of the patient receiving a regional block during surgery (whether awake or as part of a 'balanced' anaesthetic technique) and during labour

In:14.2.3 Management of the patient receiving regional techniques in the postoperative period, including liaison with surgeons, acute pain teams, and ward staff

In:14.2.4 Central nerve blocks:

In:14.2.5   spinal anaesthesia

In:14.2.6   epidural block (lumbar and sacral)

In:14.2.7   combined spinal/epidural

In:14.2.8 Major nerve block – able to perform at least one method for upper and lower limb surgery, respectively:

In:14.2.9   brachial plexus – one technique at least

In:14.2.10   [deliberate deletion]

In:14.2.11   sciatic

In:14.2.12   femoral

In:14.2.13 [*deliberate deletion*]

In:14.2.14 Minor nerve block:

In:14.2.15 superficial cervical plexus block

In:14.2.16 trunk (penile, intercostal and inguinal blocks)

In:14.2.17 upper limb (elbow and distal)

In:14.2.18 lower limb (ankle and distal)

In:14.2.19 Miscellaneous: ophthalmic blocks, topical, IVRA, infiltration and intra-articular

In:14.2.20 Recognition and management of the adverse effects of regional anaesthesia

Note: Thoracic epidural and deep cervical plexus blocks are ST Year 5, 6 and 7 competencies. A fuller range of 'major' nerve block techniques would be appropriate during these years also if the relevant training and experience are available. Cranial nerve, cervical epidural, paravertebral, lumbo sacral and autonomic block competencies are appropriate only to senior trainees working towards competency in pain and other relevant special interests. Again, there should be formal assessment, along the lines already outlined, of each block before the trainee can be judged as competent.

14.3: Attitudes and behaviour

In:14.3.1 Provides explanations of regional techniques in a way that patients can understand

In:14.3.2 Understands patients' anxieties about regional techniques, especially the stress of undergoing surgery while conscious

In:14.3.3 Recognizes need for communication with staff about use of regional block

In:14.3.4 Handles patients gently during performance of regional block

In:14.3.5 Meticulous attention to safety and sterility during performance of regional blocks

In:14.3.6 Enlists help/advice from other professionals when appropriate

14.4: Workplace training objectives

In:14.4.1 Trainees should take appropriate opportunities to use regional anaesthesia in patients undergoing a range of operations in specialties such as orthopaedics, gynaecology, urology and plastic surgery in order to demonstrate their attainment of the listed requirements. All such cases should be fully detailed in the logbook

15: Trauma and accidents

This is a 'General Unit of Training' in which it is expected that all trainees will gain appropriate intermediate level training.

Many aspects of this unit of training will be closely linked with knowledge and skills covered in other units of training. The recommendations made here are therefore broadly stated. Increasingly, anaesthetic trainees completing intermediate level training will have taken part in a course in Advanced

Trauma Life Support (ATLS or equivalent) which will have fulfilled the requirements of this unit of training. For those trainees that have not had this opportunity, it is suggested that this unit of training be modelled along similar lines.

15.1: Knowledge

In:15.1.1 Management of head injury, spinal injury and multiple trauma with major blood loss

In:15.1.2 Major incident management, triage and anaesthesia in situations outside the hospital

In:15.1.3 Transfer of the traumatized patient including emergency airway and pain management

In:15.1.4 Management of the burned patient

In:15.1.5 Immersion/drowning and near-drowning

In:15.1.6 Hypothermia

In:15.1.7 Trauma scoring systems

15.2: Skills

In:15.2.1 Many of the skills required are those also associated with other specialties, but there is the additional requirement to be able to perform rapid assessments and to prioritize patients' needs

In:15.2.2 Experience in transfers should be gained

In:15.2.3 Management of allergy

15.3: Attitudes and behaviour

In:15.3.1 Linking with other specialists to work in a team (this includes paramedic and ambulance personnel)

In:15.3.2 Understanding and adherence to, agreed protocols

In:15.3.3 Recognizing the essential requirement for stabilization prior to transfer

In:15.3.4 To be able to organize and manage the safe transfer of the intubated/ventilated patient

15.4: Workplace training objectives

In:15.4.1 The trainee should attain the ability to be an effective member of the trauma team and take an appropriate role in managing transfers

Recommended local requirements to support training

- Every hospital should have a designated consultant anaesthetist to coordinate anaesthetic services for trauma
- In hospitals designated to receive major trauma patients there should be a defined trauma team to respond immediately whenever a patient with major injuries is admitted
- Hospitals designated to receive major trauma patients should have:
  - Access to core specialities at all times

- An intensive care unit
- Facilities for high dependency care
- Any hospital designated to manage major trauma in children should have staff with paediatric training and experience. There should be an agreed set of guidelines for the treatment of children
- There should be agreed guidelines for the referral and transfer of trauma patients

16: Diagnostic imaging, anaesthesia and sedation

This is an intermediate level 'Additional Unit of Training' which may or may not be available to trainees depending on the distribution and availability of services locally.

The role of the anaesthetist in providing general anaesthesia and sedation together with physiological and pharmacological support for patients in the X-ray department is evolving rapidly. Trainees need to understand the benefits and risks particularly with regard to interventional procedures.

16.1: Knowledge

In:16.1.1 Preanaesthetic preparation
In:16.1.2 Techniques appropriate for adults and children for CT scanning, MR imaging and angiography
In:16.1.3 Post-investigation care

16.2: Skills

In:16.2.1 Pre-anaesthetic preparation
In:16.2.2 Sedation and general anaesthetic techniques for:
In:16.2.3   angiography and interventional procedures
In:16.2.4   CT scanning, adults and children
In:16.2.5   magnetic resonance imaging with respect to:
In:16.2.6 • the isolated patient
In:16.2.7 • the problems due to magnetic field
In:16.2.8 Post-investigation care

16.3: Attitudes and behaviour

In:16.3.1 Establishing good communication and an understanding of their working needs with nursing staff, radiographers and radiologists

16.4: Workplace training objectives

In:16.4.1 Trainees should understand the implications of different interventional radiological procedures in their anaesthetic care of the patient and be able to establish safe anaesthesia or sedation within the confines and limitations of the X-ray department

Recommended local requirements to support training

The provision of anaesthetic and monitoring equipment together with assistance for the anaesthetist should be to a similar standard as is provided in the operating theatres for an equivalent case.

17: Maxillo-facial/dental anaesthesia

This is an intermediate level 'Additional Unit of Training' which may or may not be available to trainees depending on the distribution and availability of services locally.

Maxillo-facial surgery covers a range of procedures from simple dental extractions to complex resections and reconstructive procedures. The age range of patients is similarly wide, from childhood to the elderly.

17.1: Knowledge

In:17.1.1 Preoperative assessment

In:17.1.2 Day-case/in-patient requirements

In:17.1.3 Resuscitation facilities

In:17.1.4 Anaesthesia for dental extractions (to include sedation and analgesic techniques)

In:17.1.5 Paediatric anaesthesia

In:17.1.6 Assessment and management of the difficult airway including fibre-optic intubation. Anaesthesia for maxillo-facial surgery including the perioperative management of the fractured jaw and other major facial injuries

In:17.1.7 Postoperative management for all patients undergoing dental or maxillo-facial procedures

17.2: Skills

Many of the skills required for this unit of training are shared with ENT surgery

In:17.2.1 Patient assessment for day-stay surgery, including children and the mentally and physically handicapped

In:17.2.2 Pre- and postoperative instructions for patients

In:17.2.3 Talking to patients and explaining the anaesthesia proposed

In:17.2.4 Choice of anaesthetic technique

In:17.2.5 Potential problems and hazards of the shared airway

In:17.2.6 Airway management including nasal masks, naso-pharyngeal airways, laryngeal mask airways, oral and nasal endotracheal intubation

In:17.2.7 Working with dental and oral surgeons and their use of mouth props and packs

In:17.2.8 Appropriate monitoring techniques and record-keeping

In:17.2.9 Recovery and patient assessment for discharge including regular audit of outcomes

In:17.2.10 Management of emergencies

In:17.2.11 Conscious sedation:

In:17.2.12 Patient selection, assessment and suitability for treatment under sedation

In:17.2.13 The techniques and drugs available including non-pharmacological methods

In:17.2.14 Administration methods – oral, inhalational, intravenous, transmucosal, patient-controlled

In:17.2.15 Monitoring and management of the sedated patient

17.3: Attitudes and behaviour

In:17.3.1 Develop an understanding of the needs of the surgeon when operating on a shared airway but the absolute importance of not compromising patient safety

In:17.3.2 To support and guide recovery and other staff taking responsibility for the unconscious patient who has undergone surgery to the airway

17.4: Workplace training objectives

In:17.4.1 Trainees should develop confidence in the anaesthetic management of adults and children undergoing surgery to the airway

Recommended local requirements to support training

- Surgery is undertaken on patients of all ages from neonates to the elderly. There must be a paediatric facility with trained paediatric nurses
- Upper airway problems are commonplace, equipment and expertise for fibreoptic intubation must be available
- Rapid access to an experienced and efficient emergency service is required
- Access to beds for intensive or high dependency care must be available when required

18: Ophthalmic anaesthesia

This is an intermediate level 'Additional Unit of Training' which may or may not be available to trainees depending on the distribution and availability of services locally.

This specialty affords potentially very valuable training for trainees at intermediate level. The age range of the patients and the wide adoption of local anaesthetic techniques are particular aspects that can be beneficial to the development of the trainee. However, it is recognized that only a proportion of trainees will be able to gain this experience in the ST Years 3 and 4.

18.1: Knowledge

In:18.1.1 Preoperative assessment with particular reference to patients with co-morbidities

In:18.1.2 Choice of local or general anaesthetic techniques in relation to the patient and surgery with particular reference to:

In:18.1.3   strabismus surgery

In:18.1.4   cataract surgery

In:18.1.5   surgery for the detached retina

In:18.1.6 Penetrating eye injury

In:18.1.7 Control of intraocular pressure

In:18.1.8 Action of anaesthetic drugs on the eye

In:18.1.9 Anatomy relevant to local anaesthetic blocks

In:18.1.10 Local analgesia

In:18.1.11   topical anaesthesia

In:18.1.12   risks of sharp needles in peribulbar and retrobulbar techniques

In:18.1.13   sub-Tenon's block

In:18.1.14 Problems of glaucoma surgery

In:18.1.15 Postoperative care

18.2: Skills

In:18.2.1 Assessment and preparation, including the use of day-care facilities

In:18.2.2 Anaesthetic management of patients for lachrymal surgery including syringing and probing and dacryocystorhinostomy

In:18.2.3 Requirements for strabismus surgery, including knowledge of the oculocardiac reflex

In:18.2.4 Control of intraocular pressure

In:18.2.5 The use of topical preparations, possible effects and interactions

In:18.2.6 Appropriate local anaesthetic methods

In:18.2.7 Techniques of general anaesthesia for ophthalmic surgery

In:18.2.8 Choice and use of appropriate method for airway maintenance under general anaesthesia

In:18.2.9 Postoperative care

18.3: Attitudes and behaviour

In:18.3.1 Understanding of the importance of the patient's general health and wishes to decisions relating to the choice of anaesthetic techniques

In:18.3.2 Being an effective communicator with elderly patients in explaining the risks and benefits of general and local anaesthesia for eye surgery

18.4: Workplace training objectives

In:18.4.1 Trainees should develop expertise in the administration of local anaesthesia for eye surgery trying to obtain competency in at least one block. They should also show the necessary medical knowledge and skill in the preoperative assessment of elderly patients

Recommended local requirements to support training

Availability of facilities, support staff including assistance for the anaesthetist and the anaesthetic and monitoring equipment must be to the standards set out in documents from the RCA and AAGBI.

19: Plastics/burns

This is an intermediate level 'Additional Unit of Training' which may or may not be available to trainees depending on the distribution and availability of services locally.

While much plastic surgery takes place in specialist centres, there are often routine lists in other hospitals, this should enable most anaesthetic trainees to gain some intermediate level experience in this specialty. However, severe burns, although initially admitted to many A&E departments will, following resuscitation, be transferred to a specialist unit. Training opportunities will therefore be limited, although the expectation is that many anaesthetists will be involved in the initial resuscitation of burns at a receiving hospital. It is recognized that training in this field will, in many cases, need to be supplemented by other teaching and instructional methods such as CD-ROM presentations.

19.1: Knowledge

In:19.1.1 Preoperative assessment

In:19.1.2 Assessment and management of the difficult airway including fibreoptic intubation

In:19.1.3 Day-case/in-patient requirements

In:19.1.4 Paediatric anaesthesia

In:19.1.5 Postoperative management for patients who have undergone plastic surgical procedures with particular reference to free flaps

In:19.1.6 Physiology of tissue blood flow

In:19.1.7 Benefits and risks of hypotensive anaesthesia

In:19.1.8 Pathophysiology of the patient with burns

In:19.1.9 Resuscitation of the patient with burns with particular reference to fluid management

In:19.1.10 Pathophysiology, assessment, diagnosis and management of injury due to heat and smoke inhalation

19.2: Skills

Plastic surgery

In:19.2.1 General and regional anaesthesia for plastic surgery including:

In:19.2.2   anaesthesia for head and neck surgery

In:19.2.3   anaesthesia for free flaps and reimplantation

In:19.2.4   anaesthesia for cleft palate repair

In:19.2.5 Specific problems of prolonged anaesthesia

In:19.2.6 Manipulation and control of blood pressure to assist surgery

In:19.2.7 Managing the acutely compromised airway including experience with trans-tracheal ventilation

In:19.2.8 Prediction and management of the difficult intubation

In:19.2.9 Selection of the appropriate method of airway maintenance, use of the LMA

In:19.2.10 Techniques for continuous local anaesthesia

Burns

In:19.2.11 Resuscitation in the management of the patient with burns

In:19.2.12 Recognition and treatment of airway problems

In:19.2.13 Institution of intravenous fluid therapy and fluid replacement

In:19.2.14 Analgesia

In:19.2.15 Transportation requirements

In:19.2.16 Temperature maintenance

In:19.2.17 Monitoring:

In:19.2.18   insertion of lines

In:19.2.19   problems with access

In:19.2.20 Responses to drugs in burned patients

In:19.2.21 Recognition and management of the airway burn and initiating appropriate treatment

19.3: Attitudes and behaviour

In:19.3.1 To be able to foresee potential problems and plan appropriately

In:19.3.2 When using elective hypotensive techniques to maintain professional independence, recognizing the absolute need to protect the patient's safety at all times and not to succumb to unreasonable pressure from the surgeon

19.4: Workplace training objectives

In:19.4.1 Trainees should develop skills in the management of the difficult airway, learn the value and limitations of hypotensive techniques and obtain a clear understanding of the priorities in the resuscitation of the patient with burns

Recommended local requirements to support training

Plastics

- The care of head and neck patients is an integral part of plastic anaesthesia. Specialist units accepting these patients need to make specific arrangements including protocols, staff training and rapid availability of facilities, especially access to HDU or ICU beds. Optimal management will improve outcome and save resources in the long term

Burns

- Emergency anaesthetic assessment and treatment of burned patients may be required in any hospital with an A&E department. Guidelines should be available concerning immediate care and transfer to an appropriate Burn Care service
- The critical care of burned patients is an integral part of burns anaesthesia services. Specialist departments accepting these patients need to make specific arrangements including protocols, staff training and rapid availability of facilities. Optimal management will improve outcome and save resources in the long term
- Major burn anaesthesia should take place only in a Burns Centre or Bums Unit. Full consultant cover should be available
- Paediatric burn cases, which constitute a major proportion of burn victims, require special facilities and staffing
- Pain relief throughout the care process and especially for interventions is an integral part of burn anaesthesia provision

20: Miscellaneous

This is an intermediate level 'Additional Unit of Training' which may or may not be available to trainees depending on the distribution and availability of services locally.

There are a number of other aspects of the practice of anaesthesia, critical care and pain management which will, to a greater or lesser extent, be available to trainees within a specific training programme. Some are itemized here, others may be added.

20.1: Knowledge

In:20.1.1 Electro-convulsive therapy (ECT)
In:20.1.2 Radiotherapy
In:20.1.3 Minimal access surgery
In:20.1.4 Perioperative management of a patient with sleep apnoea

20.2: Skills

In:20.2.1 The ways in which anaesthetic techniques need to be modified to suit the requirements of particular environments, surgical techniques and patients with uncommon but potentially dangerous problems

20.3: Attitudes and behaviour

In:20.3.1 Cooperation with other medical professionals in using anaesthetic skills to assist their work but only within the anaesthetist's responsibility to safeguard the patient
In:20.3.2 Recognizing the ethical duty that the anaesthetist has to their patient

20.4: Workplace training objectives

In:20.4.1 Trainees should demonstrate adaptability in their approach to anaesthetic practice but recognize the essential importance of not compromising the safety of the anaesthetized patient whatever the external demands that are being made

21: Applied physiology

21.1: Knowledge

Candidates are expected to be able to apply the basic knowledge of human physiology necessary to pass the Primary FRCA examination to the clinical practice of anaesthesia and intensive care medicine. While all branches of physiology are of importance, it is recognized that clinical relevance dictates the topics selected for the examination.

In:21.1.1 Haematological
In:21.1.2 Anaemia
In:21.1.3 Polycythaemia
In:21.1.4 Immunity and allergy
In:21.1.5 Inflammation
In:21.1.6 Blood groups
In:21.1.7 Alternative oxygen carrying solutions

22: Applied clinical pharmacology

22.1: Knowledge

This section requires a wider knowledge of drugs than in the Primary FRCA examination. For drugs used in anaesthesia and intensive care medicine candidates will also be expected to be aware of new drugs which are undergoing evaluation and whose human application has been reported in the mainstream anaesthetic journals. There will be emphasis on the practical application of pharmacological and pharmacokinetic knowledge, and upon an appreciation of the hazards and limitation of individual techniques.

In:22.1.16 Premedication:
In:22.1.17 • The use of anxiolytics, sedatives and antisialagogues
In:22.1.18 • Pro-kinetic and anti-emetic drugs
In:22.1.19 • H2 and proton pump antagonists
In:22.1.20 Inhalational anaesthesia:
In:22.1.21 • Control of alveolar tension during induction and recovery
In:22.1.22 • Control of anaesthetic depth and prevention of awareness
In:22.1.23 • Management of sedation techniques (including Entonox)
In:22.1.24 • Environmental effects
In:22.1.25 Intravenous anaesthesia:
In:22.1.26 • Methods for achieving specified plasma concentrations
In:22.1.27 • Bolus, infusion, and profiled administration
In:22.1.28 • Management of neuromuscular blockade:
In:22.1.29 • Techniques for the use and reversal of muscle relaxants
In:22.1.30 • Management of abnormal responses
In:22.1.31 Regional anaesthesia:
In:22.1.32 • Choice of agent and technique
In:22.1.33 • Additives
In:22.1.34 • Systemic effects
In:22.1.35 • Avoidance of toxicity
In:22.1.36 Prevention of postoperative nausea and vomiting
In:22.1.37 Application of pharmacological principles to the control of acute
        pain
In:22.1.38 (including intraoperative analgesia and postoperative pain
        management) and chronic pain
In:22.1.39 Pharmacological control of myocardial function, vascular resistance,
        heart
In:22.1.40 rate and blood pressure
In:22.1.41 Anticoagulant and thrombolytic therapies. Management of
        coagulopathies
In:22.1.42 Pharmacological control of blood sugar
In:22.1.43 Pharmacological problems in cardiopulmonary bypass.
        Cardioplegia
In:22.1.44 Therapeutic problems associated with organ transplantation: heart,
        lung, liver kidney
In:22.1.45 Management of malignant hyperthermia
In:22.1.46 Pharmacological considerations in cardiopulmonary resuscitation,
        major
In:22.1.47 trauma and exsanguinations
In:22.1.48 Pharmacological control of severe infections
In:22.1.49 Pharmacological treatment of severe asthma
In:22.1.50 Effect of renal or hepatic impairment on drug disposition

23: The statistical basis of clinical trial management

23.1: Knowledge

In:23.1.1 Candidates will be expected to understand the statistical fundamentals upon which most clinical research is based. They may be asked to suggest suitable approaches to test problems, or to comment on experimental results. They will not be asked to perform detailed calculations or individual statistical tests

23.2: Data collection and analysis

In:23.2.1 Simple aspects of study design defining the outcome measures and the uncertainty of measuring them

23.3: Application to clinical practice

In:23.3.1 Distinguishing statistical from clinical significance
In:23.3.2 Understanding the limits of clinical trials
In:23.3.3 The basics of systematic review and its pitfalls

23.4: Study design

In:23.4.1 Defining a clinical research question
In:23.4.2 Understanding bias
In:23.4.3 Controls, placebos, randomization, blinding exclusion criteria
In:23.4.4 Statistical issues, especially sample size ethical issues

24: Clinical measurement

24.1: Knowledge

The Final examination assumes knowledge of the Primary FRCA examination syllabus, with the addition of more sophisticated measurements. There is an emphasis on clinical applications of clinical measurement, such as indications, practical techniques and interpretation of acquired data. Candidates will be expected to understand the sources of error and the limitations of individual measurements.

In:24.1.1 Assessment of respiratory function
In:24.1.2 Assessment of cardiac function
In:24.1.3 The electroencephalograph (EEG) and evoked potentials
In:24.1.4 The electromyograph (EMG) and measurement of nerve conduction
In:24.1.5 Assessment of neuromuscular function, peripheral nerve stimulators
In:24.1.6 Principles and practice of in vitro blood-gas measurements. Interpretation of data
In:24.1.7 Interpretation of biochemical data
In:24.1.8 Interpretation and errors of dynamic pressure measurements including systemic, pulmonary arterial and venous pressures, intracranial, intrathoracic and intra-abdominal pressures
In:24.1.9 Methods of measurement of cardiac output and derived indices; limitations and interpretation

In:24.1.10 Principles of imaging techniques including CT, MRI and ultrasound. Doppler effect

In:24.1.11 Interpretation and errors of capnography, oximetry and ventilatory gas analysis

Table A1.2 Blueprint of workplace-based assessments mapped against intermediate level competences

Intermediate level competences	Workplace-based assessments			
	DOPS	Anaes-CEX	CBD	MSF
Generic knowledge and skills	X	X	X	
Academic/research			X	
Cardiac/thoracic anaesthesia	X	X	X	
Intensive care medicine	X	X	X	X
Neuroanaesthesia	X	X	X	X
Obstetric anaesthesia	X	X	X	X
Paediatric anaesthesia	X	X	X	X
Pain management, acute and chronic	X	X	X	X
Vascular anaesthesia	X	X	X	X
Day surgery	X	X	X	X
Ear, nose and throat (otorhinolaryngology)	X	X	X	X
General surgery/gynaecology/urology (± transplantation)		X	X	X
Orthopaedic anaesthesia	X	X	X	X
Regional anaesthesia	X	X	X	X
Trauma and accidents	X	X	X	X
Diagnostic imaging, anaesthesia and sedation	X	X	X	
Maxillo-facial/dental anaesthesia	X	X	X	X
Ophthalmic anaesthesia	X	X	X	X
Plastics/burns	X	X	X	

Table A1.2 Blueprint of workplace-based assessments mapped against intermediate level competences—cont'd

Intermediate level competences	Workplace-based assessments			
	DOPS	Anaes-CEX	CBD	MSF
Communication skills, attitudes and behaviour	X	X	X	X
The responsibilities of professional life	X		X	X
Teaching and medical education	X			X
Health care management			X	
Medical ethics and law		X	X	

Updated guidance on the practical application of these assessments can be found in the training pages of the RCoA website.

REGULATIONS: PRIMARY AND FINAL FRCA EXAMINATION REGULATIONS

These Regulations apply to Examinations commencing after 1 August 2009 (www.rcoa.ac.uk/docs/regulations2009.pdf)

Introduction

The Regulations which govern the content and conduct of the examinations leading to the award of the Fellowship of the Royal College of Anaesthetists. They specify:

- Eligibility requirements
- Application procedures
- Limitations on the number of attempts
- The requirement for guidance in the event of failure
- Procedures for making representations and appeals
- The sanctions for infringements.

Section 1: Training definitions

1 (a) For the purpose of these Regulations a trainee is someone who has received 'approved training' in the UK and/or the Republic of Ireland.

(b) For the purpose of these Regulations 'approved training' means training:

(i) which is part of a UK PMETB approved programme of training in Anaesthesia or Acute Care Common Stem (ACCS) which, if satisfactorily completed, may contribute to the award of a Certificate of Completion of Training in Anaesthesia; or

(ii) has been approved by the College of Anaesthetists of the Royal College of Surgeons in Ireland; or

(iii) in certain circumstances has been approved as part of the Overseas Doctors' Training Scheme; and

(iv) which is appropriate to the part of the examination for which the candidate is applying.

Section 2: Commencement and revocation

2 (a) These Regulations came into force on 1 August 2009 and apply to examinations commencing on or after that date.

   (b) These Examination Regulations made by the Council of the Royal College of Anaesthetists supersede any previous Regulations, which are hereby revoked.

Section 3: Examinations

3 (a) The examination for the Fellowship of the Royal College of Anaesthetists (FRCA) will be in two parts. The first part will be known as the Primary FRCA Examination and the second part will be known as the Final FRCA Examination.

   (b) There will normally be three sittings of the Primary FRCA Examination and two sittings of the Final FRCA Examination in each academic year. Council may at any time decide, subject to adequate notice, to alter the number of sittings of either or both parts in any year.

   (c) The subject matter of each part of the examination is specified in the relevant parts of The CCT in Anaesthesia; Part II: Competency Based Basic Level Training and Assessment, and Part III: Competency Based Intermediate Level Training and Assessment.

   (d) The nature of each examination, together with details of the marking systems used and the prizes which may be awarded are described in Appendices 1, 2 and 4 of these Regulations.

Primary FRCA

4 The Primary FRCA Examination is divided into three sections taken on two separate days:

   • Multiple Choice Question (MCQ) paper
   • Objective Structured Clinical Examination (OSCE)
   • Structured Oral Examination (SOE).

5 (a) Candidates must pass the MCQ paper before they can apply to sit the OSCE and SOE.

   (b) A pass in the MCQ paper will be valid for two years, after which time if the whole examination has not been passed the MCQ must be re-taken.

(c) At the first attempt the OSCE and SOE sections must be taken together. If one section is failed only that section must be retaken, subject to Regulations 5(b) and (d). If both sections are failed then they must be retaken at the same sitting.

(d) A pass in the OSCE or SOE will be valid for two years, after which time if the whole examination has not been passed, the relevant section(s) must be re-taken.

(e) Candidates will be allowed five attempts at the MCQ and four attempts at the OSCE and SOE, subject to remaining eligible under Regulation 13.

(f) Under Regulation 17(b)(i) a pass in the whole Primary FRCA Examination is valid for 10 years for entry to the Final FRCA Examination.

6   Transitional arrangements

(a) All attempts under previous Regulations count in full against attempts allowed under the 2009 Regulations.

(b) At the first attempt after 1 August 2009, candidates must sit both the OSCE and SOE sections in accordance with Regulation 5(c).

Final FRCA

7   The Final FRCA Examination is divided into two sections taken on two separate days:

1.   A written section consisting of
   • Multiple Choice Question (MCQ) paper
   • Short Answer Question (SAQ) paper
2.   Structured Oral Examination (SOE).

8   (a) Candidates must pass the written section before they can apply to sit the SOE.

(b) A pass in the written section will be valid for two years after which time, if the whole examination has not been passed, the written section must be retaken.

(c) Candidates will be allowed six attempts at each section subject to remaining eligible under Regulation 17.

9   Transitional arrangements

(a) All attempts under previous Regulations count in full against attempts allowed under the 2009 Regulations.

(b) At the first attempt after 1 August 2009, candidates must sit and pass the written section before applying to sit the SOE in accordance with Regulation 8(a).

Section 4: Prioritization of applications

10   There is no prioritization for the Primary MCQ or Final written papers, but candidates may not always get their first choice of venue.

11   (a) Subject to their being eligible in all other respects to sit the Primary OSCE/ SOE or Final FRCA SOE priority will be given to applicants who are:

(i)   trainees currently in Deanery approved training posts on a PMETB approved training programme in Anaesthesia or ACCS (as defined in these Regulations)

(ii) Specialty/Staff and Associate Specialist (SAS) Grade Doctors who meet the requirements of Regulations 13(b)(iv), 17(a)(iv) or 17(c)(iii)

(iii) trainees sponsored by the College under the Overseas Doctors' Training Scheme.

(b) The following applicants will be accepted, in the order listed, if the College has the capacity to examine them at the sitting applied for, in the Primary OSCE/SOE and Final SOE:

(i)   former UK trainees

(ii) trainees currently in approved training posts in the Republic of Ireland

(iii) former trainees in the Republic of Ireland.

Candidates in the above categories will be told as soon as possible after the published closing date for applications whether or not their applications have been accepted.

12 Specialists directed by PMETB to undergo an assessment of knowledge of Anaesthesia to support an application for entry to the Specialist Register under 'Article 14' will be admitted to the appropriate examination(s) under special arrangements.

Section 5: Eligibility for the primary FRCA MCQ examination

The College strongly recommends that candidates should not sit the Primary FRCA MCQ paper until they have passed the Initial Assessment of Competency.

13 A person is eligible to enter the Primary FRCA MCQ paper who:

(a) is eligible for full registration with the General Medical Council (United Kingdom); and

(b) (i)   is currently registered with the College as a trainee in a Deanery approved training post on a PMETB approved training programme in Anaesthesia or ACCS (as defined in these Regulations); or

(ii) is currently registered as a trainee in Anaesthesia with the College of Anaesthetists of The Royal College of Surgeons in Ireland; or

(iii) left an approved Anaesthesia or ACCS training post in the United Kingdom or Ireland no more than five years before the published start date of the sitting applied for; or

(iv) is a Specialty/SAS Grade Doctor who:

- left approved training in the United Kingdom or Ireland more than five years before the published start date of the sitting applied for

- is currently practising Anaesthesia in the UK

- is a member of the College: and has the written support of the Regional Advisor.
    - (v) is a trainee sponsored under the Overseas Doctor's Training Scheme by the Bernard Johnson Advisor (Overseas); and
  - (c) satisfies the requirements of these Regulations with regard to application procedures and other matters.
14 A person shall not be eligible to enter for the Primary MCQ paper who has already attempted and failed that paper five times.

Section 6: Eligibility for the primary FRCA OSCE and SOE

The College strongly recommends that candidates should not sit the Primary FRCA OSCE and SOE until they are at least half way through their Basic Level training programme in Anaesthesia.

15 A person is eligible to enter the Primary FRCA OSCE and SOE who:
  - (a) is eligible to enter the Primary FRCA MCQ paper as prescribed in Regulations 13, with the exception that trainees following an ACCS course of training must have been allocated to Anaesthesia as their chosen specialty
  - (b) has passed the Primary FRCA MCQ paper within 2 years before the published starting date of the sitting applied for
  - (c) (i) has passed the Initial Assessment of Competency in Anaesthesia (IAC); or
    - (ii) has passed the College of Anaesthetists RCSI equivalent of the IAC; or
    - (iii) is a Specialty/SAS grade Doctor who has not passed the IAC but has the written support of the Regional Adviser; and
    - (iv) is a trainee sponsored under the Overseas Doctor's Training Scheme who has the written support of his College Tutor.
  - (d) satisfies the requirements of these Regulations with regard to application procedures and other matters.
16 A person shall not be eligible to enter for the Primary FRCA OSCE and/or SOE who has attempted and failed:
  - (a) either the OSCE or SOE section of the Primary FRCA Examination twice, until they have attended the mandatory guidance – see Regulation 31(a).
  - (b) either the OSCE or SOE section of the Primary FRCA Examination four times.

ACCS trainees allocated to Emergency Medicine or General (Internal) Medicine (Acute) as their chosen specialties are not eligible to sit this examination. NB A pass in the CARCSI Primary MCQ Examination does not give exemption from the FRCA Primary MCQ Examination.

Section 7: Eligibility for the final FRCA examination

The College strongly recommends that candidates should not sit the Final FRCA Examination until they are at least one-third of the way through their intermediate level training programme in Anaesthesia.

17 A person is eligible to enter for the Final FRCA Examination who:

(a) (i) is currently registered with the College as a trainee in a Deanery approved training post on a PMETB approved training programme in Anaesthesia (as defined in these Regulations); or

(ii) is currently registered as a trainee in Anaesthesia with the College of Anaesthetists of The Royal College of Surgeons in Ireland; or

(iii) left an approved training post in the United Kingdom or Ireland no more than 5 years before the published starting date of the sitting applied for; or

(iv) is a Specialty/SAS Grade Doctor who left approved training more than 5 years before the published start date of the sitting applied for;

- is currently practising Anaesthesia in the UK;
- is a member of The College; and
- has the written support of the Regional Adviser; or

(v) is a holder of an exempting qualification (see Paragraph 19) and satisfies the following criteria:

- has passed the exempting qualification within the ten years before the published start date of the Final exam applied for, has joined the College's Voluntary Register,
- has been employed as an anaesthetist in an NHS post, with a clearly determined training element, for 12 months immediately prior to the date of the Final examination applied for. This post must be prospectively approved by the College's Bernard Johnson Advisor (Overseas).

(b) (i) has passed the Primary FRCA Examination within ten years before the published start date of the sitting applied for; or

(ii) satisfies the conditions stated in Regulation 19 even if they have failed any part of the Primary FRCA Examination four times; and

(c) (i) has been awarded the UK Basic Level Training Certificate, the UK SHO Training Certificate or the Irish Certificate of Completion of Basic Specialist Training; or

(ii) if they are sponsored as a trainee under the Overseas Doctor's Training Scheme, has received at least one satisfactory supervisor's report at a standard equivalent to that of a Deanery Annual Review of Competence Progression (ARCP) before the published start date of the sitting applied for; or

(iii) if they are a Specialty/SAS Grade Doctor they have the written support of the Regional Adviser; and

(d) satisfies the requirements of these Regulations with regard to application procedures and other matters.

18 A person shall not be eligible to enter either section of the Final FRCA Examination who has attempted and failed:

(a) either section of the Final FRCA Examination three times, until they have attended the mandatory guidance (see Regulation 33.(b)).

(b) either section of the Final FRCA Examination six times.

Exemptions

19 A candidate for the Final FRCA Examination shall be exempt from passing the Primary FRCA Examination who, within the ten years preceding the closing date of the sitting applied for, and only in such years as are specified, and subject to annual renewal of approval by the Council:

(a) has passed:

(i) the Primary examination for the Fellowship of the Faculty or the College of Anaesthetists of The Royal College of Surgeons in Ireland (provided it was sat in the Republic of Ireland); or

(ii) the examinations for the Fellowship of the Australian and New Zealand College of Anaesthetists; or

(iii) the examinations for the European Diploma in Anaesthesiology and Intensive Care of the European Academy of Anaesthesiology or the European Society of Anaesthesiology.

(b) has obtained any of the following qualifications:

(i) Fellowship of the Faculty or the College of Anaesthetists of the Royal College of Surgeons in Ireland;

(ii) Doctor of Medicine (Anaesthesiology) of the University of Colombo, Sri Lanka;

(iii) Master of Anaesthesia of the University of Khartoum, Sudan before December 2007;

(iv) Master of Medicine (Anaesthesia) of the National University of Singapore;

(v) Fellowship in Anaesthesiology of the College of Physicians and Surgeons Pakistan awarded in respect of success in the relevant examination since April 1998;

(vi) Doctor of Medicine (Anaesthesia) University of the West Indies since September 2003;

(vii) Fellowship of the College of Anaesthetists of South Africa;

(viii) Certificate of the American Board of Anesthesiology;

(ix) Fellowship in Anaesthesia of the Royal College of Physicians and Surgeons of Canada;

(x) Fellowship in Anaesthesia of the Bangladesh College of Physicians and Surgeons since July 1999; or

(xi) Fellowship of the Hong Kong College of Anaesthesiologists since January 2001.

Section 8: Application procedures

Applications

20 The Examination Calendar and application forms are published by the College, copies of which may be downloaded from the College website at: www.rcoa.ac.uk/docs/examcalendar.pdf

21 Applications for admission to an examination must be received by the College on or after the published opening date but not later than 5pm on the published closing date of the sitting applied for, as shown in the Examinations Calendar.

22 Applications for admission must be accompanied by the fee and any certificates required to support the application form. Late or incomplete applications will not be accepted.

23 The fees payable for admission to each part shall be those fixed by Council and published in the Examinations Calendar and should be paid by a cheque made payable to The Royal College of Anaesthetists and drawn on a United Kingdom clearing bank, or by a sterling draft or postal order.

Withdrawals

24 (a) A candidate withdrawing an application for admission to an examination before the closing date for applications may receive back the full amount of the fee paid, subject to a deduction for administrative expenses, provided the withdrawal is received in writing. A candidate who withdraws in any other circumstances (with the exception of those described in Regulation 24(b) and Section 9) or who fails to appear for an examination will not normally be entitled to any refund of fee.

(b) Candidates who have attended a guidance interview after failing either the Primary FRCA OSCE and/or SOE twice (see Regulation 33.(a)), may withdraw their next application to sit the examination and receive back the full amount of the fee paid without any deduction for administration expenses. This concession will be granted only once. Withdrawals must be made in writing and received by the Examinations Department by the Thursday before the published start date of the OSCE and SOE.

(c) Candidates who have attended a guidance interview after failing either the written or SOE sections of the Final FRCA Examination three times (see Regulation 33.(b)), may withdraw their next application to sit the examination and receive back the full amount of the fee paid without any deduction for administration expenses. This concession will be granted twice, firstly after guidance for the written examination and secondly after guidance for the SOE. Withdrawals must be made in writing and received by the Examinations Department by the Thursday before the published start date of the relevant examination.

Section 9: Pregnancy and disability

Pregnancy

25 Regulations 26 to 28 apply only to female candidates whose pregnancy or pregnancy-related illness or condition renders them unable to attend the examination. These Regulations do not apply to any other situations. This special treatment in relation to female candidates is permitted under the Sex Discrimination Act 1975.

26 Any prospective candidate should notify the Examinations Department as soon as possible of the fact of their pregnancy and the expected week of confinement. Such details should, where possible, be attached to the appropriate application form and fee.

27 A prospective candidate must submit an appropriate medical certificate which satisfies the College if:

(a) she has any pregnancy-related problems or illness; or

(b) her confinement is due shortly before or around the date of the examination; or

(c) her condition gives her sufficient discomfort for her to consider that it will have a detrimental effect upon her performance. In such circumstances, should such a candidate be unable to sit for the examination, withdrawal will be permitted and the examination fee will be refunded (subject to a deduction for administrative expenses).

28 A candidate who does not inform the Examinations Department of her pregnancy will not normally be allowed to withdraw her application after the closing date without forfeiting her examination fee. However, when the pregnancy is diagnosed after submitting an application but prior to the examination and the candidate is subsequently unable to attend for the examination due to pregnancy related reasons, then upon submission of an appropriate medical certificate which satisfies the College, the candidate may withdraw from the examination and the fee will be refunded (subject to a deduction for administrative expenses).

Disability

29 Dyslexia. The Regulations for accommodating dyslexic candidates are contained in Appendix 3.

30 All other requests for special consideration for dealing with disabilities will be considered on an individual basis. Requests must include a written statement of support from the employer's occupational health department confirming that the candidate's difficulties warrant special examination arrangements.

Section 10: Fellowship by examination

31 As stated in the Charter and Ordinances of The Royal College of Anaesthetists, a person shall be entitled to be admitted a Fellow of the College if he or she has:

(a) passed the appropriate examinations for Fellowship; and

(b) complied with such conditions as may be prescribed by the Council in the Regulations of the College.

Section 11: Failures and guidance

Failures

32 A candidate who is unsuccessful in an examination may, subject to the provisions of Sections 5, 6 and 7, and Regulation 33, enter for the next or any subsequent sitting of that examination.

Guidance

33 (a) No candidate may attempt the OSCE or SOE sections of the Primary FRCA Examination more than twice without attending a guidance interview.

(b) No candidate may attempt either section of the Final FRCA Examination more than three times without attending a guidance interview.

(c) Guidance interviews should normally be attended within six months of the date of examination failure that triggered the need for guidance.

(d) For the purpose of this Regulation, 'guidance' shall comprise:

(i) subject to the consent of the candidate, the provision to the College by their College Tutor of a confidential report on that candidate;

(ii) the attendance by the candidate at a guidance session arranged by the College; and

(iii) any other requirement that Council may from time to time authorize.

Section 12: Representations and appeals

34 A candidate wishing to make representations with regard to the conduct of an examination or to appeal against any result must address such representation or appeal to the Training and Examinations Director in writing within two months of completing the relevant examination. In no circumstances may such representations be addressed to an examiner. Representations and appeals shall be dealt with in accordance with the College's Examinations (Representations and Appeals) Regulations. Copies of these Regulations can be downloaded from the College website at: www.rcoa.ac.uk/docs/exam-appeal-regs.pdf.

Section 13: Infringements

35 The College Council may refuse to admit to an examination, or to proceed with the examination of, any candidate who infringes any of the Regulations, or who is considered by the presiding examiner to be guilty of behaviour prejudicial to the proper conduct and management of the examination or who has previously been found guilty of such behaviour. If in the opinion of Council any examination success has been secured by cheating, deception or fraud of any kind whatsoever, the Council may quash that result and any qualifications resulting from it and withdraw any diploma, certificate or other award so obtained.

APPENDICES TO REGULATIONS

These appendices are not Regulations. They are provided for the guidance of candidates and may change from time to time as decided by Council.

Appendix 1: Structure of the examinations
Primary FRCA Examination

There are three sections to the Examination; questions on data interpretation may appear in any part.

Multiple choice questions (MCQ)
- 90 MCQs in 3 hours comprising three subsections, approximately:
- 30 questions in pharmacology;
- 30 questions in physiology and biochemistry; and
- 30 questions in physics, clinical measurement and data interpretation.

The MCQ section must be passed before the OSCE and SOE sections can be attempted.

Objective structured clinical examination (OSCE)

Up to 18 stations in approximately 1 hour 50 minutes (of which only 16 count towards the result) currently comprising stations covering: resuscitation, technical skills, anatomy (general procedure), history-taking, physical examination, communication skills, anaesthetic equipment, monitoring equipment, measuring equipment, anaesthetic hazards, and the interpretation of X-rays. One or more of the stations may involve the use of a medium fidelity simulator.

Structured oral examination (SOE)

There are two sub-sections to the SOE section comprising:
- 30 minutes consisting of three questions in pharmacology, and three questions in physiology and biochemistry; followed by
- 30 minutes consisting of three questions in physics, clinical measurement, equipment and safety, and three questions on clinical topics (including a critical incident).

Final FRCA Examination

There are two sections to the examination.

Written

There are two sub-sections to the written examination comprising:
(a) MCQ paper: 90 MCQs in 3 hours comprising approximately:
  - 20 questions in medicine and surgery;
  - 40 questions in anaesthesia and pain management including applied basic sciences (mainly pharmacology and physiology);
  - 10 questions in clinical measurement; and
  - 20 questions in intensive therapy.
(b) Short answer question (SAQ) paper: 12 compulsory questions in three hours on the principles and practice of clinical anaesthesia.

Structured Oral Examination (SOE)

There are two sub-sections to the SOE comprising:

- Clinical anaesthesia: 50 minutes duration comprising ten minutes to view clinical material, 20 minutes devoted to three questions based on the clinical material and 20 minutes devoted to three questions on clinical anaesthesia unrelated to the clinical material; followed by:
- Clinical science: 30 minutes duration consisting of four questions on the application of basic science to anaesthesia, intensive care medicine and pain management.

Appendix 2: The marking systems

All sections have to be passed to pass the whole Examination at Primary and Final levels.

In all sections of the examination, the performance of borderline candidates is reviewed by the examiners before the final marks are awarded.

If, in the opinion of the examiners, a candidate's answers in the SOEs have been dangerous then the candidate's performance is reviewed by all the examiners before the marks are confirmed.

Primary FRCA

MCQ

One mark will be awarded for each correct answer. Negative marking is not used for wrong answers. The pass mark will be set by the examiners using a combination of linear and Angoff referencing.

A candidate's performance in each of the three subsections is taken into consideration when calculating the overall mark. Candidates who perform very poorly in one or more sub-sections will fail the MCQ paper.

Candidates who make ambiguous marks on their optically read mark sheet will not be given the benefit of any doubt.

OSCE

Each station is marked out of 20 with the pass mark for each station being determined by the examiners before the examination, using modified Angoff referencing. The pass marks for each of the 16 stations are summed to obtain the pass mark for the whole examination.

Up to two additional stations may be included in an examination to test new questions. Neither the candidates nor the examiners will know which stations these are and the results will not contribute to the final mark.

SOE

Two examiners are present for each part of the SOE. Each examiner marks every question independently. All the marks are totalled and the pass mark is determined using a modified Rothman system.

Final FRCA written section

The marks for the MCQ and the SAQ papers are added to give a total mark. The pass mark for the written section is the sum of the pass marks of the two papers.

MCQ

One mark will be awarded for each correct answer. Negative marking is not used for wrong answers. The pass mark will be set by the examiners using a combination of linear and Angoff referencing.

SAQ paper

All 12 questions must be attempted; candidates will fail the written section if one or more questions on the SAQ paper are not attempted.

Candidates who get poor fails in three or more questions will have their examination papers reviewed by the examiners.

If a candidate answers a question in the wrong answer book normally that answer will not be marked by the examiners (and the candidate will fail the written section).

Each question is marked out of 20 with the pass mark for each question being determined by the examiners collectively before the examination using modified Angoff referencing. The pass marks for the 12 questions are summed to obtain the pass mark for the whole paper.

SOE

Two examiners are present for each part of the SOE. Each examiner marks every question independently. All the marks are totalled and the pass mark is determined using a modified Rothman system.

Appendix 3: Dyslexic candidates

1. The following guidelines specify the procedure and provisions for special arrangements. Please note that special consideration will only be allowed if the application and appropriate documentation is received by the closing date of the sitting applied for.

2. To qualify for special consideration candidates must supply:
   (a) a written assessment from an educational psychologist (dated within 5 years), which includes a statement confirming that the candidate's difficulties warrant special examination arrangements and that such special arrangements have been required on previous occasions in similar circumstances; and
   (b) a letter of support from their College Tutor or Regional Adviser (or supervising consultant of equivalent standing if applying from overseas); and
   (c) confirmation in writing from the candidate that, in the Multiple Choice Question (MCQ) paper he/she agrees to his/her answers being transferred onto the answer sheet by a member of College staff (see provisions below).

3. Such an application will be considered by the Chairman of the relevant examination, who will bear in mind the occupational requirements of the specialty. If a candidate is not able to supply the above documents before the commencement of the examination, the candidate may choose to:
   (a) withdraw without penalty as per the standard procedure, or
   (b) proceed without special arrangements.

Provisions

4. The following provisions will be allowed:
   (a) MCQ papers: No additional time will be allowed in the examination room BUT such candidates may mark the question booklet only and submit their booklet for the transfer of marks onto the answer sheet by a member of College staff. Additional time is therefore provided by not transferring answers onto an answer sheet.
   (b) SAQ papers: Dyslexic candidates will be seated in the examination room 15 minutes before the admission of other candidates in order to read the questions and make any notes on rough paper within this time. After 15 minutes, the question paper will be removed and the other candidates will be seated. After the instructions have been given, the written papers will be distributed and the examination will commence. Dyslexic candidates will be given an extra 15 minutes to write their answers i.e. three hours 15 minutes.
   (c) SOEs: No special arrangements will be considered.

Appendix 4: Prizes

The following prizes may, at the discretion of Council, be awarded to candidates who perform outstandingly in all the sections of the relevant examination at their first attempt:

Nuffield prize

Awarded for outstanding achievement in the Primary FRCA Examination.

Macintosh prize

Awarded for outstanding achievement in the summer sitting of the Final FRCA Examination.

Magill prize

Awarded for outstanding achievement in the autumn sitting of the Final FRCA Examination.

Index

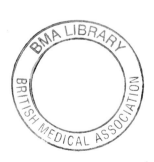
Lightning Source UK Ltd.
Milton Keynes UK
UKOW020108110112

185122UK00010B/3/P